T0226687

Gout and Calcium Crystal Related Arthropathies

Editor

TUHINA NEOGI

RHEUMATIC DISEASE CLINICS OF NORTH AMERICA

www.rheumatic.theclinics.com

Consulting Editor
MICHAEL H. WEISMAN

May 2014 • Volume 40 • Number 2

ELSEVIER

1600 John F. Kennedy Boulevard • Suite 1800 • Philadelphia, Pennsylvania, 19103-2899
http://www.theclinics.com

RHEUMATIC DISEASE CLINICS OF NORTH AMERICA Volume 40, Number 2
May 2014 ISSN 0889-857X, ISBN 13: 978-0-323-26680-2

Editor: Jennifer Flynn-Briggs
Developmental Editor: Casey Jackson

© 2014 Elsevier Inc. All rights reserved.

This periodical and the individual contributions contained in it are protected under copyright by Elsevier, and the following terms and conditions apply to their use:

Photocopying
Single photocopies of single articles may be made for personal use as allowed by national copyright laws. Permission of the Publisher and payment of a fee is required for all other photocopying, including multiple or systematic copying, copying for advertising or promotional purposes, resale, and all forms of document delivery. Special rates are available for educational institutions that wish to make photocopies for non-profit educational classroom use. For information on how to seek permission visit www.elsevier.com/permissions or call: (+44) 1865 843830 (UK)/ (+1) 215 239 3804 (USA).

Derivative Works
Subscribers may reproduce tables of contents or prepare lists of articles including abstracts for internal circulation within their institutions. Permission of the Publisher is required for resale or distribution outside the institution. Permission of the Publisher is required for all other derivative works, including compilations and translations (please consult www.elsevier.com/permissions).

Electronic Storage or Usage
Permission of the Publisher is required to store or use electronically any material contained in this periodical, including any article or part of an article (please consult www.elsevier.com/permissions). Except as outlined above, no part of this publication may be reproduced, stored in a retrieval system or transmitted in any form or by any means, electronic, mechanical, photocopying, recording or otherwise, without prior written permission of the Publisher.

Notice
No responsibility is assumed by the Publisher for any injury and/or damage to persons or property as a matter of products liability, negligence or otherwise, or from any use or operation of any methods, products, instructions or ideas contained in the material herein. Because of rapid advances in the medical sciences, in particular, independent verification of diagnoses and drug dosages should be made.

Although all advertising material is expected to conform to ethical (medical) standards, inclusion in this publication does not constitute a guarantee or endorsement of the quality or value of such product or of the claims made of it by its manufacturer.

Rheumatic Disease Clinics of North America (ISSN 0889-857X) is published quarterly by Elsevier Inc., 360 Park Avenue South, New York, NY 10010-1710. Months of issue are February, May, August, and November. Business and editorial offices: 1600 John F. Kennedy Boulevard, Suite 1800, Philadelphia, PA 19103-2899. Periodicals postage paid at New York, NY and additional mailing offices. Subscription prices are USD 335.00 per year for US individuals, USD 579.00 per year for US institutions, USD 165.00 per year for US students and residents, USD 395.00 per year for Canadian individuals, USD 722.00 per year for Canadian institutions, USD 465.00 per year for international individuals, USD 722.00 per year for international institutions, and USD 230.00 per year for Canadian and foreign students/residents. To receive student/resident rate, orders must be accompanied by name of affiliated institution, date of term, and the *signature* of program/residency coordinator on institution letterhead. Orders will be billed at individual rate until proof of status received. Foreign air speed delivery is included in all *Clinics* subscription prices. All prices are subject to change without notice. **POSTMASTER:** Send address changes to *Rheumatic Disease Clinics of North America,* Elsevier Health Sciences Division, Subscription Customer Service, 3251 Riverport Lane, Maryland Heights, MO 63043. **Customer Service: 1-800-654-2452 (US and Canada). From outside of the US and Canada: 314-447-8871. Fax: 314-447-8029. For print support, e-mail: JournalsCustomerService-usa@elsevier.com. For online support, e-mail: JournalsOnline Support-usa@elsevier.com.**

Reprints. For copies of 100 or more of articles in this publication, please contact the Commercial Reprints Department, Elsevier Inc., 360 Park Avenue South, New York, New York, 10010-1710; Tel.: +1-212-633-3874, Fax: +1-212-633-3820, and E-mail: reprints@elsevier.com.

Rheumatic Disease Clinics of North America is covered in *MEDLINE/PubMed (Index Medicus), Current Contents/Clinical Medicine, Science Citation Index, ISI/BIOMED,* and *EMBASE/Excerpta Medica.*

Printed and bound by CPI Group (UK) Ltd, Croydon, CR0 4YY

Contributors

CONSULTING EDITOR

MICHAEL H. WEISMAN, MD
Director, Division of Rheumatology, Professor of Medicine, Cedars-Sinai Medical Center, Los Angeles, California

EDITOR

TUHINA NEOGI, MD, PhD, FRCPC
Associate Professor of Medicine and Epidemiology, Clinical Epidemiology Research and Training Unit, and Rheumatology, Boston University School of Medicine, Boston, Massachusetts

AUTHORS

ABHISHEK ABHISHEK, MBBS, MD, MRCP, PhD
Department of Rheumatology, Addenbrookes Hospital, Cambridge; Academic Rheumatology, University of Nottingham, Nottingham, United Kingdom

MICHAEL A. BECKER, MD
Professor of Medicine (Emeritus), Section of Rheumatology, The University of Chicago, Chicago, Illinois

FERDIA BOLSTER, MD
Specialist Registrar Radiology, Department of Radiology, Mater Misericordiae University Hospital, Dublin, Ireland

EDWIN CASTILLO, MD
Division of Rheumatology, Hospital Universitario Cruces, Baracaldo, Spain

YASHAAR CHAICHIAN, MD
Rheumatology Fellow, Section of Rheumatology, The University of Chicago, Chicago, Illinois

ASHIKA CHHANA, PhD
Bone & Joint Research Group, Department of Medicine, Faculty of Medical & Health Sciences, University of Auckland, Auckland, New Zealand

SANDRA P. CHINCHILLA, MD
Division of Rheumatology, Hospital Universitario Cruces, Baracaldo, Spain

SAIMA CHOHAN, MD
Assistant Professor of Medicine, Section of Rheumatology, The University of Chicago, Chicago, Illinois

HYON K. CHOI, MD, DrPH
Professor of Medicine, Section of Rheumatology and Clinical Epidemiology Unit, Boston University School of Medicine, Boston, Massachusetts

NICOLA DALBETH, MBChB, MD, FRACP
Associate Professor in Rheumatology, Bone & Joint Research Group, Department of Medicine, Faculty of Medical & Health Sciences, University of Auckland; Consultant Rheumatologist, Auckland District Health Board, Department of Rheumatology, Greenlane Clinical Centre, Auckland, New Zealand

MICHAEL DOHERTY, MD, FRCP
Academic Rheumatology, University of Nottingham, Nottingham, United Kingdom

ANTHONY DOYLE, MBChB, FRANZCR, ABR
Associate Professor, Department of Anatomy and Radiology, University of Auckland; Consultant Radiologist, Auckland District Health Board, Department of Radiology, Auckland City Hospital, Auckland, New Zealand

LAURA DURCAN, MD
Specialist Registrar Rheumatology, Division of Rheumatology, Mater Misericordiae University Hospital, Dublin, Ireland

HANG-KORNG EA, MD, PhD
Associate Professor of Cell Biology, AP-HP, hôpital Lariboisière, Service de rhumatologie (centre Viggo Petersen), pôle appareil locomoteur; Sorbonne Paris Cité, University Paris Diderot (UFR de Médecine); INSERM, UMR-S 1132, Hopital Lariboisière, Paris, France

N. LAWRENCE EDWARDS, MD, FACP, FACR
Professor and Vice Chairman, Department of Medicine, University of Florida College of Medicine, Gainesville, Florida

ANGELO L. GAFFO, MD, MSPH
Section of Rheumatology, Veterans Affairs Medical Center; Division of Clinical Immunology and Rheumatology, Department of Medicine, School of Medicine, University of Alabama, Birmingham, Alabama

ANA M. HERRERO-BEITES, MD
Division of Physical Medicine, Hospital de Górliz, Spain

EOIN C. KAVANAGH, MB BCh, FRCSI
Clinical Associate Professor of Medicine, Department of Radiology, Mater Misericordiae University Hospital, Dublin, Ireland

FRÉDÉRIC LIOTÉ, MD, PhD
Professor of Rheumatology, AP-HP, hôpital Lariboisière, Service de rhumatologie (centre Viggo Petersen), pôle appareil locomoteur; Sorbonne Paris Cité, University Paris Diderot (UFR de Médecine); INSERM, UMR-S 1132, Hopital Lariboisière, Paris, France

GERALDINE M. MCCARTHY, MD, FRCPI
Clinical Professor of Medicine, Division of Rheumatology, Mater Misericordiae University Hospital, Dublin, Ireland

FIONA M. MCQUEEN, MBChB, MD, FRACP
Professor of Rheumatology, Department of Molecular Medicine and Pathology, University of Auckland; Consultant Rheumatologist, Auckland District Health Board, Department of Rheumatology, Greenlane Clinical Centre, Auckland, New Zealand

TONY R. MERRIMAN, PhD
Department of Biochemistry, University of Otago, Dunedin, New Zealand

FERNANDO PEREZ-RUIZ, MD, PhD
Division of Rheumatology, BioCruces Health Institute, Hospital Universitario Cruces, Baracaldo, Spain

EDWARD RODDY, DM, FRCP
Senior Lecturer in Rheumatology, Research Institute for Primary Care and Health Sciences, Keele University, Keele, Staffordshire, United Kingdom

ANN K. ROSENTHAL, MD
Will and Cava Ross Professor of Medicine, Division of Rheumatology, Department of Medicine, Zablocki VA Medical Center and The Medical College of Wisconsin, Milwaukee, Wisconsin

LAWRENCE M. RYAN, MD
Professor of Medicine, Division of Rheumatology, Department of Medicine, Zablocki VA Medical Center and The Medical College of Wisconsin, Milwaukee, Wisconsin

SEBASTIAN E. SATTUI, MD
Division of Clinical Immunology and Rheumatology, Department of Medicine, School of Medicine, University of Alabama, Birmingham, Alabama

NAOMI SCHLESINGER, MD
Professor of Medicine, Chief, Division of Rheumatology, Department of Medicine, Rutgers – Robert Wood Johnson Medical School, New Brunswick, New Jersey

JASVINDER A. SINGH, MBBS, MPH
Medicine Service, Center for Surgical Medical Acute Care Research and Transitions (C-SMART), Birmingham VA Medical Center; Division of Clinical Immunology and Rheumatology, Department of Medicine, School of Medicine, University of Alabama, Birmingham, Alabama; Department of Orthopedic Surgery, Mayo Clinic College of Medicine, Rochester, Minnesota

ALEXANDER SO, PhD, FRCP
Professor, Service de Rhumatologie, CHUV, Lausanne, Switzerland

Contents

> Gout is the most prevalent inflammatory arthritis in men. The findings of several epidemiologic studies from a diverse range of countries suggest that the prevalence of gout has risen over the past few decades. Although incidence data are scarce, data from the United States suggests that the incidence of gout is also rising. Evidence from prospective epidemiologic studies has confirmed dietary factors (animal purines, alcohol, and fructose), obesity, the metabolic syndrome, hypertension, diuretic use, and chronic kidney disease as clinically relevant risk factors for hyperuricemia and gout. Low-fat dairy products, coffee, and vitamin C seem to have a protective effect.

> Calcium pyrophosphate crystal deposition (CPPD) is common and mainly associates with increasing age and osteoarthritis (OA). Recent studies suggest that CPPD occurs as the result of a generalized articular predisposition and may also associate with low cortical bone mineral density. The epidemiology of basic calcium phosphate (BCP) crystal deposition is poorly understood. Although periarticular BCP crystal deposits occurs at all ages and in both sexes, intra-articular BCP crystal deposition tends to associate with increasing age and OA. Calcium pyrophosphate and BCP crystals frequently coexist in joints with OA.

> Gout has been academically considered to be a step-up disease consisting of different stages: acute gout, intercritical gout, and chronic gout. This simple approach may lead to misinterpretation and misdiagnosis. In clinical practice, we should consider gout as a single disease with either or both acute (most commonly, episodes of acute inflammation) and persistent clinical manifestations, but not restricted to chronic synovitis. In this article, an innovative, practical, and rational approach to the clinical manifestations and diagnosis of gout is presented, which may be supportive for clinicians involved in everyday care and management of patients with gout.

others being involved in glycolysis. Whereas much is understood about the genetic control of serum urate levels, little is known about the genetic control of inflammatory responses to MSU crystals. Extending knowledge in this area depends on recruitment of large, clinically ascertained gout sample sets suitable for GWAS.

This article summarizes the structural damage that is observed in advanced gout and current understanding of the mechanisms by which this damage occurs. Interactions between monosodium urate crystals and cells within the joint are described as well as knowledge gained from imaging studies. Future research directions and potential therapeutic strategies for the prevention and treatment of joint damage in gout are also discussed.

Calcium pyrophosphate dihydrate and basic calcium phosphate (BCP) crystals are the most common calcium-containing crystals associated with rheumatic disease. Clinical manifestations of calcium crystal deposition include acute or chronic inflammatory and degenerative arthritides and certain forms of periarthritis. The intra-articular presence of BCP crystals correlates with the degree of radiographic degeneration. Calcium crystal deposition contributes directly to joint degeneration. Vascular calcification is caused by the deposition of calcium hydroxyapatite crystals in the arterial intima. These deposits may contribute to local inflammation and promote further calcification, thus aggravating the atherosclerotic process. Calcium crystal deposition results in substantial structural consequence in humans.

This article presents an overview of the treatment of acute gout. Nonpharmacologic and pharmacologic treatments, monotherapy versus combination therapy, suggested recommendations, guidelines for treatment, and drugs under development are discussed.

Calcium crystal arthritis is often unrecognized, poorly managed, and few effective therapies are available. The most common types of calcium crystals causing musculoskeletal syndromes are calcium pyrophosphate (CPP) and basic calcium phosphate (BCP). Associated syndromes have different clinical presentations and divergent management strategies. Acute CPP arthritis is treated similarly to acute gouty arthritis, whereas chronic CPP and BCP arthropathy may respond to strategies used for osteoarthritis. Calcific tendonitis is treated with a variety of interventions designed to dissolve BCP crystals. A better understanding of the causes and larger well-planned trials of current therapies will lead to improved care.

Gout is a common disorder with clinical signs and symptoms resulting from inflammatory responses to monosodium urate crystals deposited in tissues from extracellular fluids saturated for urate. Long-term management of gout focuses on nonpharmacologic and pharmacologic means to achieve and maintain serum urate levels in a subsaturating range. Despite a firm understanding of gout pathophysiology, means to achieve certain diagnosis, and a variety of effective therapies, treatment outcomes remain suboptimal. In this review, available nonpharmacologic and pharmacologic therapies for chronic gout are discussed and a framework is provided for successful achievement and maintenance of goal-range serum urate levels.

Over the past decade much has been learned about the mechanisms of crystal-induced inflammation and renal excretion of uric acid, which has led to more specific targeting of gout therapies and a more potent approach to future management of gout. This article outlines agents being developed for more aggressive lowering of urate and more specific anti-inflammatory activity. The emerging urate-lowering therapies include lesinurad, arhalofenate, ulodesine, and levotofisopam. Novel gout-specific anti-inflammatories include the interleukin-1β inhibitors anakinra, canakinumab, and rilonacept, the melanocortins, and caspase inhibitors. The historic shortcomings of current gout treatment may, in part, be overcome by these novel approaches.

RHEUMATIC DISEASE CLINICS
OF NORTH AMERICA

RELATED INTEREST

Clinics in Sports Medicine, July 2013 (Volume 32, Issue 3; p. 577–597)
Arthritis Mimicking Sports-Related Injuries
Donald J. Flemming, MD, and Stephanie A. Bernard, MD, *Editors*

DOWNLOAD
Free App!

Review Articles
THE CLINICS

NOW AVAILABLE FOR YOUR iPhone and iPad

Foreword

Gout and Crystal Arthropathies

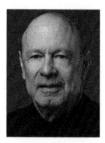

Michael H. Weisman, MD
Consulting Editor

Dr Tuhina Neogi has put a new face on an ancient disease in this excellent little issue. The epidemiology of gout is a frightening story. In a disease where we have a known pathogenesis and effective treatment along with prevention strategies, we find the problem is increasing! Why is this happening and is it reversible? Dr Neogi tells us straight away that gout is now the most common form of inflammatory arthritis in the United States, yet our medical schools and house officer-training programs likely are not responsive to this important fact. We have learned from this issue that gout has multiple phases, and the asymptomatic phase is becoming increasingly recognized as important, especially in terms of associated comorbidities. Advanced imaging has now given us a window into newer pathologic mechanisms for joint damage. Structural damage in gout appears to be multifactorial and the story is unfolding regarding the importance of urate-lowering treatment especially in the asymptomatic phase of the disease. Finally, it is surprising how little we know about CPPD deposition diseases—this is a call to arms for our research establishment. The role of calcium deposition in its various forms appears to be a major player in initiating and sustaining inflammation leading to joint destruction. This very timely issue is welcome and Tuhina has done an excellent job.

Michael H. Weisman, MD
Division of Rheumatology
Cedars-Sinai Medical Center
8700 Beverly Boulevard
Los Angeles, CA 90024, USA

E-mail address:
michael.weisman@cshs.org

Rheum Dis Clin N Am 40 (2014) xiii
http://dx.doi.org/10.1016/j.rdc.2014.03.001
0889-857X/14/$ – see front matter © 2014 Published by Elsevier Inc.

Preface

Gout and Crystal Arthropathies

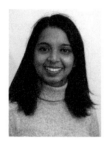

Tuhina Neogi, MD, PhD, FRCPC
Editor

Gout is now the most common form of inflammatory arthritis in the United States, with a recent resurgence of research interest in its cause and management. Calcium crystal–related arthritis has also attracted renewed attention, with new nomenclature having been recently elaborated, aiding contemporary research efforts. Novel insights regarding risk factors for gout and calcium crystal–related arthritis, including dietary, lifestyle, and genetic factors, have been elucidated in the past decade, providing new management options and treatment targets for drug development. Patients with crystal-related arthropathies are also recognized to have higher prevalence of certain comorbidities that themselves require specific management efforts.

With improved understanding of the biologic basis for the acute inflammatory response in acute gout, new pharmacologic agents for the management of acute gout are being developed and tested, providing additional therapeutic options for patients suffering from gout. New treatments for hyperuricemia have also been developed, including some that are directed at pathways not previously targeted by the traditionally used urate-lowering therapies. One of the major consequences of inadequately managed hyperuricemia is the occurrence of tophi. It is now better understood that tophi are not inert deposits of urate, but rather are biologically active and contribute to joint destruction, affecting the integrity of both bone and cartilage. Calcium crystal deposition is also increasingly being recognized as a potential etiologic factor contributing to the onset and progression of joint damage, including osteoarthritis. Advances in imaging technology are providing new insights into the nature and extent of both calcium and urate crystal deposition and will enable greater insights into their effects on joint damage. Such imaging modalities may also offer new avenues for testing the efficacy of new pharmacologic agents in crystal-related arthropathies, complementing the biochemical and patient-reported outcomes used presently. In summary, there have been tremendous advances in understanding the epidemiology, biology, imaging, structural consequences, and management of crystal-related arthropathies, but much work remains to be done.

Rheum Dis Clin N Am 40 (2014) xv–xvi
http://dx.doi.org/10.1016/j.rdc.2014.02.001   **rheumatic.theclinics.com**
0889-857X/14/$ – see front matter © 2014 Elsevier Inc. All rights reserved.

The articles in this issue provide in-depth reviews of the current state of these scientific advances and lay out a framework for a research agenda that will eventually advance the care of millions of patients with crystal-related arthropathies worldwide.

Tuhina Neogi, MD, PhD, FRCPC
Clinical Epidemiology Research and Training Unit, and Rheumatology
Boston University School of Medicine
650 Albany Street
Clin Epi Unit, Suite X200
Boston, MA 02118, USA

E-mail address:
tneogi@bu.edu

Epidemiology of Gout

Edward Roddy, DM, FRCP[a],*, Hyon K. Choi, MD, DrPH[b]

KEYWORDS

- Gout • Hyperuricemia • Prevalence • Incidence • Etiology • Epidemiology

KEY POINTS

- Gout has become more prevalent over the past few decades, affecting over 3% of adults in the United States. The limited incidence data in the United States suggest a similarly increasing trend.
- Excessive consumption of meat, seafood, sugar-sweetened soft drinks, fructose, and alcohol increases the risk of developing hyperuricemia and gout, whereas low-fat dairy products, coffee, and vitamin C seem to be protective against these conditions.
- Obesity, hypertension, the metabolic syndrome, chronic renal failure, and use of diuretics, β-blockers, as well as angiotensin II (AII) receptor antagonists (other than losartan) are independent risk factors for the development of hyperuricemia and gout, whereas diabetes mellitus, calcium channel blockers, and losartan seem to reduce the risk of developing these conditions.

INTRODUCTION

Gout is a crystal deposition disease that arises when supersaturation of body tissues with urate occurs, leading to the formation of monosodium urate (MSU) crystals in and around joints. Gout is the most prevalent inflammatory arthritis in men and is associated with impaired quality of life.[1] Clinical manifestations include excruciatingly painful acute attacks of gouty arthritis, formation of tophaceous MSU crystal deposits in joints and other body tissues, chronic joint damage, renal stone formation, and potential renal insufficiency.

This article reviews trends in the prevalence and incidence of gout and the epidemiologic evidence underpinning our understanding of etiologic factors for its development including hyperuricemia, dietary factors, comorbidities (metabolic syndrome, renal disease, and osteoarthritis [OA]), and medications. The burden of comorbidity associated with and caused by gout is discussed elsewhere in this issue. Where possible, priority has been given to population-based prospective epidemiologic studies (Table 1).

[a] Research Institute for Primary Care and Health Sciences, Keele University, Keele, Staffordshire ST5 5BG, UK; [b] Section of Rheumatology and Clinical Epidemiology Unit, Boston University School of Medicine, 650 Albany Street, Suite 200, Boston, MA 02118, USA
* Corresponding author.
E-mail address: e.roddy@keele.ac.uk

Rheum Dis Clin N Am 40 (2014) 155–175
http://dx.doi.org/10.1016/j.rdc.2014.01.001
0889-857X/14/$ – see front matter © 2014 Elsevier Inc. All rights reserved.

rheumatic.theclinics.com

Table 1
Epidemiologic studies of risk factors for gout

Study	Design	Population	Total Sample	Age Range (y)	% Male	Duration of Follow-Up (y)	Method of Gout Ascertainment and Number of Incident Gout	Risk Factors Studied	Adjustment For
Framingham Heart Study	Cohort	Framingham, Massachusetts	4427	29–62	44	28	Clinical diagnosis; 200 in men, 104 in women	Hyperuricemia, age, education level, BMI, alcohol intake, diuretics, hypertension, glucose, cholesterol	Age, education level, BMI, alcohol intake, hypertension, diuretics, blood glucose level, blood cholesterol level, menopausal status
Health Professionals Follow-up Study	Cohort	Male health professionals	51,529	40–75	100	12	ARA criteria; 730	Dietary purines, dairy products, caffeinated drinks, soft drinks, fructose, vitamin C, alcoholic drinks, BMI, hypertension, diuretics, renal failure	Age, energy intake, BMI, diuretic use, hypertension, renal failure, dietary factors
Nurses' Health Study	Cohort	Female nurses	89,433	30–55	0	26	ARA criteria; 896	Caffeinated drinks, soft drinks, fructose	Age, energy intake, BMI, menopause, postmenopausal hormone use, diuretics, hypertension, dietary factors

ARIC	Cohort	Population-based study in 4 US communities	10,872	45–64	43	9	Self-reported physician diagnosis; 274	Gender, race, BMI, hypertension, alcohol intake, eGFR	Age, gender, race, BMI, diabetes, hypertension, diuretics, menopause, meat intake, alcohol intake, eGFR
THIN	Case-control	UK general practice	1,775,505	20–89	73	5.2	GP diagnosis; 24,768 cases	Alcohol intake, BMI, hypertension, diuretics, antihypertensives, chronic renal failure	Age, gender, calendar year, alcohol intake, BMI, ischemic heart disease, hypertension, hyperlipidemia, diabetes, chronic renal impairment, diuretics, antihypertensives

Abbreviations: ARA, American Rheumatism Association; ARIC, Atherosclerosis Risk in Communities; BMI, body mass index; eGFR, estimated glomerular filtration rate; GP, general practitioner; THIN, The Health Improvement Network.

Table 2
Prevalence of gout

Country	Author	Year	Data Source	Gout Definition	Prevalence Estimate
United States	Wallace et al	1990	Medical claims database	Claim for gout or ULT in 1 y	2.9/1000
		1999			5.2/1000
	Lawrence et al	1969	National Health Interview Surveys	Self-reported 1-y period prevalence	4.8/1000
		1976			7.8/1000
		1980			8.3/1000
		1983 to 1985			9.9/1000
		1988			8.5/1000
		1992			8.4/1000
		1996			9.4/1000
	Juraschek et al	1988–1994	NHANES III	Self-reported lifetime physician diagnosis	26.4/1000
		2007–2010	NHANES 2007–2010	Self-reported lifetime physician diagnosis	37.6/1000
United Kingdom	Currie	1975	GP records	GP diagnosis (lifetime prevalence)	2.6/1000
	Steven	1987	GP records (Scotland)	GP diagnosis (lifetime prevalence)	3.4/1000
	Harris et al	1993	GP records (England)	GP diagnosis (lifetime prevalence)	9.5/1000
	Mikuls et al	1999	General Practice Research Database	GP diagnosis (1-y consultation prevalence)	13.9/1000
	Annemans et al	2000–2005	IMS Disease Analyzer	GP diagnosis (5.5-year consultation prevalence)	14.0/1000
	Elliott et al	2001	RCGP weekly returns service	GP diagnosis (1-y consultation prevalence)	4.3/1000
		2002			4.2/1000
		2003			4.9/1000
		2004			4.7/1000
		2005			4.8/1000
		2006			4.9/1000
		2007			4.7/1000

New Zealand	Lennane et al	1958	Random community sample	Personal interview and examination (lifetime prevalence)	European 3/1000 Maori 27/1000
	Prior and Rose[15]	1966	Random community sample	Personal interview and examination (lifetime prevalence)	European 9/1000 Maori 60/1000
	Klemp et al	1992	Random community sample	Personal interview and examination, ARA criteria (lifetime prevalence)	European 29/1000 Maori 64/1000
	Winnard et al	2009	ANZHT	Hospital discharge records (1988–2009) or prescription for allopurinol/colchicine (2001–2009)	European 32/1000 Maori 61/1000 Pacific 71/1000
China	Nan et al	2002	Random community sample	Interview and questionnaire, self-report, confirmed in medical record	3.6/1000
	Miao et al	2004	Random community sample	Interview, questionnaire and examination, ARA criteria	5.3/1000

Abbreviations: ANZHT, Aotearoa New Zealand Health Tracker; ARA, American Rheumatism Association; GP, general practitioner; NHANES, National Health and Nutrition Examination Survey; RCGP, Royal College of General Practitioner; ULT, urate-lowering therapy.

PREVALENCE OF GOUT

Data from several countries suggest that gout is becoming more prevalent (**Table 2**). In the United States, the National Health Interview Surveys asked participants about members of their household having gout within the preceding year. The 1-year period prevalence of self-reported gout increased from 4.8 per 1000 in 1969 to 7.8 per 1000 in 1976, increasing further to 8.3 per 1000 in 1980.[2] Since then, the prevalence has remained fairly stable at 8.4–9.9 per 1000,[3] with the most recently published estimate being 9.4 per 1000 in 1996.[4] Similarly, the National Health and Nutrition Examination Survey (NHANES) found that the self-reported lifetime prevalence of physician-diagnosed gout increased from 26.4 per 1000 in NHANES III (1988–1994) to 37.6 per 1000 in NHANES 2007–2010.[5] Furthermore, serum uric acid level (the key causal precursor of gout and primary end-point recommended by the US Food and Drug Administration for gout drug approval) has increased over the interval between the 2 NHANES studies.[6] Gout-related claims in an administrative claims database increased from 2.9 per 1000 in 1990 to 5.2 per 1000 in 1999.[7]

In the United Kingdom, the estimated lifetime prevalence of gout was 2.6 per 1000 in 1975, 3.4 per 1000 in 1987, and 9.5 per 1000 in 1993.[8–10] In the General Practice Research Database (GPRD), the 1-year consultation prevalence of gout was 13.9 per 1000 in 1999.[11] A similar consultation prevalence of 14.0 per 1000 was seen in the IMS Disease Analyzer between 2000 and 2005.[12] Subsequently, the Royal College of General Practitioners Weekly Returns Service (RCGP-WRS) found that the annual prevalence seemed to increase slightly from 4.3 per 1000 in 2001 to 4.7 per 1000 in 2007.[13]

Comparison of data from successive surveys undertaken in New Zealand using similar methods shows a marked increase in the prevalence of gout in both European and Maori subjects.[14–16] Lifetime prevalence estimates in 1958, 1966, and 1992 were 3 per 1000, 9 per 1000, and 29 per 1000 in European subjects, respectively. The corresponding estimates in Maori subjects were 27 per 1000, 60 per 1000, and 64 per 1000, respectively. More recently, a nationwide study that used different methods of sampling and case ascertainment showed similar prevalence estimates (ie, 32 per 1000 for European subjects and 61 per 1000 for Maori subjects).[17]

Data from China also suggest that gout is becoming more prevalent. Successive random population surveys in the city of Qingdao found the prevalence of gout to be 3.6 per 1000 in 2002, increasing to 5.3 per 1000 in 2004.[18,19]

There is notable variation in the prevalence of gout obtained in these studies. This variation is likely explained by a combination of differing methods used for sampling, case ascertainment, and definition; different time periods for prevalence estimation (ie, confined-period prevalence vs lifetime prevalence); demographics; and differences in genetic, lifestyle, and comorbid risk factor profiles in different geographic populations. However, comparison of estimates within the same countries and within the same data sets reduces the impact of this methodological and clinical heterogeneity and provides sufficient evidence that gout has become increasingly more common over the past few decades.

INCIDENCE OF GOUT

There are fewer studies examining the incidence of gout. In the United States, the John Hopkins Precursors Study recruited 1216 male medical students (mean age 22.2 years) between 1948 and 1964, following them up for a mean period of 29 years.[20] A total of 60 men developed gout, corresponding to an incidence of 1.73 per 1000 person-years. The Health Professionals Follow-Up Study (HPFS)[21] followed up

47,150 male health professionals for 12 years, identifying 730 cases of incident gout (incidence, 1.50 per 1000 person-years, using the American College of Rheumatology [ACR] survey criteria).[22] In an analysis nested within the Framingham Heart Study, 1951 men and 2476 women aged between 29 and 62 years and free of gout at recruitment in 1947 were followed up for a median of 28 years.[23] The incidence of gout per 1000 person-years was 4.0 in men and 1.4 in women. Serial investigations of computerized medical records from the Rochester Epidemiology Project showed that the incidence of gout without diuretic exposure (using the ACR survey criteria[22]) doubled from 20.2 per 100,000 in 1977–1978 to 45.9 per 100,000 in 1995–1996, whereas the proportion of gout associated with diuretic use decreased significantly during this period.[24]

In contrast to the Rochester Epidemiology Project, data from 3 primary care consultation database studies in the United Kingdom do not suggest that the incidence of gout is changing. Gout incidence remained fairly stable in the GPRD in the 1990s, ranging from 11.9 per 10,000 person-years in 1991 to 18.0 per 10,000 person-years in 1994, before decreasing back to 13.1 per 10,000 person-years in 1999.[11] A study using the Health Improvement Network (THIN) UK primary care database followed up 1,775,505 individuals, aged 20 to 89 years and free of gout at baseline, for an average of 5.2 years between January 2000 and December 2007.[25] A total of 24,768 cases of incident gout were identified, equating to a crude incidence rate of 2.68 per 1000 person-years (incidence per 1000 person-years was 4.42 in men and 1.32 in women), and the incidence remained stable over the study period (in 2000–2001, the rate was 2.67 per 1000 patient-years, and in 2006–2007, the rate was 2.52 per 1000 patient-years). Although the incidence of gout seems to be higher in the later THIN study than the earlier GPRD study, data from the RCGP-WRS found the mean annual incidence of gout to be 12.4 cases per 10,000 person-years between 1994 and 2007, without evidence of changing incidence over this period.[13]

HYPERURICEMIA

It has been well-established that hyperuricemia is the key causal precursor to the development of gout. Population studies have demonstrated and quantified a direct positive (linear to exponential) relation between serum urate levels and a future risk of gout, as summarized here. The Normative Aging Study followed up 2046 healthy male veterans aged 21 to 81 years over a period of 14.9 years, identifying 84 new cases of acute gouty arthritis.[26] The incidence of gout per 1000 person-years in people with serum urate levels less than 6.0 mg/dL, 6.0 to 6.9 mg/dL, 7.0 to 7.9 mg/dL, 8.0 to 8.9 mg/dL, 9.0 to 9.9 mg/dL, and 10.0 mg/dL or more was 0.8, 0.9, 4.1, 8.4, 43.2, and 70.2, respectively. In the Framingham Heart Study, there was a similar marked dose-dependent increase in both incidence and relative risk (RR) of developing gout with serum urate level (**Fig. 1**).[23] A study from Italy undertaken in the Health Search/Longitudinal Patient Primary Care database also found a dose-response relationship between serum urate levels at baseline and incident gout.[27] Compared to those with a serum urate level less than 6 mg/dL, the odds of incident gout were 1.75 (95% confidence interval [CI], 1.44–2.12) with serum urate levels 6 to 7 mg/dL, rising to 6.20 (95% CI, 5.32–7.24) and 15.31 (95% CI, 12.51–18.75) in those with serum urate levels of 7 to 9 mg/dL and 9 mg/dL or more, respectively. In the Kinmen Study from Taiwan, 42 of 223 men with hyperuricemia but no history of gout at baseline in 1991 had developed gout when reexamined in 1996–1997, corresponding to a 5-year cumulative incidence of 18.8%.[28] The 5-year cumulative incidence was 10.8% in those with a serum urate level of 7.0 to 7.9 mg/dL, 27.7% in those with a serum urate level of 8.0 to 8.9 mg/dL, and 61.1% in those with a serum urate level 9.0 mg/dL or more. These studies,

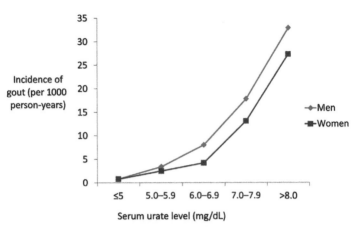

Fig. 1. Increasing incidence of gout in men and women with serum urate level. (*Data from* Bhole V, de Vera M, Rahman MM, et al. Epidemiology of gout in women: fifty-two-year followup of a prospective cohort. Arthritis Rheum 2010;62:1069–76.)

together with the fact that effective management of hyperuricemia prevents gout, provide convincing evidence that hyperuricemia is a necessary casual component for the development of gout.

DIETARY FACTORS

Although an association between gout and dietary factors, particularly purine-rich foods and alcoholic beverages, has been recognized for centuries, it is only recently that robust epidemiologic evidence of such association has emerged (**Table 3**). The most comprehensive assessment of the association between gout and diet has been undertaken in the HPFS. In this large prospective study, a semiquantitative food frequency questionnaire was administered to 51,529 male health professionals at baseline and at 4- and 8-year follow-ups. Over a 12-year period, 730 cases of incidence of gout were identified. In addition to confirming the historical observations that excessive consumption of purine-rich foods and alcoholic drinks are independent risk factors for gout, evidence has been provided for more novel dietary associations: namely, that fructose and sugar-sweetened soft drinks increase the risk of developing gout, whereas dairy products, coffee, and vitamin C seem to be protective against the development of gout.

Purine-rich foods theoretically predispose to gout by providing exogenous substrate for purine metabolism, the end product of which is uric acid in humans (**Fig. 2**). Compared with men in the lowest quintile, men in the highest quintiles of total meat and seafood intake had an increased risk of incident gout of 41% and 51%, respectively, adjusting for age; energy intake; BMI, calculated as the weight in kilograms divided by the height in meters squared; diuretic use; hypertension; renal failure; and dietary factors including alcohol (see **Table 3**).[21] Consumption of purine-rich vegetables was not a risk factor for incident gout. Men in the highest quintile of consumption of dairy products, particularly low-fat dairy products, had almost half the risk of incident gout compared to those in the lowest quintile. High-fat dairy consumption had no protective effect. The multivariate RRs per additional daily serving were 1.21 (95% CI, 1.04–1.41) for total meat, 1.07 (95% CI, 1.01–1.12) for seafood, 0.82 (95% CI, 0.75–0.90) for total dairy, and 0.79 (95% CI, 0.71–0.87) for low-fat dairy. A recent

Table 3
Dietary factors and risk of incident gout

Dietary Factor	Study	Exposure Group	Referent Group	Multivariate Risk Estimate (95% Confidence Interval)
Total Meat	HPFS	Highest quintile	Lowest quintile	RR, 1.41 (1.07–1.86)
Seafood	HPFS	Highest quintile	Lowest quintile	RR, 1.51 (1.17–1.95)
Purine-rich vegetables	HPFS	Highest quintile	Lowest quintile	RR, 0.96 (0.79–1.19)
Dairy products	HPFS	Highest quintile	Lowest quintile	RR, 0.56 (0.42–0.74)
Low-fat dairy	HPFS	Highest quintile	Lowest quintile	RR, 0.58 (0.45–0.76)
High-fat dairy	HPFS	Highest quintile	Lowest quintile	RR, 1.00 (0.77–1.29)
Coffee	HPFS	≥6 cups/d	None	RR, 0.41 (0.19–0.88)
	Nurses' Health Study	≥4 cups/d	None	RR, 0.43 (0.30–0.61)
Decaffeinated coffee	HPFS	≥4 cups/d	None	RR, 0.73 (0.46–1.17)
	Nurses' Health Study	>1 cups/d	None	RR, 0.77 (0.63–0.95)
Tea	HPFS	≥4 cups/d	None	RR, 0.82 (0.38–1.75)
	Nurses' Health Study	≥4 cups/d	None	RR, 1.55 (0.98–2.47)
Total caffeine	HPFS	Highest quintile	Lowest quintile	RR, 0.83 (0.64–1.08)
	Nurses' Health Study	Highest quintile	Lowest quintile	RR, 0.52 (0.41–0.68)
Sugar-sweetened soft drinks	HPFS	≥2 servings/d	<1 serving/mo	RR, 1.85 (1.08–3.16)
	Nurses' Health Study	≥2 servings/d	<1 serving/mo	RR, 2.39 (1.34–4.26)
Diet soft drinks	HPFS	≥2 servings/d	<1 serving/mo	RR, 1.12 (0.82–1.52)
	Nurses' Health Study	≥2 servings/d	<1 serving/mo	RR, 1.18 (0.87–1.58)
Free fructose	HPFS	Highest quintile	Lowest quintile	RR, 2.02 (1.49–2.75)
	Nurses' Health Study	Highest quintile	Lowest quintile	RR, 1.62 (1.20–2.19)
Vitamin C	HPFS	≥1500 mg/d	<250 mg/d	RR, 0.55 (0.38–0.80)
Alcohol	ARIC	"High" alcohol intake	Not defined	HR, 2.00 (1.42–2.82)
	THIN	>42 units/wk	None	OR, 3.00 (2.66–3.38)
	HPFS	≥50 g/d	None	RR, 2.53 (1.73–3.70)
	Framingham Heart (men)	≥7 oz/wk	0–1 oz/wk	RR, 2.21 (1.56–3.14)
	Framingham Heart (women)	≥7 oz/wk	0–1 oz/wk	RR, 3.10 (1.69–5.68)
Beer	HPFS	>2 servings/d	<1 serving/mo	RR, 2.51 (1.77–3.55)
Spirits	HPFS	>2 servings/d	<1 serving/mo	RR, 1.60 (1.19–2.16)
Wine	HPFS	>2 servings/d	<1 serving/mo	RR, 1.05 (0.64–1.72)

Abbreviations: ARIC, Atherosclerosis Risk in Communities; HR, hazards ratio; OR, odds ratio; RR, relative risk; THIN, the Health Improvement Network.

randomized controlled trial (RCT) has found that intact milk intake has an acute urico-suric urate lowering effect.[29] Proteins contained in milk, such as casein, lactalbumin, and orotic acid, may exert their uricosuric effects without the concomitant purine load contained in other animal protein sources such as meat and seafood.[29,30] Another

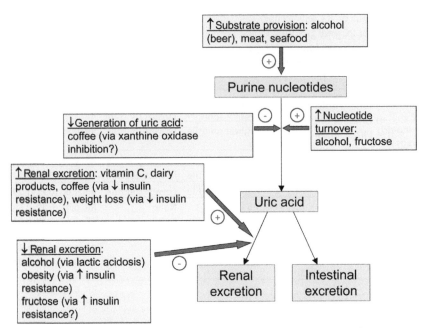

Fig. 2. Proposed mechanism of action of lifestyle factors in the etiology of hyperuricemia and gout. ↑, Increased; ↓, decreased.

RCT has suggested that skimmed milk powder derivatives have antiinflammatory effects against acute gout flares among patients with preexisting gout.[31]

Excessive consumption of purine-rich foods has been shown to trigger recurrent gout attacks in a novel internet-based case-crossover study in which each participant acts as his or her own control, thereby allowing the effect of transient exposures on an acute event to be studied while eliminating confounding due to individual characteristics that do not change during the study period.[32] In an analysis of 1247 recurrent gout attacks occurring over a 1-year period in 633 participants, the multivariate odds ratios (ORs) for recurrent gout attacks for each increasing quintile of purine consumption were 1.17 (95% CI, 0.88–1.55), 1.38 (95% CI, 1.02–1.87), 2.21 (95% CI, 1.62–3.01), and 4.76 (95% CI, 3.37–6.74), respectively, compared with the lowest quintile over a 2-day period and adjusted for use of alcohol, diuretics, allopurinol, colchicine, and nonsteroidal antiinflammatory drugs.

Coffee is thought to reduce serum uric acid levels by several mechanisms (see **Fig. 2**). Coffee is rich in antioxidants, such as the phenol chlorogenic acid, which are thought to increase insulin sensitivity[33,34] and in turn enhance renal urate excretion.[35] Caffeine is itself a methylxanthine and may therefore be a competitive inhibitor of xanthine oxidase,[36] the major enzyme in purine metabolic pathways. In a subsequent HPFS analysis, a dose-dependent inverse relationship between the number of cups of coffee consumed per day and incident gout was seen (0 cups; RR, 1.00 referent; <1 cup; RR, 0.97; 95% CI, 0.78–1.20; 1–3 cups; RR, 0.92; 95% CI, 0.75–1.11; 4–5 cups; RR, 0.60; 95% CI, 0.41–0.87; ≥6 cups; RR, 0.41; 95% CI, 0.19–0.88).[37] A similar more modest inverse association was seen between consumption of decaffeinated coffee and incident gout, whereas no association was seen for either tea consumption or total caffeine intake. The association between coffee consumption and incident gout in women has been examined in the Nurses' Health

Study.[38] A total of 89,433 female nurses who were gout free before baseline were followed up for 26 years, during which 896 incident gout cases occurred. A similar inverse relationship was found between coffee consumption and risk of gout. Compared with women who drank no coffee, women who drank 948 mL or more of coffee per day had less than half the risk of incident gout, after adjustment for age, total energy intake, BMI, menopause, use of hormonal replacement, diuretic use, hypertension, and dietary factors (see **Table 3**). As with men in the HPFS,[37] there was a modest inverse relationship with decaffeinated coffee and no association with tea. In contrast to men in the HPFS, there was a negative association between total caffeine intake and incident gout. Women consuming 359 to 497 mg/d and 498 mg/d or more had 23% and 48% reduced risk, respectively, compared with women consuming 131 mg/d or less (see **Table 3**).

Fructose acts as a substrate for uric acid production by enhancing degradation of purine nucleotides (see **Fig. 2**).[39] Consumption of sugar-sweetened soft drinks has also been shown to increase the risk of incident gout in a dose-dependent manner in the HPFS.[40] Compared to men who consumed sugar-sweetened soft drinks less frequently than once per month, the multivariate RR of incident gout was 1.29 (95% CI, 1.00–1.68) in those consuming 5 to 6 servings per week, 1.45 (95% CI, 1.02–2.08) in those with once daily consumption, and 1.85 (95% CI, 1.08–3.16) in those consuming 2 or more servings per day. Consumption of diet soft drinks was not a risk factor for incident gout. A positive dose-dependent relationship was also seen between free fructose intake and incident gout (quintile 1, referent; quintile 2; RR, 1.29; 95% CI, 1.02–1.64; quintile 3; RR, 1.41; 95% CI, 1.09–1.82; quintile 4; RR, 1.84; 95% CI, 1.40–2.41; quintile 5; RR, 2.02; 95% CI, 1.49–2.75). In the Nurses' Health Study, women drinking 1 serving of sugar-sweetened soft drink per day and 2 or more servings per day were at a 74% and 139% higher risk of incident gout, respectively, compared to those consuming less than 1 serving per month (see **Table 3**).[41] Compared to women in the lowest quintile of free fructose intake, the multivariate RRs of incident gout in the highest and second highest quintiles were 1.62 (95% CI, 1.20–2.19) and 1.34 (95% CI, 1.01–1.76), respectively.

Vitamin C has recognized uricosuric properties (see **Fig. 2**),[42] and high vitamin C intake has been shown to be protective against the development of gout in the HPFS.[43] The multivariate RR of incident gout was 0.97 (95% CI, 0.85–1.12) for total vitamin C consumption of 250 to 499 mg/d; 0.83 (95% CI, 0.71–0.97), for 500 to 999 mg/d; 0.66 (95% CI, 0.52–0.86), for 1000 to 1499 mg/d; and 0.55 (95% CI, 0.38–0.80), for 1500 mg/d or more, compared with the RR of those consuming less than 250 mg/d.

Cherries and cherry extract have recognized urate-lowering properties and hence have attracted much interest as a potential treatment of gout. However, epidemiologic evidence of the association between cherry consumption and gout is sparse. In the internet-based case-crossover study described earlier, intake of cherries (multivariate OR, 0.65; 95% CI, 0.50–0.85) and cherry extract (OR, 0.55; 95% CI, 0.30–0.98) over the preceding 2-day period both seemed to be protective against recurrent gout attacks.[44]

ALCOHOL CONSUMPTION

Several studies have examined the long-recognized observation that alcohol consumption is a risk factor for the development of gout (see **Table 3**). Alcohol consumption is thought to predispose to gout by providing substrate for purine metabolism in the form of guanosine (particularly beer), enhancing nucleotide turnover and impairing renal urate excretion via lactic acidosis (see **Fig. 2**).[45] The Atherosclerosis Risk in Communities (ARIC) study was a population-based prospective cohort study that recruited 15,792 individuals aged 45 to 64 years between 1987 and 1989. In a subanalysis undertaken in 10,872 participants who did not have gout before baseline, 274 people developed gout over the 9-year follow-up period.[46] Those who fulfilled an unspecified definition of "high" alcohol intake had twice the risk of incident gout, adjusted for sex, race, BMI, alcohol intake, and estimated glomerular filtration rate. In a case-control study nested within the THIN primary care database study, 24,768 people with incident gout were compared with 50,000 control subjects without gout who were frequency matched for age, gender, and calendar year.[25] There was a dose-response relationship between incident gout and prior alcohol consumption. Compared with those who did not drink alcohol, the multivariate ORs of incident gout in those drinking 1 to 9, 10 to 24, 25 to 42, and more than 42 units of alcohol per week were 1.06 (95% CI, 1.01–1.11), 1.56 (95% CI, 1.49–1.65), 2.45 (95% CI, 2.27–2.63), and 3.00 (95% CI, 2.66–3.38), respectively, adjusting for age, calendar year, general practitioner (GP) visits, BMI, ischemic heart disease, hypertension, hyperlipidemia, diabetes, chronic renal failure, and use of diuretics (1 unit = 10 mL of pure ethanol or 8 g of alcohol). In the HPFS, increasing alcohol intake was associated with increasing risk of incident gout.[47] Compared with men who did not drink alcohol, the multivariate RRs were 1.09 (95% CI, 0.85–1.40) for daily alcohol consumption of 0.1 to 4.9 g, 1.25 (95% CI, 0.95–1.64), for 5.0 to 9.9 g; 1.32 (95% CI, 0.99–1.75), for 10.0 to 14.9 g; 1.49 (95% CI, 1.14–1.94), for 15.0 to 29.9 g; 1.96 (95% CI, 1.48–2.60), for 30.0 to 49.9 g; and 2.53 (95% CI, 1.73–3.70) for 50 g or more. The multivariate RR per 10-g increase in daily alcohol consumption was 1.17 (95% CI, 1.11–1.22). Compared with men drinking each type of drink less than once per month, those imbibing 2 or more drinks per day had 2.5 times the risk of incident gout for beer, 1.6 times for spirits, and no increased risk associated with wine (see **Table 3**). The multivariate RR per serving per day was 1.49 (95% CI, 1.32–1.70) for beer, 1.15 (95% CI, 1.04–1.28) for spirits, and 1.04 (95% CI, 0.88–1.22) for wine. The Framingham Heart Study has shown excessive alcohol consumption to be an independent risk factor for gout in both women and men.[23] Women who drank 7 oz or more of alcohol per week had more than 3 times the risk of incident gout and men drinking this amount had more than twice the risk, compared with those who drank less than 0 to 1 oz per week (see **Table 3**). Moderate consumption (2–6 oz/wk) was not associated with incident gout in either gender. In the internet-based case-crossover study described earlier,[48] alcohol consumption was found to trigger recurrent gout attacks (multivariate OR, 2.5; 95% CI, 1.1–5.9; ≥ 7 alcoholic drinks consumed in the previous 2 days, compared with no consumption; adjusted for purine intake and diuretic use).

OBESITY AND THE METABOLIC SYNDROME

Gout is commonly associated with comorbidity, including the metabolic syndrome. In a large cross-sectional study undertaken in NHANES III, the prevalence of the metabolic syndrome in people with gout was 62.8% compared with 25.4% among people without gout (OR, 3.05; 95% CI, 2.01–4.61; adjusted for age and gender).[49]

Several individual components of the metabolic syndrome have been shown to be independent risk factors for the development of gout (**Table 4**). A dose-dependent effect between increasing BMI and risk of incident gout has been demonstrated in several large prospective epidemiologic studies. In the THIN database case-control study, individuals with a BMI between 25 and 29 kg/m^2 had a multivariate OR of 1.62 (95% CI, 1.55–1.70) for incident gout and those with BMI of 30 kg/m^2 or more

Table 4
Medical conditions and risk of incident gout

Risk Factor	Study	Exposure Group	Referent Group	Multivariate Risk Estimate (95% Confidence Interval)
BMI	THIN	BMI 25–29 kg/m^2	BMI 20–24 kg/m^2	OR, 1.62 (1.55–1.70)
	THIN	BMI ≥30 kg/m^2	BMI 20–24 kg/m^2	OR, 2.34 (2.22–2.47)
	HPFS	BMI 25–29.9 kg/m^2	BMI 21–22.9 kg/m^2	RR, 1.95 (1.44–2.65)
	HPFS	BMI 30–34.9 kg/m^2	BMI 21–22.9 kg/m^2	RR, 2.33 (1.62–3.36)
	HPFS	BMI ≥35 kg/m^2	BMI 21–22.9 kg/m^2	RR, 2.97 (1.73–5.10)
	ARIC (women)	BMI 30–34.9 kg/m^2	BMI <25 kg/m^2	RR, 2.76 (1.40–5.44)
	ARIC (women)	BMI ≥35 kg/m^2	BMI <25 kg/m^2	RR, 3.90 (1.95–7.82)
	Framingham Heart (men)	BMI 25–29.9 kg/m^2	BMI <25 kg/m^2	RR, 1.76 (1.22–2.54)
	Framingham Heart (men)	BMI ≥30 kg/m^2	BMI <25 kg/m^2	RR, 2.90 (1.89–4.44)
	Framingham Heart (women)	BMI 25–29.9 kg/m^2	BMI <25 kg/m^2	RR, 1.44 (0.88–2.37)
	Framingham Heart (women)	BMI ≥30 kg/m^2	BMI <25 kg/m^2	RR, 2.74 (1.65–4.58)
Hypertension	THIN	Hypertension	No hypertension	OR, 1.18 (1.13–1.23)
	HPFS	Hypertension	No hypertension	RR, 2.31 (1.96–2.72)
	ARIC	Hypertension	No hypertension	HR, 2.00 (1.52–2.61)
	Framingham Heart (men)	Hypertension	No hypertension	RR, 1.59 (1.12–2.24)
	Framingham Heart (women)	Hypertension	No hypertension	RR, 1.82 (1.06–3.14)
Diabetes mellitus	THIN (men)	Diabetes mellitus	No diabetes mellitus	RR, 0.59 (0.55–0.64)
	THIN (women)	Diabetes mellitus	No diabetes mellitus	RR, 0.90 (0.80–1.00)
	THIN	Type I diabetes mellitus	No diabetes mellitus	RR, 0.33 (0.24–0.46)
	THIN	Type II diabetes mellitus	No diabetes mellitus	RR, 0.69 (0.64–0.73)
Chronic renal failure	THIN	Chronic renal failure	No chronic renal failure	OR, 2.48 (2.19–2.81)
	HPFS	Chronic renal failure	No chronic renal failure	RR, 3.61 (1.60–8.14)

had an OR of 2.34 (95% CI, 2.22–2.47) when compared with those with a BMI 20 to 24 kg/m^2.[25] In the HPFS, compared with those with a BMI of 21 to 22.9 kg/m^2, the multivariate RR of incident gout in men was 0.85 in those with a BMI less than 21 kg/m^2, increasing to 1.40 in those with BMI 23 to 24.9 kg/m^2, 1.95 in those with BMI 25 to 29.9 kg/m^2, 2.33 in those with BMI 30 to 34.9 kg/m^2, and 2.97 in those with a BMI of 35 kg/m^2 or more.[50] Furthermore, risk of incident gout was increased in men who had gained 20 to 29 lbs (multivariate RR, 1.57; 95% CI, 1.15–2.14) and 30 lbs or more (RR, 2.47; 95% CI, 1.86–3.28) in weight since the age of 21 years compared with those whose weight was stable. In contrast, weight loss of 10 lbs or more since baseline reduced the risk of incident gout by 39% (multivariate RR, 0.61; 95% CI, 0.40–0.92).

An analysis undertaken in the ARIC study provides similar data for women (see **Table 4**).[51] A total of 6263 women aged 45 to 64 years with no history of gout before baseline were followed up for 9 years, identifying 106 cases of incident gout. When compared with women with a BMI less than 25 kg/m^2 at baseline, the adjusted RR of incident gout was 1.63 (95% CI, 0.84–3.18) with a BMI of 25 to 29.9 kg/m^2, 2.76 (95% CI, 1.40–5.44) with a BMI of 30 to 34.9 kg/m^2, and 3.90 (95% CI, 1.95–7.82) with a BMI of 35 kg/m^2 or more. In women with a BMI of 25 to 29.9 kg/m^2 and BMI 30 kg/m^2 or more at the age of 25 years, the multivariate RRs for incident gout were 3.36 (95% CI, 2.09–5.41) and 2.84 (95% CI, 1.33–6.09), respectively, when compared with those with a BMI less than 25 kg/m^2 at the age of 25 years. Women with the highest tertile of weight gain ($\geq$16.3 kg) from the age of 25 years to baseline had twice the risk of incident gout compared with individuals in the lowest tertile (multivariate RR, 2.05; 95% CI, 1.06–3.96).

Evidence of a dose-dependent effect of increasing BMI on risk of incident gout in men and women is provided by the Framingham Heart Study (see **Table 4**).[23] Compared to those with a BMI less than 25 kg/m^2, the multivariate RR of incident gout was 1.44 (95% CI, 0.88–2.37) in women with a BMI of 25 to 29.9 kg/m^2, rising to 2.74 (95% CI, 1.65–4.58) in those with a BMI of 30 kg/m^2 or more. In men, the corresponding RRs were 1.76 (95% CI, 1.22–2.54) and 2.90 (95% CI, 1.89–4.44), respectively. Increasing BMI has also been found to be an independent risk factor for gout flare in the THIN database (BMI 15–19 kg/m^2: hazard ratio [HR] in men 0.77, HR in women 0.79; BMI 25–29 kg/m^2: HR in men 1.07, HR in women 1.10; BMI$\geq$30 kg/m^2: HR in men 1.12, HR in women 1.43) when compared with those with a BMI in the range 20 to 24 kg/m^2.[52]

Several large prospective epidemiologic studies have examined the association between hypertension and gout (see **Table 4**). Hypertension was found to be an independent risk factor for incident gout in the THIN database case-control study, although the magnitude of increased risk was small.[25] In contrast, in both HPFS and ARIC, the risk of incident gout in those with hypertension was twice that of those without hypertension.[46,50] The findings of these 2 studies suggest that hypertension has a greater effect on risk of incident gout in women than in men. In the Framingham Heart Study, the multivariate RR of incident gout associated with hypertension was 1.59 (95% CI, 1.12–2.24) in men and 1.82 (95% CI, 1.06–3.14) in women, although there was considerable overlap of the confidence intervals.[23] However, in the THIN database, narrower confidence intervals suggest that hypertension has a greater influence on gout flares in women (multivariate RR, 1.45; 95% CI, 1.30–1.62) than in men (RR, 1.08; 95% CI, 1.02–1.13).[52]

Although hyperglycemia and insulin resistance are recognized components of the metabolic syndrome, the role of diabetes mellitus as a risk factor for the development for gout has received relatively little attention. In the THIN database case-control study, individuals with diabetes had a 33% lower risk of developing gout than those without diabetes (multivariate RR, 0.67; 95% CI, 0.63–0.71).[53] This finding was more marked in men than in women (see **Table 4**). The risk of developing gout reduced with increasing duration of diabetes: duration 0 to 3 years, RR, 0.81 (95% CI, 0.74–0.90); 4 to 9 years, RR, 0.67 (95% CI, 0.61–0.73); and 10 years or longer, RR, 0.52 (95% CI, 0.46–0.58). Risk was also less with type I than with type II diabetes (see **Table 4**). Although these findings may seem counterintuitive, the predisposition to hyperuricemia and gout induced by hyperinsulinemia and insulin resistance in the prediabetic state is thought to be reversed by the uricosuric effects of glycosuria once frank diabetes develops.[54–56]

A less-well-established putative risk factor for gout is obstructive sleep apnea, which is commonly associated with components of both the metabolic syndrome and hyperuricemia.[57–59] Hypoxia enhances nucleotide turnover thereby generating purines that are metabolized to uric acid,[60,61] providing a biologically plausible mechanism by which obstructive sleep apnea might predispose to gout. In a small cross-sectional study undertaken in a GP consultation database, gout was associated with sleep disorders (OR, 1.39; 95% CI, 1.06–1.81; adjusted for age, gender, practice, diabetes, hypertension, diuretic use, and ischemic heart disease).[62] There was no association with obstructive sleep apnea, although the study was underpowered. Larger prospective epidemiologic studies are required to examine this proposed association in more detail.

MEDICATIONS

Several medications and substances have been implicated in the etiology of gout[63]; however, diuretics have received the greatest attention. A recent systematic review examined the risk of gouty arthritis in patients using diuretics,[64] identifying 2 RCTs and 11 epidemiologic studies. In one RCT, the rate ratio of gout for use of bendroflua-zide versus placebo was 11.8, whereas the other RCT found a rate ratio of 6.3 for use of hydrochlorothiazide plus triamterene versus placebo. A total of 3 cohort studies[28,50,65] and 4 case-control studies[66–69] found an increased occurrence of gout in diuretic users. The 2 largest cohort studies identified by this systematic review adjusted for medications,[65] comorbidities,[50,65] and lifestyle factors,[50] finding RRs of 1.77 for incident gout in the HPFS (95% CI, 1.42–2.20)[50] and 1.99 for initiation of antig-out medication (95% CI, 1.21–3.26).[65] The Framingham Heart Study was not included in this review but reported multivariate RRs for diuretic use of 2.39 (95% CI, 1.53–3.74) in women and 3.41 (95% CI, 2.38–4.89) in men.[23] In the THIN case-control study, the RR for incident gout among those currently using diuretics was 2.36 (95% CI, 2.21–2.52) in people with hypertension and 3.01 (95% CI, 2.72–3.33) in those without hypertension, after adjustment for GP visits, BMI, alcohol use, ischemic heart disease, hypertension, hyperlipidemia, renal failure, and use of other antihypertensive drugs.[70] Furthermore, among current diuretic users, the risk of developing gout increased with both the duration of diuretic therapy and increased dosage, providing evidence of a dose-dependent effect. Finally, the aforementioned internet-based case-crossover study has also shown consistent findings for the risk of recurrent gout.[67] These studies collectively confirm the well-recognized clinical entity of diuretic-induced gout, also known as secondary gout.

Aspirin has long-been recognized to have effects on renal tubular urate handling. In the 1950s, high-dose aspirin was found to be uricosuric, while low doses were urate retaining.[71] However, only recently has epidemiologic evidence of the clinical significance of this association come to light. In the internet-based case-crossover study, use of low-dose aspirin (≤325 mg/d) in the previous 2 consecutive days was associated with an increased risk of recurrent gout attacks (OR, 1.81; 95% CI, 1.30–2.51).[72] Concurrent use of allopurinol removed the increased risk of recurrent gout attacks associated with low-dose aspirin (adjusted OR, 0.89; 95% CI, 0.55–1.44) suggesting that urate-lowering therapy may mitigate the risk of recurrent acute gout exacerbated by use of low-dose aspirin.

Several classes of antihypertensive drugs are known to influence serum urate levels. β-Blockers increase serum urate levels, whereas both calcium channel blockers and losartan have urate-lowering properties.[63,73] In addition to examining the risk of gout associated with diuretic use, the THIN primary care database case-control study described above also investigated the risk of incident gout conferred by a wide range of antihypertensive drugs including calcium channel blockers, losartan, β-blockers, angiotensin-converting enzyme (ACE) inhibitors, and nonlosartan AII receptor blockers.[70] Among those with hypertension, current use of β-blockers (RR, 1.48; 95% CI, 1.40–1.57), ACE inhibitors (RR, 1.24; 95% CI, 1.17–1.32), and nonlosartan AII receptor blockers (RR, 1.29; 95% CI, 1.16–1.43) was more common in those with incident gout, whereas current use of calcium channel blockers (RR, 0.87; 95% CI, 0.82–0.93) and losartan (RR, 0.81; 95% CI, 0.70–0.94) was less common.

RENAL DISEASE

The association between gout and renal disease is complex and could be bidirectional, that is, although renal disease predisposes to the development of gout, gout and its treatment are themselves thought to lead to renal impairment and chronic kidney disease. Such associations have been recognized for many years, yet early studies were undertaken in specialist secondary care populations,[74–76] which may not be representative of most patients with gout who are managed exclusively in primary care. More recently, 2 population-based epidemiologic studies have provided convincing evidence that renal disease is a risk factor for gout. In the HPFS, the multivariate RR of incident gout in men with chronic renal failure compared with those without chronic renal failure was 3.61 (95% CI, 1.60–8.14).[50] In the THIN case-control study, prior history of chronic renal failure was strongly associated with incident gout (OR, 2.48; 95% CI, 2.19–2.81).[25] Renal failure was also associated with risk of gout flare (HR, 1.33; 95% CI, 1.20–1.48).[52] Furthermore, in the ARIC study, participants with a low estimated glomerular filtration rate (<60 mL/min) had twice the risk of incident gout compared with those with a normal estimated glomerular filtration rate (>90 mL/min) (multivariate HR, 2.43; 95% CI, 1.50–3.94).[46]

OA

Although hyperuricemia is a very strong risk factor for gout, many hyperuricemic individuals do not develop gout. It is not fully understood why some people with hyperuricemia seem to form and deposit MSU crystals more readily than others; however, it is thought that MSU crystals may deposit more easily in osteoarthritic cartilage.[77] This hypothesis has also been suggested to explain the striking predilection of gout for the first metatarsophalangeal (MTP) joint, which is also a target joint for OA.[78] Both radiographic and clinical cross-sectional studies have shown that attacks of gout occur at joints already affected by OA. A hospital-based study of 262 subjects with gout found a significant correlation between the occurrence of acute attacks of gout and radiographic OA at the first MTP joints, tarsal joints, and knees.[79] More recently, a community-based study of 164 subjects with gout found a strong association between sites of acute attacks of gout and the presence of clinical OA (multivariate OR, 7.94; 95% CI, 6.27–10.05), adjusted for age, gender, BMI, and diuretic use.[80] However, nodal OA was not more frequent in gout subjects than in 656 control subjects without gout.[81] Such cross-sectional studies cannot determine causality or temporal aspects of this association; hence further prospective studies are required.

SUMMARY

Several epidemiologic studies from a diverse range of countries suggest that gout has increased in prevalence over the past few decades, making it the most common inflammatory arthritis, particularly among men. Incidence data are scarce; however, the Rochester Epidemiology Project found that the incidence of gout without diuretic exposure has doubled in the United States between the 1970s and the 1990s.

Evidence from prospective epidemiologic studies has confirmed purported dietary factors, obesity, the metabolic syndrome, hypertension, use of diuretics, and chronic kidney disease as clinically relevant risk factors for hyperuricemia and gout, whereas low-fat dairy products, coffee, and vitamin C seem to be protective against these conditions. Furthermore, the use of β-blockers and AII receptor antagonists (other than losartan) are independent risk factors for the development of hyperuricemia and gout, whereas calcium channel blockers and losartan seem to reduce the risk of developing these conditions. While further prospective studies are necessary to explore putative risk factors such as obstructive sleep apnea, OA, and more novel observations concerning antihypertensive medications in more depth, the immediate challenge is to translate the key findings of these epidemiologic observations into simple messages to improve the prevention and management of this prevalent but often undertreated condition.

REFERENCES

1. Chandratre P, Roddy E, Clarson L, et al. Health-related quality of life in gout: a systematic review. Rheumatology (Oxford) 2013;52(11):2031–40.
2. Lawrence RC, Hochberg MC, Kelsey JL, et al. Estimates of the prevalence of selected arthritic and musculoskeletal diseases in the United States. J Rheumatol 1989;16:427–41.
3. Lawrence RC, Helmick CG, Arnett FC, et al. Estimates of the prevalence of arthritis and selected musculoskeletal disorders in the United States. Arthritis Rheum 1998;41:778–99.
4. Lawrence RC, Felson DT, Helmick CG, et al. Estimates of the prevalence of arthritis and other rheumatic conditions in the United States. Part II. Arthritis Rheum 2008;58:26–35.
5. Juraschek SP, Miller ER 3rd, Gelber AC. Body mass index, obesity, and prevalent gout in the United States in 1988–1994 and 2007–2010. Arthritis Care Res (Hoboken) 2013;65:127–32.
6. Zhu Y, Pandya BJ, Choi HK. Prevalence of gout and hyperuricemia in the US general population: the National Health and Nutrition Examination Survey 2007–2008. Arthritis Rheum 2011;63:3136–41.
7. Wallace KL, Riedel AA, Joseph-Ridge N, et al. Increasing prevalence of gout and hyperuricemia over 10 years among older adults in a managed care population. J Rheumatol 2004;31:1582–7.
8. Currie WJ. Prevalence and incidence of the diagnosis of gout in Great Britain. Ann Rheum Dis 1979;38:101–6.
9. Steven MM. Prevalence of chronic arthritis in four geographical areas of the Scottish Highlands. Ann Rheum Dis 1992;51:186–94.
10. Harris CM, Lloyd DC, Lewis J. The prevalence and prophylaxis of gout in England. J Clin Epidemiol 1995;48:1153–8.
11. Mikuls TR, Farrar JT, Bilker WB, et al. Gout epidemiology: results from the UK General Practice Research Database, 1990–1999. Ann Rheum Dis 2005;64: 267–72.
12. Annemans L, Spaepen E, Gaskin M, et al. Gout in the UK and Germany: prevalence, comorbidities and management in general practice 2000–2005. Ann Rheum Dis 2008;67:960–6.
13. Elliot AJ, Cross KW, Fleming DM. Seasonality and trends in the incidence and prevalence of gout in England and Wales 1994–2007. Ann Rheum Dis 2009; 68:1728–33.

14. Lennane GA, Rose BS, Isdale IC. Gout in the Maori. Ann Rheum Dis 1960;19: 120–5.
15. Prior IA, Rose BS. Uric acid, gout and public health in the South Pacific. N Z Med J 1966;65:295–300.
16. Klemp P, Stansfield SA, Castle B, et al. Gout is on the increase in New Zealand. Ann Rheum Dis 1997;56:22–6.
17. Winnard D, Wright C, Jackson G, et al. Gout, diabetes and cardiovascular disease in the Aotearoa New Zealand adult population: co-prevalence and implications for clinical practice. N Z Med J 2012;126:53–64.
18. Nan H, Qiao Q, Dong Y, et al. The prevalence of hyperuricemia in a population of the coastal city of Qingdao, China. J Rheumatol 2006;33:1346–50.
19. Miao Z, Li C, Chen Y, et al. Dietary and lifestyle changes associated with high prevalence of hyperuricaemia and gout in the Shandong coastal cities of Eastern China. J Rheumatol 2008;35:1859–64.
20. Roubenoff R, Klag MJ, Mead LA, et al. Incidence and risk factors for gout in white men. JAMA 1991;266:3004–7.
21. Choi HK, Atkinson K, Karlson EW, et al. Purine-rich foods, dairy and protein intake, and the risk of gout in men. N Engl J Med 2004;350:1093–103.
22. Wallace SL, Robinson H, Masi AT, et al. Preliminary criteria for the classification of the acute arthritis of primary gout. Arthritis Rheum 1977;20:895–900.
23. Bhole V, de Vera M, Rahman MM, et al. Epidemiology of gout in women: fifty-two-year followup of a prospective cohort. Arthritis Rheum 2010;62:1069–76.
24. Arromdee E, Michet CJ, Crowson CS, et al. Epidemiology of gout: is the incidence rising? J Rheumatol 2002;29:2403–6.
25. Cea Soriano L, Rothenbacher D, Choi HK, et al. Contemporary epidemiology of gout in the UK general population. Arthritis Res Ther 2011;13:R39.
26. Campion EW, Glynn RJ, DeLabry LO. Asymptomatic hyperuricemia. Risks and consequences in the Normative Aging Study. Am J Med 1987;82:421–6.
27. Trifirò G, Morabito P, Cavagna L. Epidemiology of gout and hyperuricaemia in Italy during the years 2005-2009: a nationwide population-based study. Ann Rheum Dis 2013;72:694–700.
28. Lin KC, Lin HY, Chou P. The interaction between uric acid level and other risk factors on the development of gout among asymptomatic hyperuricemic men in a prospective study. J Rheumatol 2000;27:1501–5.
29. Dalbeth N, Wong S, Gamble GD, et al. Acute effect of milk on serum urate concentrations: a randomised controlled crossover trial. Ann Rheum Dis 2010;69: 1677–82.
30. Garrel DR, Verdy M, PetitClerc C, et al. Milk- and soy-protein ingestion: acute effect on serum uric acid concentration. Am J Clin Nutr 1991;53:665–9.
31. Dalbeth N, Ames R, Gamble GD, et al. Effects of skim milk powder enriched with glycomacropeptide and G600 milk fat extract on frequency of gout flares: a proof-of-concept randomised controlled trial. Ann Rheum Dis 2012;71:929–34.
32. Zhang Y, Chen C, Choi H, et al. Purine-rich foods intake and recurrent gout attacks. Ann Rheum Dis 2012;71:1448–53.
33. Bruce CR, Carey AL, Hawley JA, et al. Intramuscular heat shock protein 72 and heme oxygenase-1 mRNA are reduced in patients with type 2 diabetes: evidence that insulin resistance is associated with a disturbed antioxidant defense mechanism. Diabetes 2003;52:2338–45.
34. Thirunavukkarasu V, Anuradha CV. Influence of α-lipoic acid on lipid peroxidation and antioxidant defence system in blood of insulin-resistant rats. Diabetes Obes Metab 2004;6:200–7.

35. Ter Maaten JC, Voorburg A, Heine RJ, et al. Renal handling of urate and sodium during acute physiological hyperinsulinaemia in healthy subjects. Clin Sci (Lond) 1997;92:51–8.
36. Kela U, Vijayvargiya R, Trivedi CP. Inhibitory effects of methylxanthines on the activity of xanthine oxidase. Life Sci 1980;27:2109–19.
37. Choi HK, Willett W, Curhan G. Coffee consumption and risk of incident gout in men: a prospective study. Arthritis Rheum 2007;56:2049–55.
38. Choi HK, Curhan G. Coffee consumption and risk of incident gout in women: the Nurses' Health Study. Am J Clin Nutr 2010;92:922–7.
39. Raivio KO, Becker A, Meyer LJ, et al. Stimulation of human purine synthesis de novo by fructose infusion. Metabolism 1975;24:861–9.
40. Choi HK, Curhan G. Soft drinks, fructose consumption, and the risk of gout in men: prospective cohort study. BMJ 2008;336:309–12.
41. Choi HK, Willett W, Curhan G. Fructose-rich beverages and risk of gout in women. JAMA 2010;304:2270–8.
42. Juraschek SP, Miller ER 3rd, Gelber AC. Effect of oral vitamin C supplementation on serum uric acid: a meta-analysis of randomized controlled trials. Arthritis Care Res (Hoboken) 2011;63:1295–306.
43. Choi HK, Gao X, Curhan G. Vitamin C intake and the risk of gout in men: a prospective study. Arch Intern Med 2009;169:502–7.
44. Zhang Y, Neogi T, Chen C, et al. Cherry consumption and decreased risk of recurrent gout attacks. Arthritis Rheum 2012;64:4004–11.
45. Fam AG. Gout, diet, and the insulin resistance syndrome. J Rheumatol 2002;29:1350–5.
46. McAdams-DeMarco MA, Maynard JW, Baer AN, et al. Hypertension and the risk of incident gout in a population-based study: the atherosclerosis risk in communities cohort. J Clin Hypertens (Greenwich) 2012;14:675–9.
47. Choi HK, Atkinson K, Karlson EW, et al. Alcohol intake and risk of incident gout in men: a prospective study. Lancet 2004;363:1277–81.
48. Zhang Y, Woods R, Chaisson CE, et al. Alcohol consumption as a trigger of recurrent gout attacks. Am J Med 2006;119:800–8.
49. Choi HK, Ford ES, Li C, et al. Prevalence of the metabolic syndrome in patients with gout: the Third National Health and Nutrition Examination Survey. Arthritis Rheum 2007;57:109–15.
50. Choi HK, Atkinson K, Karlson EW, et al. Obesity, weight change, hypertension, diuretic use, and risk of gout in men: the health follow-up study. Arch Intern Med 2005;165:742–8.
51. Maynard JW, McAdams DeMarco MA, Baer AN, et al. Incident gout in women and association with obesity in the Atherosclerosis Risk in Communities (ARIC) study. Am J Med 2012;125:717.e9–17.
52. Rothenbacher D, Primatesta P, Ferreira A, et al. Frequency and risk factors of gout flares in a large population-based cohort of incident gout. Rheumatology (Oxford) 2011;50:973–81.
53. Rodríguez G, Soriano LC, Choi HK. Impact of diabetes against the future risk of developing gout. Ann Rheum Dis 2010;69:2090–4.
54. Herman JB, Goldbourt U. Uric acid and diabetes: observations in a population study. Lancet 1982;2:240–3.
55. Choi HK, Ford ES. Haemoglobin A1c, fasting glucose, serum C-peptide and insulin resistance in relation to serum uric acid levels–the Third National Health and Nutrition Examination Survey. Rheumatology (Oxford) 2008;47:713–7.

56. Cook DG, Shaper AG, Thelle DS, et al. Serum uric acid, serum glucose and diabetes: relationships in a population study. Postgrad Med J 1986;62:1001–6.
57. Parish JM, Adam T, Facchiano L. Relationship of metabolic syndrome and obstructive sleep apnea. J Clin Sleep Med 2007;3:467–72.
58. Kono M, Tatsumi K, Saibara T, et al. Obstructive sleep apnea syndrome is associated with some components of metabolic syndrome. Chest 2007;131: 1387–92.
59. Ruiz García A, Sánchez Armengol A, Luque Crespo E, et al. Blood uric acid levels in patients with sleep-disordered breathing. Arch Bronconeumol 2006; 42:492–500.
60. Glantzounis GK, Tsimoyiannis EC, Kappas AM, et al. Uric acid and oxidative stress. Curr Pharm Des 2005;11:4145–51.
61. Hasday JD, Grum CM. Nocturnal increase of urinary uric acid: creatinine ratio. A biochemical correlate of sleep-associated hypoxemia. Am Rev Respir Dis 1987; 135:534–8.
62. Roddy E, Muller S, Hayward R, et al. The association of gout with sleep disorders: a cross-sectional study in primary care. BMC Musculoskelet Disord 2013;14:119.
63. Choi HK, Mount DB, Reginato AM, et al. Pathogenesis of gout. Ann Intern Med 2005;143:499–516.
64. Hueskes BA, Roovers EA, Mantel-Teeuwisse AK, et al. Use of diuretics and the risk of gouty arthritis: a systematic review. Semin Arthritis Rheum 2012;41: 879–89.
65. Gurwitz JH, Kalish SC, Bohn RL, et al. Thiazide diuretics and the initiation of anti-gout therapy. J Clin Epidemiol 1997;50:953–9.
66. Hanly JG, Skedgel C, Sketris I, et al. Gout in the elderly - a population health study. J Rheumatol 2009;36:822–30.
67. Hunter DJ, York M, Chaisson CE, et al. Recent diuretic use and the risk of recurrent gout attacks: the online case-crossover gout study. J Rheumatol 2006;33: 1341–5.
68. Stamp L, Ha L, Searle M, et al. Gout in renal transplant recipients. Nephrology (Carlton) 2006;11:367–71.
69. Suppiah R, Dissanayake A, Dalbeth N. High prevalence of gout in patients with Type 2 diabetes: male sex, renal impairment, and diuretic use are major risk factors. N Z Med J 2008;121:43–50.
70. Choi HK, Soriano LC, Zhang Y, et al. Antihypertensive drugs and risk of incident gout among patients with hypertension: population based case-control study. BMJ 2012;344:d8190.
71. Yü TF, Gutman AB. Study of the paradoxical effects of salicylate in low, intermediate and high dosage on the renal mechanisms for excretion of urate in man. J Clin Invest 1959;38:1298–315.
72. Zhang Y, Neogi T, Chen C, et al. Low-dose aspirin use and recurrent gout attacks. Ann Rheum Dis 2014;73(2):385–90.
73. Reyes AJ. Cardiovascular drugs and serum uric acid. Cardiovasc Drugs Ther 2003;17:397–414.
74. Berger L, Yü TF. Renal function in gout. IV. An analysis of 524 gouty subjects including long-term follow-up studies. Am J Med 1975;59:605–13.
75. Fessel WJ. Renal outcomes of gout and hyperuricemia. Am J Med 1979;67: 74–82.
76. Yü TF, Berger L. Impaired renal function in gout. Its association with hypertensive vascular disease and intrinsic renal disease. Am J Med 1982;72:95–100.

77. Roddy E, Doherty M. Gout and osteoarthritis: a pathogenetic link? Joint Bone Spine 2012;79:425–7.
78. Roddy E. Revisiting the pathogenesis of podagra: why does gout target the foot? J Foot Ankle Res 2011;4:13.
79. Kawenoki-Minc E, Eyman E, Leo W, et al. Osteoarthrosis and spondylosis in gouty patients. Analysis of 262 cases of gout. Reumatologia 1974;12:267–77.
80. Roddy E, Zhang W, Doherty M. Are joints affected by gout also affected by osteoarthritis? Ann Rheum Dis 2007;66:1374–7.
81. Roddy E, Zhang W, Doherty M. Gout and nodal osteoarthritis: a case–control study. Rheumatology 2008;7:732–3.

Epidemiology of Calcium Pyrophosphate Crystal Arthritis and Basic Calcium Phosphate Crystal Arthropathy

Abhishek Abhishek, MBBS, MD, MRCP, PhD[a,b,*],
Michael Doherty, MD, FRCP[b]

KEYWORDS

- Calcium pyrophosphate crystal deposition • Calcium pyrophosphate crystal
- Basic calcium phosphate crystal • Epidemiology

KEY POINTS

- Calcium pyrophosphate (CPP) and basic calcium phosphate (BCP) crystal deposition may be asymptomatic, or cause arthritis, commonly in the elderly.
- CPP deposition (CPPD) is common, and strongly associates with age and osteoarthritis (OA), although it does not seem to associate with OA progression.
- Hyperparathyroidism, hemochromatosis, hypomagnesemia, and hypophosphatasia are other recognized risk factors for CPPD.

INTRODUCTION

Calcium pyrophosphate (CPP) and basic calcium phosphate (BCP) crystal deposition may be asymptomatic, or cause arthritis, commonly in the elderly. Although CPP crystals predominantly deposit intra-articularly, abnormal BCP crystal deposition occurs in both intra-articular and periarticular locations. However, it is difficult to study their epidemiology because their presence is frequently asymptomatic. Any estimate of incidence and prevalence is further impaired by the fact that synovial fluid aspiration is required to definitively establish their presence. Moreover, BCP crystals are identified with confidence only by sophisticated techniques such as electron microscopy and x-ray diffraction, which are not available routinely. Thus, the epidemiologic studies of CPP and BCP crystal deposition use radiographic calcification as a surrogate.

Disclosures: None.
[a] Department of Rheumatology, Box 204, Addenbrookes Hospital, Hills Road, Cambridge CB2 0QQ, UK; [b] Academic Rheumatology, University of Nottingham, Nottingham NG5 1PB, UK
* Corresponding author. Department of Rheumatology, Box 204, Addenbrookes Hospital, Hills Road, Cambridge CB2 0QQ, UK.
E-mail address: docabhishek@gmail.com

Rheum Dis Clin N Am 40 (2014) 177–191
http://dx.doi.org/10.1016/j.rdc.2014.01.002
0889-857X/14/$ – see front matter © 2014 Elsevier Inc. All rights reserved.

rheumatic.theclinics.com

Within these limitations, the epidemiology of CPP deposition (CPPD) and BCP deposition are described in this review.

Epidemiology of CPPD

The first description of articular cartilage calcification is attributed to Robert Adams, a Dublin surgeon (c. 1854).[1] Radiographic articular cartilage calcification (chondrocalcinosis [CC]) was first described in the late 1920s,[2,3] and was identified as the cardinal manifestation of a distinct disease entity (chondrocalcinosis articularis) by Zitnan and Sitaj.[4] In 1962, McCarty and colleagues[5] identified CPP crystals in joints of patients with apparently acute gouty arthritis with or without coexistent CC. Subsequently, other calcium phosphate crystals (such as hydroxyapatite, brushite, and octacalcium phosphate) were shown in joints with CC, suggesting that CC is not exclusively caused by CPPD.

Over the last 50 years, the clinical classification of CPPD has evolved from a complex system based on phenotypic similarity with several other conditions (eg, pseudogout, pseudo-rheumatoid arthritis, pseudo-osteoarthritis), to a simple system that recognizes the key manifestations of CPPD (**Box 1**).[6] Of these manifestations, the epidemiology of CC, and osteoarthritis (OA) with CC have been relatively well studied. The epidemiology of acute CPP crystal arthritis, chronic CPP crystal inflammatory arthritis, and other pseudosyndromes associated with CPPD have not been examined formally.

Joints affected by CPPD

CPPD occurs in the knees, wrists/symphysis pubis, and hips, in descending order of frequency.[7–9] Studies are conflicting as to whether the wrist or the symphysis pubis is the second most commonly affected joint. Although previous studies reported that it is rare to have CC at other joints in the absence of knee involvement, a recent cross-sectional plain radiographic study suggested that up to 40% of participants with CC do not have knee involvement.[10]

Incidence

The incidence of CPPD has not been studied in the general population. However, in middle-aged and older adults with knee OA without knee CC at baseline and followed up for 8 to 12 years, the estimated annual incidence of radiographic knee CC was 0.8% to 2.1%, and that of CPPD (CPP crystals or CC) at the knee was 2.7% to 5.5%.[11–14]

Box 1
Classification of CPPD

Asymptomatic CPPD: CPPD with no apparent clinical consequence (ie, isolated CC)

OA with CPPD: CPPD in a joint that also shows changes of OA, on imaging or histologic examination

Acute CPP crystal arthritis: acute-onset, self-limiting synovitis with CPPD (previously pseudogout)

Chronic CPP crystal inflammatory arthritis: chronic inflammatory arthritis associated with CPPD

Data from Zhang W, Doherty M, Bardin T, et al. European League Against Rheumatism recommendations for calcium pyrophosphate deposition. Part I: terminology and diagnosis. Ann Rheum Dis 2011;70(4):563–70.

Prevalence

The prevalence of CPPD has been studied in several community-based radiographic studies, using CC as a surrogate (**Table 1**). The prevalence of CC depends on the joint radiographed and the age of the population. In the 3 studies of middle-aged and older people from Europe and the United States, the prevalence of CC was 7.0% to 8.1% if just knees were examined, 10.0% if knees, wrists, and hands were radiographed, and 10.4% if knees and hips were radiographed.[9,16,17] In an Italian study involving community-dwelling adults older than 18 years, CPPD was the fourth most prevalent condition after OA, rheumatoid arthritis (RA), and gout, with a prevalence (95% confidence interval [CI]) of 0.42 (0.33–0.58)%.[15] Studies restricted to older people,[18,21] or hospital-based studies, report a higher prevalence of CPPD ($\leq$34.0%).[22]

CPPD has been reported in people from all ethnic backgrounds. However, CPPD seems to be more common in whites than in Asians. For example, the prevalence of CC is lower in Beijing, China than in Framingham, MA.[19] A suggested environmental cause for this difference is the 15-fold higher concentration of calcium in the tap water in Beijing, which can suppress parathyroid hormone secretion.[19]

As expected, the incidence and prevalence of CPPD depends on the method used for its identification. Standard plain radiographs underestimate the prevalence of CPPD.[23,24] For example, 17% patients without radiographic knee CC had CPP crystals at the time of total knee replacement for OA.[23] Other studies also suggest that between one-quarter and half of OA knees with CPP crystals do not have radiographic CC.[25,26] However, because it is not feasible to perform arthrocentesis in population studies, it is likely that epidemiologic studies using ultrasonography (which is more sensitive for detection of CC) would better define the epidemiology of CPPD.[27,28]

CPPD: a systemic predisposition or a local abnormality?

A recent study suggests that common sporadic CPPD also results from a generalized predisposition.[29] In a cross-sectional radiographic study,[29] joints with CC clustered together more often than would be expected by chance alone. This clustering was present in patients with and without OA. In addition, CC at 1 joint associated with CC at distant joints, and bilateral CC at 1 joint area associated with CC at distant joints compared with unilateral CC.[29] These associations were independent of age, sex,

Table 1 Prevalence of CPPD			
Study	**Age Range (y)**	**Joints**	**CC Prevalence (%)**
Salaffi et al,[15] 2005	18–91	Symptomatic joints	0.42
Neame et al,[16] 2003	40–86	Knee	7.0
Felson et al,[17] 1989	63–93	Knee	8.1
Ramonda et al,[9] 2009	>65	Knee, pelvis	10.4
Sanmarti et al,[8] 1993	60–88	Wrist, hand, knee	10.0
Bergstrom et al,[7] 1986	70–79	Wrist, hand, knee	11.5
Bergstrom et al,[18] 1986	79	Wrist, hand, knee	16.0
Zhang et al,[19] 2006	>60	Wrist	0.7
Zhang et al,[19] 2006	>60	Knee	1.79[a], 2.67[b]
Al-Arfaj & Al-Boukai,[20] 2002	50–93	Wrist, hand, knee	3.9[c]

[a] Male.
[b] Female.
[c] 6.7% in patients >60 y.

body mass index (BMI), and OA at the distant joint. This finding further supports the view that CC at least in part results from a systemic predisposition. Although polyarticular CC is well recognized, this was the first systematic study confirming systemic predisposition to CC.[29] A smaller ultrasonographic study also suggested that most patients with CPPD have oligoarticular or polyarticular rather than monoarticular CC.[30]

Risk factors

There are several established risk factors for CPPD (**Box 2**).

Age The prevalence of CPPD increases with age. In a community-based study in Nottinghamshire, United Kingdom, the prevalence of knee CC increased from 3.7% at age 55 to 59 years to 17.5% at age 80 to 84 years (**Fig. 1**).[16] Similarly, in the Framingham study, there was more than a doubling in the prevalence of knee CC with each 10-year increase in age after the age of 60 years (relative risk [RR] [95% CI] 2.40 [1.97–2.91]).[17] Similarly, in Swedish studies, the prevalence of knee CC at age 70, 75, and 79 years was 6.8%, 8.0%, and 12.3%, respectively; whereas that of CC at knee, wrist, or hand was 7.5%, 10.1%, and 16.0%, respectively.[7,18]

Sex Large community-based studies[16,17,31] suggest that sex does not predispose to CPPD. However, some smaller community-based studies and 1 large study from China have reported a higher prevalence of CC in women.[8,18,19] A recent meta-analysis suggested that sex does not predispose to CPPD (odds ratio [OR] [95% CI] 0.89 [0.58–1.38]).[6]

Heredity Rarely, CPPD is inherited as a monogenic autosomal-dominant characteristic, and most instances of such hereditary CPPD have been attributed to mutations in the *ANKH* gene.[32–34] Familial CPPD can also occur as part of a severe dysplastic OA phenotype associated with mutations in procollagen type 2[35] and CCAL1[36] genes. Although small hospital-based cross-sectional studies suggest that up to a quarter of CPPD cases are inherited,[37–39] there seems to be either no or only a small contribution of genetic predisposition to prevalent sporadic CPPD. For example, the prevalence of CC in 122 siblings of index cases with knee CC and OA awaiting total joint replacement was similar to that of 1727 community-dwelling adults after adjusting for age, sex, BMI, and OA (adjusted OR [aOR] [95% CI] 1.16 [0.58–2.29]).[40] Similarly, only 1 case of familial CPPD and premature OA was identified (E490del mutation in *ANKH*) in a study of 95 UK whites with apparently sporadic CC.[41] However, the genetic contribution to sporadic CPPD is supported by a UK-based case-control study, which reported that the -4 bp G to A single nucleotide polymorphism (SNP) in the 5'-UTR

Box 2
Risk factors for CPPD

Increasing age

OA

Meniscectomy and joint injury

Metabolic diseases: hyperparathyroidism, hemochromatosis[a], hypomagnesemia, hypophosphatasia, chronic kidney disease stage 5[b]

Hereditary: mutations in *ANKH*, part of severe dysplastic OA phenotype

[a] Associates with structural arthropathy.
[b] Risk factor for acute CPP crystal arthritis.

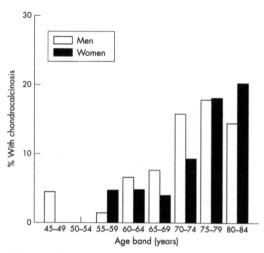

Fig. 1. Prevalence of knee CC by age and sex. (*Reproduced from* Neame RL, Carr AJ, Muir K, et al. UK community prevalence of knee chondrocalcinosis: evidence that correlation with osteoarthritis is through a shared association with osteophyte. Ann Rheum Dis 2003;62(6):514; with permission.)

of *ANKH* associates with CPPD (OR [95% CI] for CPPD in homozygous state = 6.00 [2.2–16.5]).[42] SNPs in plasma cell glycoprotein 1 and tissue nonspecific alkaline phosphatase do not seem to associate with sporadic CPPD.[43]

OA OA associates with CPPD.[16,17,44] This finding is independent of age.[16,17,44] Although OA associates with CPPD at knees, wrists, scaphotrapezoid joint, and metacarpophalangeal joints (MCPJs),[44–47] recent studies suggest that hip OA does not associate with CPPD.[9,29,31] In a large case-control study, knee OA associated with CC at wrists, hips, and knees, whereas hip OA did not associate with CC at any joint.[29]

The prevalence of CPPD at an index joint depends on the severity of OA. For example, the prevalence of knee CC + OA in community-dwelling adults is 3.4%,[40] whereas in clinic-based studies of knee OA, the prevalence of knee CPPD varies between 8% and 33%,[11,14,25,48,49] increasing to 30% to 53% in end-stage knee OA.[23,50]

Although small hospital-based case series and case-control studies have suggested that CPPD associates with a rapidly progressive destructive form of OA,[51,52] larger prospective community-based studies have shown that at least at the knee, CC either protects against or does not associate with knee OA progression. The adjusted RR (aRR) (95% CI) for progression of knee OA was 0.4 (0.2–0.7) in the Boston OA Knee Study and 0.9 (0.6–1.5) in the Health ABC Study.[48] Another study did not find any evidence for an association between CC and progression of knee OA.[53] In addition, knee CC does not associate with incident knee OA (aRR [95% CI] 1.20 [0.50–2.70]), suggesting that CC is at least in part a consequence, and not a cause, of OA.[54] The key facts concerning the association between OA and CPPD are summarized in **Box 3**.

Other musculoskeletal conditions Hospital-based case-control studies have suggested that CC associates with gout[55] but not with hyperuricemia.[56] This finding suggests that the association between CC and gout may be mediated by a generalized predisposition to crystal formation, or by epitaxy (the formation of 1 crystal type on another). Current evidence suggests that there is either a negative[56–58] or

> **Box 3**
> **Association between OA and CPPD: key facts**
>
> - Association between OA and CC is independent of age
> - OA associates with CC except at the hip
> - Prevalence of CC increases with severity of OA
> - Presence of CC does not seem to associate with OA progression
> - CC does not associate with incident OA

no[9] association between CPPD and RA. However, defleshed skeletal studies have suggested a possible association between CPPD and both RA and spondyloarthropathy.[59] A retrospective hospital-based case series also reported a high (25.8%) prevalence of CPP crystals in RA synovial fluid aspirates.[60] However, this study lacked a control group, and the high prevalence of CPP crystal may be caused by older age (mean age: 64.5 years), and long disease duration (mean: 12 years), which may result in secondary OA.[60] A recent meta-analysis of published studies supported a strong negative association between RA and CPPD (pooled OR [95% CI] 0.18 [0.08–0.41]).[6] There is no association between Paget disease and CC.[61]

Meniscectomy/Joint injury Meniscectomy is a risk factor for knee CC.[62,63] In an early study of people who had undergone unilateral meniscectomy more than 25 years before, knee CC was 5-fold more likely in the operated knee than in the contralateral unoperated knee.[62] Similarly, some case reports have suggested that recurrent joint injury caused by joint hypermobility can also result in CPPD.[64]

Knee alignment In a cross-sectional study of UK adults, self-reported constitutional varus knee alignment in the third decade (20s) associated with subsequent knee CC (aOR [95% CI] 1.77 [1.05, 2.98]). This finding was independent of age, sex, BMI in the 20s, and knee OA.[65] However, current knee malalignment did not associate with knee CC, supporting a causal association between early life knee malalignment and CC.

Metabolic diseases Several metabolic diseases are reported to associate with CC.[66] Although the association between diabetes and CC may be confounded by age, other reported associations between rare diseases such as Wilson disease and ochronosis are based on case reports of florid CC in young patients.[67] One case-control study reported no association between hypothyroidism and CC.[68] Hemochromatosis, hyperparathyroidism, hypomagnesemia, and hypophosphatasia are recognised risk factors for CC, and these should be screened for specifically in young (<55 years) patients, especially those with polyarticular CPPD.[67,69]

Hemochromatosis The association between hemochromatosis and CPPD was first reported by Schumacher.[70] Subsequent hospital-based case series reported that structural arthropathy with CC was present at the knees, wrists, hips, pubic symphysis, or MCPJs in 12 of 32 cases with hemochromatosis.[71] CC was present in 1 in 3 patients with hemochromatosis in a recent large hospital-based study.[72] As with sporadic CPPD, knees and wrists were the commonest sites of CC in those with hemochromatosis.[72] Large population-based studies have not identified any association between C282Y homozygosity and CPPD.[73] However, homozygosity for H63D, which carries a smaller risk of iron overload, has been associated with knee and hip CC in those younger than 65 years (OR [95% CI] 4.7 [1.2–18.5]).[73] This situation may be caused by variable penetrance of *HFE* mutations, channeling bias, or the possibility that factors unrelated to iron overload predispose to CPPD in hemochromatosis.

Hyperparathyroidism The association between CC and hyperparathyroidism is supported by several studies. One age-matched and sex-matched case-control study found CC to be 9 times more likely in those with hyperparathyroidism than in those without (30.7% vs 3.4%).[74] Furthermore, hyperparathyroid patients with CC tend to be younger than those with CC in the absence of hyperparathyroidism; however, as expected, the association between CC and hyperparathyroidism is not independent of age, because hyperparathyroid patients with CC are older than hyperparathyroid patients without CC.[75,76] A meta-analysis of published literature carried out by a European League Against Rheumatism (EULAR) task force in 2011 confirmed a strong association between hyperparathyroidism and CPPD (pooled OR [95% CI] 3.03 [1.15–8.02]).[6]

A recent case-control study found an association between low metacarpal index (a measure of cortical bone mineral density) and CC (aOR [95% CI] 1.41 [1.06–1.89]), and this was independent of age, sex, BMI, OA, and vascular and soft tissue calcification.[77] There was no association between calcaneal bone mineral density measured using dual-energy X-ray absorptiometry and CC (aOR [95% CI] 1.15 [0.76–1.73]). The differential association between metacarpal index, calcaneal bone mineral density, and CC raises the possibility that this may be mediated by subclinical hyperparathyroidism.[77]

Hypomagnesemia A case of postparathyroidectomy acute CPP crystal synovitis with acute hypomagnesemia was first described in 1966.[78] Subsequently, several cases of CC were described in patients with idiopathic hypomagnesemia[79] and hypomagnesemia caused by renal loss.[80,81] CPPD was identified as a manifestation of the Gitelman variant of Bartter syndrome.[82–84] Hypomagnesemia caused by gastrointestinal loss also leads to CPPD. In a cross-sectional study, prevalence of CC was investigated in patients with intestinal failure, and age-matched and sex-matched controls. The prevalence of CC was higher in patients with intestinal failure (OR [95% CI] 7.0 [1.45–66.1]) and was significantly higher in patients with lower serum magnesium levels (OR [95% CI] 13.5 [2.76–127.3]).[85]

The reported association between diuretic use and knee CC has been hypothesized to be mediated by diuretic-induced hypomagnesemia.[16] Although severe hypomagnesemia associates with CC, it is unclear if there is a role of mild hypomagnesemia in the pathogenesis of CPPD, because serum magnesium levels are similar in people with apparently sporadic CPPD and matched controls.[9,79,86]

Hypophosphatasia The association between hypophosphatasia and CC is based on several case reports of florid polyarticular CC at a young age.[67] However, low alkaline phosphatase levels do not seem to play a role in the occurrence of sporadic CPPD, because there is no difference in serum alkaline phosphatase levels in those with and without CPPD in the absence of a history of hypophosphatasia.[79,86,87] Although some laboratory-based studies have reported low synovial fluid alkaline phosphatase levels in joints with CPP crystals,[88] others have reported no difference in synovial fluid alkaline phosphatase levels in those with and without CPPD.[89–92] Although gross hypophosphatasia associates with CPPD, these studies do not support a role of low alkaline phosphatase activity in the cause of CPPD at a population level.

Risk factors for acute CPP crystal arthritis A recent population-based age-matched and sex-matched case-control study using data from the THIN (The Health Improvement Network) database reported that hyperparathyroidism (aOR [95% CI] 4.87 [2.10,

11.3]), OA (aOR [95% CI] 2.91 [2.48, 3.43]), and loop diuretic use (aOR [95% CI] 1.35 [1.09, 1.67]) were independent associations for acute CPP crystal arthritis.[93] Patients with stage 5 chronic kidney disease were also more likely to have acute CPP crystal arthritis (aOR [95% CI] 2.29 [1.30–4.01]).[93] As with gout, it is possible that risk factors for crystal deposition may differ from those that predispose to acute crystal-induced synovitis, which is generally considered to be caused by crystal shedding from pre-formed deposits within cartilage.

Epidemiology of BCP Crystal Deposition

BCP crystals are the umbrella term for several BCP crystals including carbonate-substituted hydroxyapatite, octacalcium and tricalcium phosphates, and whitlockite. Of these crystals, hydroxyapatite is the most abundant in man. The current under-standing of calcium crystal deposition suggests that Robert Adams' first pathologic description of joint calcification could have been at least in part caused by BCP crystal deposition. Subsequently, calcific periarthritis of the shoulder and radiographic periar-ticular shoulder calcification were identified in 1870 and 1907, respectively. In 1966, McCarty and Gatter[94] identified hydroxyapatite crystals in such calcific material, and in 1976, Dieppe and colleagues[95] identified BCP crystals in synovial fluid from OA knees. Soon after this, McCarty and colleagues[96] and Halverson and colleagues[97] identified apatite-associated destructive arthropathy (AADA) or Milwaukee shoulder as a distinct clinical entity. A formal classification of articular and periarticular syn-dromes associated with BCP crystal deposition has never been devised. A simple clin-ical classification system similar to that proposed by the EULAR task force for CPPD is presented in **Box 4**.

The epidemiology of BCP crystal deposition is less well understood, and there are scant data, particularly on BCP crystal-associated arthropathy. Calcific periarthritis occurs in all age groups and in both sexes. Hospital-based case series have sug-gested that it is more common in women, and occurs at all ages,[98] including child-hood.[99] Pseudopodagra caused by calcific periarthritis seems to be especially common in women.[100] The best epidemiologic data on calcific periarthritis comes from a US study of more than 12,000 shoulder radiographs undertaken as part of an insurance medical assessment. This study showed a crude adult prevalence of calcific periarticular deposits at the shoulder of 3%.[101] Most calcifications were asymptomatic, with just more than one-third of these having shoulder symptoms.[101] Calcifications were more common in women, and unlike other crystal deposition (urate, CPPD), the prevalence was highest in those younger than 40 years.[101] Calcific shoulder periarthritis is 3-fold more common in people with type II diabetes mellitus than in age-matched and sex-matched controls.[102,103] Calcific shoulder periarthritis

---

Box 4
Proposed classification of BCP crystal deposition

Asymptomatic BCP crystal deposition: BCP crystal deposits with no apparent clinical consequences

OA with BCP crystal deposition: BCP deposition in a joint that also shows changes of OA on imaging or histologic examination

Acute BCP crystal periarthritis: acute-onset, self-limiting synovitis with CPPD

Apatite-associated destructive arthropathy: destructive arthropathy associated with BCP crystals

associates with long-standing and poorly controlled diabetes, hyperlipidemia, minor trauma, and hypomagnesemia.[102,103] A hospital-based case-control study suggested that diabetics with shoulder calcification were more likely to have renal and retinal complications of diabetes.[104] Periarticular calcification is also common in connective tissue diseases and may result in acute calcific periarthritis.[105]

In contrast to calcific periarthritis, AADA seems to be more common in elderly women.[106] AADA seems to target the shoulders, knees, hips, elbows, and ankles.[106] In a comprehensive review using data from more than 72 patients with Milwaukee shoulder syndrome, the mean (range) age of patients was 72 (50–90) years, and there was a 4:1 female preponderance.[107] The dominant shoulder was more commonly affected and usually had more severe disease.[107] Trauma/overuse, neurologic involvement, dialysis, and CPPD were the identifiable risk factors, whereas no risk factors were apparent in a large proportion of patients.[107] Patients with knee arthropathy along with Milwaukee shoulder syndrome were more likely to have valgus than varus knees.[107] Further studies are required to better identify and define the subset of patients with AADA at other joints, and then to study its epidemiology.

The prevalence of intra-articular BCP crystal deposition in OA joints has been relatively well studied. In 2 recent studies, BCP crystals were present in all end-stage OA joints, suggesting that BCP crystal deposition is integral to the process of end-stage OA.[108,109] BCP crystals frequently coexist with CPP crystals in OA joints. In hospital-based studies of symptomatic knee OA, BCP crystals (or alizarin red positivity) coexists with CPP crystals in 16% to 40% of cases.[12,23–26,50,110] Just as for CPPD, BCP crystals become more prevalent with increasing severity of OA. In a prospective study involving sequential analysis of knee OA synovial fluids,[12] BCP crystals developed as the disease progressed. For example, BCP crystals were identified in less than a quarter of patients at first aspiration but were present in more than half of patients at final aspiration (mean interval 3.6 years). However, large prospective studies are required to identify the epidemiology of BCP crystal deposition diseases, and to confirm if BCP crystals result in progression of OA.

CPP and BCP crystal deposition diseases are common. Research over the last 50 years has helped understand the prevalence and disease associations of CPPD. This research has translated into routine clinical practice. For example, polyarticular CPPD, especially in those younger than 50 years, triggers screening to identify metabolic diseases and familial predisposition. On the contrary, CPPD in the context of severe OA at the index joint, or in commonly affected joints in the elderly, should not result in detailed metabolic screening. However, the epidemiology of clinical manifestations of CPPD like chronic CPP crystal inflammatory arthritis, acute CPP crystal arthritis, and that of clinical syndromes associated with BCP crystal deposition is poorly understood. Further research using noninvasive imaging modalities like ultrasonography, which is able to identify both intra-articular and periarticular calcium deposits with greater sensitivity than plain radiographs, may be able to better define the epidemiology of chronic CPP crystal inflammatory arthritis or clinical features associated with BCP crystal deposition.

IMPORTANT POINTS AND OBJECTIVES FOR RECALL

- CPPD is common and strongly associates with age and OA, although it does not seem to associate with OA progression.
- Hyperparathyroidism, hemochromatosis, hypomagnesemia, and hypophosphatasia are other recognized risk factors for CPPD. Rare familial forms of CPPD have been reported in many countries, mainly presenting as young-onset

polyarticular CPPD. Local biomechanical risk factors specifically for knee CC include previous meniscectomy, joint injury, and constitutional knee malalignment.

- The epidemiology of BCP crystal deposition is poorly understood. Nonetheless, periarticular BCP crystal deposits occur at all ages and in both sexes. Intra-articular BCP crystal deposition tends to associate with increasing age and OA; they are present in all hips and knees with end-stage OA.
- Apatite-associated destructive arthropathy (Milwaukee shoulder syndrome) seems to be more common in older women.

REFERENCES

1. Dieppe P, Doherty M. The first descriptions of chondrocalcinosis. Arthritis Rheum 1989;32(10):1339–40.
2. Mandl F. Pathologie und Therapie der Zwischenknorpelerkrankugen des Knie-gelenkes. Arch Klin Chir 1927;146:149–214.
3. Werwath S. Abnorme Kalkablagerungen innerhalb des Kniegelenkes, ein Betrag zur Frage der Primen Meniskopathie. Fortschr Roentgenstr Nuclearmed 1928;37:169.
4. Zitnan D, Sitaj S. Chondrocalcinosis polyarticularis (familiaris): roentgenological and clinical analysis. Cesk Rentgenol 1960;14:27–34.
5. McCarty DJ, Kohn NH, Faires JS. The significance of calcium phosphate crystals in the synovial fluid of arthritic patients: the 'pseudogout syndrome': I. Clinical aspects. Ann Intern Med 1962;56(5):711–37 [Original Research].
6. Zhang W, Doherty M, Bardin T, et al. European League Against Rheumatism recommendations for calcium pyrophosphate deposition. Part I: terminology and diagnosis. Ann Rheum Dis 2011;70(4):563–70.
7. Bergstrom G, Bjelle A, Sundh V, et al. Joint disorders at ages 70, 75 and 79 years–a cross-sectional comparison. Br J Rheumatol 1986;25(4):333–41.
8. Sanmarti R, Panella D, Brancos MA, et al. Prevalence of articular chondrocalcinosis in elderly subjects in a rural area of Catalonia. Ann Rheum Dis 1993;52(6):418–22.
9. Ramonda R, Musacchio E, Perissinotto E, et al. Prevalence of chondrocalcinosis in Italian subjects from northeastern Italy. The Pro.V.A. (PROgetto Veneto Anziani) study. Clin Exp Rheumatol 2009;27(6):981–4.
10. Abhishek A, Doherty S, Maciewicz R, et al. Chondrocalcinosis is common in the absence of knee involvement. Arthritis Res Ther 2012;14(5):R205.
11. Reuge L, Van Linthoudt D, Gerster JC. Local deposition of calcium pyrophosphate crystals in evolution of knee osteoarthritis. Clin Rheumatol 2001;20(6):428–31.
12. Nalbant S, Martinez JA, Kitumnuaypong T, et al. Synovial fluid features and their relations to osteoarthritis severity: new findings from sequential studies. Osteoarthritis Cartilage 2003;11(1):50–4.
13. Hernborg J, Linden B, Nilsson BE. Chondrocalcinosis: a secondary finding in osteoarthritis of the knee. Geriatrics 1977;32(9):123–4, 126.
14. Massardo L, Watt I, Cushnaghan J, et al. Osteoarthritis of the knee joint: an eight year prospective study. Ann Rheum Dis 1989;48(11):893–7.
15. Salaffi F, De Angelis R, Grassi W. Prevalence of musculoskeletal conditions in an Italian population sample: results of a regional community-based study. I. The MAPPING study. Clin Exp Rheumatol 2005;23(6):819–28.
16. Neame RL, Carr AJ, Muir K, et al. UK community prevalence of knee chondrocalcinosis: evidence that correlation with osteoarthritis is through a shared association with osteophyte. Ann Rheum Dis 2003;62(6):513–8.

17. Felson DT, Anderson JJ, Naimark A, et al. The prevalence of chondrocalcinosis in the elderly and its association with knee osteoarthritis: the Framingham Study. J Rheumatol 1989;16(9):1241–5.
18. Bergstrom G, Bjelle A, Sorensen LB, et al. Prevalence of rheumatoid arthritis, osteoarthritis, chondrocalcinosis and gouty arthritis at age 79. J Rheumatol 1986;13(3):527–34.
19. Zhang Y, Terkeltaub R, Nevitt M, et al. Lower prevalence of chondrocalcinosis in Chinese subjects in Beijing than in white subjects in the United States: the Beijing Osteoarthritis Study. Arthritis Rheum 2006;54(11):3508–12.
20. Al-Arfaj AS, Al-Boukai AA. Articular chondrocalcinosis in Saudi Arabia. Saudi Med J 2002;23(5):577–9.
21. Ellman MH, Levin B. Chondrocalcinosis in elderly persons. Arthritis Rheum 1975;18(1):43–7.
22. Wilkins E, Dieppe P, Maddison P, et al. Osteoarthritis and articular chondrocalcinosis in the elderly. Ann Rheum Dis 1983;42(3):280–4.
23. Viriyavejkul P, Wilairatana V, Tanavalee A, et al. Comparison of characteristics of patients with and without calcium pyrophosphate dihydrate crystal deposition disease who underwent total knee replacement surgery for osteoarthritis. Osteoarthritis Cartilage 2007;15(2):232–5.
24. Gibilisco PA, Schumacher HR Jr, Hollander JL, et al. Synovial fluid crystals in osteoarthritis. Arthritis Rheum 1985;28(5):511–5.
25. Ledingham J, Regan M, Jones A, et al. Radiographic patterns and associations of osteoarthritis of the knee in patients referred to hospital. Ann Rheum Dis 1993; 52(7):520–6.
26. Pattrick M, Hamilton E, Wilson R, et al. Association of radiographic changes of osteoarthritis, symptoms, and synovial fluid particles in 300 knees. Ann Rheum Dis 1993;52(2):97–103.
27. Barskova VG, Kudaeva FM, Bozhieva LA, et al. Comparison of three imaging techniques in diagnosis of chondrocalcinosis of the knees in calcium pyrophosphate deposition disease. Rheumatology (Oxford) 2013;52(6):1090–4.
28. Filippou G, Frediani B, Gallo A, et al. A "new" technique for the diagnosis of chondrocalcinosis of the knee: sensitivity and specificity of high-frequency ultrasonography. Ann Rheum Dis 2007;66(8):1126–8.
29. Abhishek A, Doherty S, Maciewicz R, et al. Evidence of a systemic predisposition to chondrocalcinosis and association between chondrocalcinosis and osteoarthritis at distant joints: a cross-sectional study. Arthritis Care Res (Hoboken) 2013;65(7):1052–8.
30. Filippou G, Filippucci E, Tardella M, et al. Extent and distribution of CPP deposits in patients affected by calcium pyrophosphate dihydrate deposition disease: an ultrasonographic study. Ann Rheum Dis 2013;72(11):1836–9.
31. Musacchio E, Ramonda R, Perissinotto E, et al. The impact of knee and hip chondrocalcinosis on disability in older people: the ProVA Study from northeastern Italy. Ann Rheum Dis 2011;70(11):1937–43.
32. Andrew LJ, Brancolini V, de la Pena LS, et al. Refinement of the chromosome 5p locus for familial calcium pyrophosphate dihydrate deposition disease. Am J Hum Genet 1999;64(1):136–45.
33. Doherty M, Hamilton E, Henderson J, et al. Familial chondrocalcinosis due to calcium pyrophosphate dihydrate crystal deposition in English families. Br J Rheumatol 1991;30(1):10–5.
34. Hughes AE, McGibbon D, Woodward E, et al. Localisation of a gene for chondrocalcinosis to chromosome 5p. Hum Mol Genet 1995;4(7):1225–8.

35. Netter P, Bardin T, Bianchi A, et al. The ANKH gene and familial calcium pyrophosphate dihydrate deposition disease. Joint Bone Spine 2004;71(5):365–8.
36. Baldwin CT, Farrer LA, Adair R, et al. Linkage of early-onset osteoarthritis and chondrocalcinosis to human chromosome 8q. Am J Hum Genet 1995;56(3): 692–7.
37. Balsa A, Martin-Mola E, Gonzalez T, et al. Familial articular chondrocalcinosis in Spain. Ann Rheum Dis 1990;49(7):531–5.
38. Fernandez Dapica MP, Gomez-Reino JJ. Familial chondrocalcinosis in the Spanish population. J Rheumatol 1986;13(3):631–3.
39. Rodriguez-Valverde V, Tinture T, Zuniga M, et al. Familial chondrocalcinosis. Prevalence in Northern Spain and clinical features in five pedigrees. Arthritis Rheum 1980;23(4):471–8.
40. Zhang W, Neame R, Doherty S, et al. Relative risk of knee chondrocalcinosis in siblings of index cases with pyrophosphate arthropathy. Ann Rheum Dis 2004; 63(8):969–73.
41. Pendleton A, Johnson MD, Hughes A, et al. Mutations in ANKH cause chondrocalcinosis. Am J Hum Genet 2002;71(4):933–40.
42. Zhang Y, Johnson K, Russell RG, et al. Association of sporadic chondrocalcinosis with a -4-basepair G-to-A transition in the 5'-untranslated region of ANKH that promotes enhanced expression of ANKH protein and excess generation of extracellular inorganic pyrophosphate. Arthritis Rheum 2005;52(4): 1110–7.
43. Zhang Y, Brown MA, Peach C, et al. Investigation of the role of ENPP1 and TNAP genes in chondrocalcinosis. Rheumatology (Oxford) 2007;46(4):586–9.
44. Sanmarti R, Kanterewicz E, Pladevall M, et al. Analysis of the association between chondrocalcinosis and osteoarthritis: a community based study. Ann Rheum Dis 1996;55(1):30–3.
45. Al-Arfaj AS. The relationship between chondrocalcinosis and osteoarthritis in Saudi Arabia. Clin Rheumatol 2002;21(6):493–6.
46. Bourqui M, Vischer TL, Stasse P, et al. Pyrophosphate arthropathy in the carpal and metacarpophalangeal joints. Ann Rheum Dis 1983;42(6):626–30.
47. Peter A, Simmen BR, Bruhlmann P, et al. Osteoarthritis of the scaphoidtrapezium joint: an early sign of calcium pyrophosphate dihydrate disease. Clin Rheumatol 2001;20(1):20–4.
48. Neogi T, Nevitt M, Niu J, et al. Lack of association between chondrocalcinosis and increased risk of cartilage loss in knees with osteoarthritis: results of two prospective longitudinal magnetic resonance imaging studies. Arthritis Rheum 2006;54(6):1822–8.
49. Dougados M, Gueguen A, Nguyen M, et al. Longitudinal radiologic evaluation of osteoarthritis of the knee. J Rheumatol 1992;19(3):378–84.
50. Derfus BA, Kurian JB, Butler JJ, et al. The high prevalence of pathologic calcium crystals in pre-operative knees. J Rheumatol 2002;29(3):570–4.
51. Gerster JC, Vischer TL, Boussina I, et al. Joint destruction and chondrocalcinosis in patients with generalised osteoarthrosis. Br Med J 1975;4(5998):684.
52. Gerster JC, Vischer TL, Fallet GH. Destructive arthropathy in generalized osteoarthritis with articular chondrocalcinosis. J Rheumatol 1975;2(3):265–9.
53. Ledingham J, Regan M, Jones A, et al. Factors affecting radiographic progression of knee osteoarthritis. Ann Rheum Dis 1995;54(1):53–8.
54. Felson DT, Zhang Y, Hannan MT, et al. Risk factors for incident radiographic knee osteoarthritis in the elderly: the Framingham Study. Arthritis Rheum 1997;40(4):728–33.

55. Stockman A, Darlington LG, Scott JT. Frequency of chondrocalcinosis of the knees and avascular necrosis of the femoral heads in gout: a controlled study. Ann Rheum Dis 1980;39(1):7–11.
56. Hollingworth P, Williams PL, Scott JT. Frequency of chondrocalcinosis of the knees in asymptomatic hyperuricaemia and rheumatoid arthritis: a controlled study. Ann Rheum Dis 1982;41(4):344–6.
57. Doherty M, Dieppe P, Watt I. Low incidence of calcium pyrophosphate dihydrate crystal deposition in rheumatoid arthritis, with modification of radiographic features in coexistent disease. Arthritis Rheum 1984;27(9):1002–9.
58. Brasseur JP, Huaux JP, Devogelaer JP, et al. Articular chondrocalcinosis in seropositive rheumatoid arthritis. Comparison with a control group. J Rheumatol 1987;14(1):40–1.
59. Rothschild B. CPPD complicating other forms of inflammatory arthritis. Clin Rheumatol 2007;26(7):1130–1.
60. Gerster JC, Varisco PA, Kern J, et al. CPPD crystal deposition disease in patients with rheumatoid arthritis. Clin Rheumatol 2006;25(4):468–9.
61. Boussina I, Gerster J, Epiney J, et al. A study of the incidence of articular chondrocalcinosis in Paget's disease of bone. Scand J Rheumatol 1976;5(1):33–5.
62. Doherty M, Watt I, Dieppe PA. Localised chondrocalcinosis in post-meniscectomy knees. Lancet 1982;1(8283):1207–10.
63. de Lange EE, Keats TE. Localized chondrocalcinosis in traumatized joints. Skeletal Radiol 1985;14(4):249–56.
64. Bird HA, Tribe CR, Bacon PA. Joint hypermobility leading to osteoarthrosis and chondrocalcinosis. Ann Rheum Dis 1978;37(3):203–11.
65. Abhishek A, Doherty S, Maciewicz RA, et al. Self-reported knee malalignment in early adult life as an independent risk for knee chondrocalcinosis. Arthritis Care Res (Hoboken) 2011;63(11):1550–7.
66. Hamilton EB. Diseases associated with CPPD deposition disease. Arthritis Rheum 1976;19(Suppl 3):353–7.
67. Jones AC, Chuck AJ, Arie EA, et al. Diseases associated with calcium pyrophosphate deposition disease. Semin Arthritis Rheum 1992;22(3):188–202.
68. Chaisson CE, McAlindon TE, Felson DT, et al. Lack of association between thyroid status and chondrocalcinosis or osteoarthritis: the Framingham Osteoarthritis Study. J Rheumatol 1996;23(4):711–5.
69. Richette P, Bardin T, Doherty M. An update on the epidemiology of calcium pyrophosphate dihydrate crystal deposition disease. Rheumatology (Oxford) 2009;48(7):711–5.
70. Schumacher HR Jr. Hemochromatosis and arthritis. Arthritis Rheum 1964;7:41–50.
71. Hamilton E, Williams R, Barlow KA, et al. The arthropathy of idiopathic haemochromatosis. Q J Med 1968;37(145):171–82.
72. Sahinbegovic E, Dallos T, Aigner E, et al. Musculoskeletal disease burden of hereditary hemochromatosis. Arthritis Rheum 2010;62(12):3792–8.
73. Alizadeh BZ, Njajou OT, Hazes JM, et al. The H63D variant in the HFE gene predisposes to arthralgia, chondrocalcinosis and osteoarthritis. Ann Rheum Dis 2007;66(11):1436–42.
74. Rynes RI, Merzig EG. Calcium pyrophosphate crystal deposition disease and hyperparathyroidism: a controlled, prospective study. J Rheumatol 1978;5(4):460–8.
75. Pritchard MH, Jessop JD. Chondrocalcinosis in primary hyperparathyroidism. Influence of age, metabolic bone disease, and parathyroidectomy. Ann Rheum Dis 1977;36(2):146–51.

76. Yashiro T, Okamoto T, Tanaka R, et al. Prevalence of chondrocalcinosis in patients with primary hyperparathyroidism in Japan. Endocrinol Jpn 1991;38(5): 457–64.
77. Abhishek A, Doherty S, Maciewicz R, et al. Association between low cortical bone mineral density, soft-tissue calcification, vascular calcification and chondrocalcinosis: a case-control study. Ann Rheum Dis 2013. http://dx.doi.org/10. 1136/annrheumdis-2013-203400.
78. Melvin KE. Articular chondrocalcinosis, hyperparathyroidism and pseudogout: hypomagnesaemic crisis. Proc R Soc Med 1966;59(7):595–6.
79. McCarty DJ, Silcox DC, Coe F, et al. Diseases associated with calcium pyrophosphate dihydrate crystal deposition. Am J Med 1974;56(5):704–14.
80. Runeberg L, Collan Y, Jokinen EJ, et al. Hypomagnesemia due to renal disease of unknown etiology. Am J Med 1975;59(6):873–81.
81. Ellman MH, Brown NL, Porat AP. Laboratory investigations in pseudogout patients and controls. J Rheumatol 1980;7(1):77–81.
82. Munoz-Fernandez S, Pantoja L, Martin Mola E, et al. Chondrocalcinosis associated with Bartter's syndrome and hypomagnesemia. J Rheumatol 1994;21(9): 1782–3.
83. Smilde TJ, Haverman JF, Schipper P, et al. Familial hypokalemia/hypomagnesemia and chondrocalcinosis. J Rheumatol 1994;21(8):1515–9.
84. Gitelman HJ, Graham JB, Welt LG. A new familial disorder characterized by hypokalemia and hypomagnesemia. Trans Assoc Am Physicians 1966;79:221–35.
85. Richette P, Ayoub G, Lahalle S, et al. Hypomagnesemia associated with chondrocalcinosis: a cross-sectional study. Arthritis Rheum 2007;57(8):1496–501.
86. Alexander GM, Dieppe PA, Doherty M, et al. Pyrophosphate arthropathy: a study of metabolic associations and laboratory data. Ann Rheum Dis 1982; 41(4):377–81.
87. Huaux JP, Geubel A, Koch MC, et al. The arthritis of hemochromatosis. A review of 25 cases with special reference to chondrocalcinosis, and a comparison with patients with primary hyperparathyroidism and controls. Clin Rheumatol 1986; 5(3):317–24.
88. Yaron M, Zurkowski P, Weiser HI, et al. Pseudogout with low values of alkaline phosphatase in the synovial fluid. Ann Intern Med 1970;73(5):751–6.
89. Rachow JW, Ryan LM. Adenosine triphosphate pyrophosphohydrolase and neutral inorganic pyrophosphatase in pathologic joint fluids. Elevated pyrophosphohydrolase in calcium pyrophosphate dihydrate crystal deposition disease. Arthritis Rheum 1985;28(11):1283–8.
90. McCarty DJ, Solomon SD, Warnock ML, et al. Inorganic pyrophosphate concentrations in the synovial fluid of arthritic patients. J Lab Clin Med 1971;78(2): 216–29.
91. Jacobelli S, Kettlun AM, Sapag-Hagar M. Inorganic pyrophosphatase activity of the synovial fluid. Kinetic and clinical study. Arthritis Rheum 1978;21(4):447–52.
92. Altman RD, Muniz OE, Pita JC, et al. Articular chondrocalcinosis. Microanalysis of pyrophosphate (PPi) in synovial fluid and plasma. Arthritis Rheum 1973;16(2): 171–8.
93. Rho YH, Zhu Y, Zhang Y, et al. Risk factors for pseudogout in the general population. Rheumatology (Oxford) 2012;51(11):2070–4.
94. McCarty DJ Jr, Gatter RA. Recurrent acute inflammation associated with focal apatite crystal deposition. Arthritis Rheum 1966;9(6):804–19.
95. Dieppe PA, Crocker P, Huskisson EC, et al. Apatite deposition disease. A new arthropathy. Lancet 1976;1(7954):266–9.

96. McCarty DJ, Halverson PB, Carrera GF, et al. "Milwaukee shoulder"–association of microspheroids containing hydroxyapatite crystals, active collagenase, and neutral protease with rotator cuff defects. I. Clinical aspects. Arthritis Rheum 1981;24(3):464–73.

97. Halverson PB, Cheung HS, McCarty DJ, et al. "Milwaukee shoulder"–association of microspheroids containing hydroxyapatite crystals, active collagenase, and neutral protease with rotator cuff defects. II. Synovial fluid studies. Arthritis Rheum 1981;24(3):474–83.

98. Lehmer LM, Ragsdale BD. Calcific periarthritis: more than a shoulder problem: a series of fifteen cases. J Bone Joint Surg Am 2012;94(21):e157.

99. Rush PJ, Wilmot D, Shore A. Hydroxyapatite deposition disease presenting as calcific periarthritis in a 14-year-old girl. Pediatr Radiol 1986;16(2):169–70.

100. Fam AG, Rubenstein J. Hydroxyapatite pseudopodagra. A syndrome of young women. Arthritis Rheum 1989;32(6):741–7.

101. Bosworth BM. Calcium deposits in the shoulder and subacromial bursitis. A survey of 12,222 shoulders. JAMA 1941;116:2477–82.

102. Mavrikakis ME, Sfikakis PP, Kontoyannis SA, et al. Clinical and laboratory parameters in adult diabetics with and without calcific shoulder periarthritis. Calcif Tissue Int 1991;49(4):288–91.

103. Mavrikakis ME, Drimis S, Kontoyannis DA, et al. Calcific shoulder periarthritis (tendinitis) in adult onset diabetes mellitus: a controlled study. Ann Rheum Dis 1989;48(3):211–4.

104. Sattar MA, Luqman WA. Periarthritis: another duration-related complication of diabetes mellitus. Diabetes Care 1985;8(5):507–10.

105. Fam AG, Pritzker KP. Acute calcific periarthritis in scleroderma. J Rheumatol 1992;19(10):1580–5.

106. Dieppe PA, Doherty M, Macfarlane DG, et al. Apatite associated destructive arthritis. Br J Rheumatol 1984;23(2):84–91.

107. McCarty DJ. Milwaukee shoulder syndrome. Trans Am Clin Climatol Assoc 1991;102:271–83 [discussion: 83–4].

108. Fuerst M, Niggemeyer O, Lammers L, et al. Articular cartilage mineralization in osteoarthritis of the hip. BMC Musculoskelet Disord 2009;10:166.

109. Fuerst M, Bertrand J, Lammers L, et al. Calcification of articular cartilage in human osteoarthritis. Arthritis Rheum 2009;60(9):2694–703.

110. Halverson PB, McCarty DJ. Patterns of radiographic abnormalities associated with basic calcium phosphate and calcium pyrophosphate dihydrate crystal deposition in the knee. Ann Rheum Dis 1986;45(7):603–5.

Clinical Manifestations and Diagnosis of Gout

Fernando Perez-Ruiz, MD, PhD[a],*, Edwin Castillo, MD[b],
Sandra P. Chinchilla, MD[b], Ana M. Herrero-Beites, MD[c]

KEYWORDS

• Gout • Diagnosis • Clinical manifestations • Tophi • Damage

KEY POINTS

• Gout has been academically considered, from the clinical point of view, to be a step-up disease consisting of different stages: acute gout, intercritical gout, and chronic gout.
• In clinical practice, clinicians should consider gout as a single disease with either or both acute (most commonly, episodes of acute inflammation) and persistent clinical manifestations, but not restricted to chronic synovitis.
• Monosodium urate crystal (MSUC) deposition and subclinical inflammation related to MSUCs are also to be considered as (asymptomatic) gout, in contrast to asymptomatic hyperuricemia with no deposition.

Gout is to be considered as the nucleation and aggregation of monosodium urate crystals (MSUCs) in tissues, mostly cartilage, synovial structures, bone, and skin, independently of the presence or absence of clinical manifestations. Further addition of descriptive terms may help to characterize the burden of disease.

INTRODUCTION: CONCEPTUAL ISSUES

Although most textbooks state that gout comprises the clinical manifestations of MSUC deposition, recent investigation using high-resolution and highly specific imaging techniques has shown that deposition and chronic inflammation may be present in

Disclosures: F. Perez-Ruiz: consultancies for Astra-Zeneca, Menarini, Metabolex, Novartis, Pfizer, SOBI. Speaker for Menarini International. Educational programs for Savient and Menarini. Investigation grants: Asociación de Reumatólogos del Hospital de Cruces; Ministerio de Sanidad (Gobierno de España); Fundación Española de Reumatología; E. Castillo, S. Chinchilla: nothing to disclose and A.M. Herrero-Beites: Investigation grants: Asociación de Reumatólogos del Hospital de Cruces.
[a] Division of Rheumatology, BioCruces Health Institute, Hospital Universitario Cruces, Pza Cruces sn, Baracaldo 48903, Spain; [b] Division of Rheumatology, Hospital Universitario Cruces, Pza Cruces sn, Baracaldo 48903, Spain; [c] Division of Physical Medicine, Hospital de Górliz, Astondo Ibiltoki, km. 2, Górliz 48630, Spain
* Corresponding author. Servicio de Reumatología, Hospital Universitario Cruces, Pza Cruces sn, Baracaldo 48903, Spain.
E-mail address: fernando.perezruiz@osakidetza.net

http://dx.doi.org/10.1016/j.rdc.2014.01.003
0889-857X/14/$ – see front matter © 2014 Elsevier Inc. All rights reserved.
rheumatic.theclinics.com

many individuals before the first symptom[1,2] and that they persist after symptoms of acute inflammation have completely subsided.[3] Therefore, MSUC deposition and subclinical inflammation related to MSUCs are also to be considered as (asymptomatic) gout, in contrast to asymptomatic hyperuricemia with no deposition. If this physiopathologic sequence is accepted, gout is to be defined as the presence of MSUCs in tissues as a consequence of long-standing hyperuricemia, despite the absence or the presence of acute or persistent clinical manifestations. To show this issue, consider that hemochromatosis, a well-known deposition disease, is defined as evidence of iron overload in the target organ, independently of the presence or absence of signs, symptoms, or organ dysfunction.

Academically, gout has been reported frequently as acute gout, intercritical gout, and chronic gout, as if these are different and an obligatory sequence of the stages of the natural history of the disease or even different diseases. We would like to take a more comprehensive approach, considering only acute clinical manifestations (mostly episodes of acute inflammation [EAIs]) and persistent clinical manifestations (chronic signs and symptoms). Again, as an example, it is not appropriate to talk about asymptomatic diabetes, acute diabetes, intercritical diabetes, or chronic diabetes but of acute and chronic clinical manifestations of diabetes. We suggest considering gout as the deposition of MSUCs in tissues (a true chronic deposition disease) with either or both acute and persistent, but even with absent clinical, manifestations.[4]

From a clinical point of view, gout has either acute (most commonly, but not restricted to, acute inflammatory episodes) or persistent clinical manifestations (including palpable tophi, joint limitation, persistent inflammation, and joint deformity). Gout should be considered a chronic disease from the beginning.

ACUTE CLINICAL MANIFESTATIONS OF GOUT
EAIs

Crystal-induced acute inflammation is the hallmark of gout and is well recognized by both patients and clinicians. Nomenclature of EAIs is variable, referred to as gout flares, gout attacks, gouty bouts, gouty arthritis, and so on. EAIs could be defined as the appearance of signs and symptoms of acute inflammation induced by MSUCs in any structure of the musculoskeletal system.

The time from the onset of hyperuricemia to tissue nucleation and growth of MSUCs is not known. The time from the onset of hyperuricemia to the development of clinical manifestations of gout seems to be directly related to the level of hyperuricemia and to the time that the individual is exposed to the hyperuricemic state.[5]

EAIs involve mainly synovial structures of joints, tendons, and bursae, thereby inducing acute arthritis, tendonitis, and bursitis. According to topographic distribution, the peripherally located structures are more commonly involved than those structures centrally located, and those of the lower limbs more frequently than that of the upper limbs. Nevertheless, in patients with long-standing gout, involvement of centrally located joints[6] and even the joints of the axial skeleton is possible. However, an absence of association between spinal pain and computed tomography (CT) of the spine showing changes suggesting gout has been reported,[7] despite the infrequent occurrence of spinal location as a presentation of gout.[8]

Therefore, involvement of the most peripheral structures of the lower limbs, such as the first metatarsophalangeal (MTP) joint, classic podagra, is a hallmark of, although not restricted to, gout. EAIs involving the first MTP joint are the presenting location in close to half, and they are involved in up to or more than 80% of untreated patients, including those without target therapeutic serum urate levels.

Tarsal, ankle, and knee structures follow in frequency of involvement and are frequent locations for the first EAIs. The most common location in the upper limb is the olecranon bursa. No difference between men and women has been observed regarding joint distribution[9] or between patients with or without chronic kidney disease.[10]

Involvement of the structures of the hands is not infrequent in patients with untreated gout of long duration,[11] but the hands are not common presenting locations, except in older women with hand osteoarthritis.[12] However, it may be the site of the first clinical presentation in patients with rapid deposition of MSUCs, as may occur in patients with the highest levels of hyperuricemia, such as heart or renal transplant patients,[13,14] because these patients frequently have chronic kidney disease and are prescribed loop diuretics.

The number of joints involved in EAIs is variable; it is more common to observe single structure involvement (monoarticular distribution), especially early in the disease. Nevertheless, oligoarticular and even polyarticular EAIs may appear, especially in patients with long-lasting, severe, untreated (or inefficiently treated) disease, and when urate-lowering treatment (ULT) induces sharp and striking reductions in serum urate levels. EAIs involving 2 or more joints were observed in 5.5% of patients, in 39% of them at presentation, and in 83%, the EAIs were located in the joints of the lower limbs.[15] A recent survey showed that in more than 90% of patients, gout presented as a single joint involvement, and less than 1% presented with EAIs involving more than 4 joints.[10]

Overt acute inflammatory clinical manifestations may be preceded by premonitory symptoms, popularly known as gouty "aura", consisting of mild pain, discomfort, and limitation.[16] Early recognition of these prodromal symptoms may facilitate early initiation of the treatment of the EAIs. Provocative factors have been well recognized in the literature, especially local trauma or changes in serum (and therefore synovial) urate concentrations, when sharp and intense changes in serum urate level occur (such as in surgery, absolute or severe dietary restriction, or initiation of full-dose urate-lowering medications). These circumstances may facilitate the disaggregation of MSUCs from solid aggregates and the shedding of preformed MSUCs into the synovial fluid. Diet transgressions, such as high purine intake, have been classically associated with an increase in the risk of initiating EAIs; a recent study in which more than half were untreated and individuals had a high purine intake reported an increased risk with increasing purine intake.[17]

The typical EAI in gout, which may be impossible to clinically distinguish from other synovial neutrophil-induced acute inflammation such as acute pyrophosphate arthritis or infectious arthritis, is most commonly of abrupt onset, with a rapid increase in inflammatory signs and symptoms (pain, swelling, function disturbance) and the utmost excruciating pain being appreciated in the first 12 to 24 hours. The presence of local redness (erythema), uncommon in other causes of acute inflammation of articular structures, can be seen in crystal-induced arthritis and infectious (septic) arthritis, typically limited to small peripheral joints or superficial bursae or tendon sheaths.

Local symptoms and signs accompanying acute inflammation of articular and periarticular joint structures such as soft tissue edema and erythema of overlying skin may vary widely, from mild to severe, with the latter often mimicking cellulitis or even phlebitis.[16] Systemic symptoms and signs may also be present, such as malaise and low-grade fever (usually well tolerated and even unnoticed by the patient).

For most patients, EAIs subside spontaneously sooner or later; they subside sooner especially if treatment is implemented early in the development of signs and symptoms of inflammation. In patients with severe disease, EAIs may recur before the previous episode has completely subsided.

Alleviation of signs and symptoms of inflammation with local cold-packs[18] or the administration of colchicine,[19] especially at the onset of symptoms, has been considered to be useful in differentiating EAIs caused by crystal deposition (including gout and acute pyrophosphate arthritis) from other causes of inflammation of joint structures.

Other Acute Clinical Manifestations

Rupture of popliteal (Baker) cysts may occur in gout as in any other arthritis, and especially in patients with previous recurrent swelling of the knee joint. Occasionally, joint blockade caused by intra-articular tophi (**Fig. 1**) may mimic meniscal derangements or osteochondritis.

Very infrequent manifestations, rarely mentioned in reviews, but observed in clinical practice, include the rupture of intradermal tophi, which may lead to the appearance of subepidermic collections, which may be misdiagnosed as an infectious pustule (**Fig. 2**A). Also, some patients with rupture of acral tophi inducing intense inflammatory response with compartment overpressure may develop necrosis of the fingerpad (see **Fig. 2**B).

Persistent clinical manifestations of gout may appear as a result of the increase of MSUC deposition in untreated gout, including the appearance of tophi, joint limitation, joint swelling, and deformity. Although mostly related to gout, other intercurrent processes may also be the cause.

PERSISTENT CLINICAL MANIFESTATIONS

Persistent, that is, nonacute, nonlimited clinical manifestations in gout are referred to as chronic gouty arthritis or chronic gouty arthropathy. A recent clinical survey showed

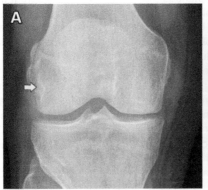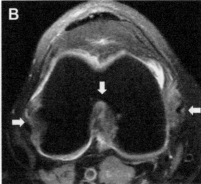

Fig. 1. A 56-year-old man referred for evaluation of persistent pain, swelling, limitation, and inflammation of the right knee joint; joint replacement was under consideration. (*A*) Plain radiograph does not show significant structural damage; an extensive erosion and soft tissue mass (*arrow*) had passed unnoticed. (*B*) Gadolinium-enhanced MRI T1-weighted sequence shows extensive masses under both collateral and cruciate ligaments (*arrows*), along with synovial membrane enhancement; other significant structural damage responsible for joint limitation was observed. Treatment with anakinra was associated with improvement in pain and swelling, but joint motion started to improve after only 6 months of control of serum urate <5 mg/dL. (*Courtesy of* F. Perez-Ruiz, MD, PhD, Baracaldo, Spain; with permission.)

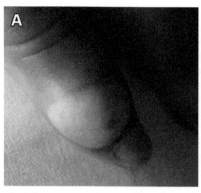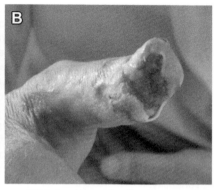

Fig. 2. Infrequent acute manifestations of gout. (*A*) Subepidermal collection of MSUCs as the first acute manifestation of gout in a renal transplant patient. (*B*) Patient admitted to hospital because of acute fingerpad necrosis; we were consulted for the presence of acute swelling of the knee joint. Extensive MSUC deposition was noted in a smear of the necrotic tissues; cultures were negative. The finger recovered completely, with a small scar remaining, on ULT. (*Courtesy of* F. Perez-Ruiz, MD, PhD, Baracaldo, Spain; with permission.)

that only half of the patients who were supposed to have chronic gouty arthropathy showed structural damage on radiographs.[10] We suggest a different clinical approach to those persistent clinical manifestations of gout.

Palpable Tophi

A tophus can be defined as a macroscopic aggregate of MSUCs. It can be appreciated on physical examination through inspection and palpation. What is frequently considered a subcutaneous tophus includes articular, intradermal, tendinous, and bursal tophi (**Fig. 3**), located sufficiently superficially to be physically apparent; they should be considered palpable tophi. Extensive intradermal tophaceous deposition has been related to self-prescription of corticosteroids.[20]

Most commonly, tophi develop after long-standing untreated gout, but infrequently may be the first clinical manifestation, even before any EAI is apparent to the patient.[21] A careful physical examination may frequently show superficial tophi that have not been perceived by the patient.

The presence of palpable tophi in physical examination directly correlates with higher frequency of periarticular tophi in bone and joint structures, which may not

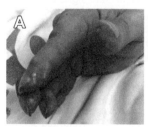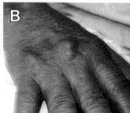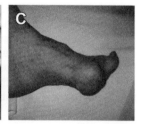

Fig. 3. (*A*) Rapid development of extended intradermal tophi in the fingerpads in a patient with serum urate level >12 mg/dL caused by chronic kidney disease and chronic heart failure on high-dose diuretics; (*B*) tophaceous deposit in an extensor tendon of the hand; (*C*) extensive deposition in synovial bursae of the toe. (*Courtesy of* F. Perez-Ruiz, MD, PhD, Baracaldo, Spain; with permission.)

be apparent on physical examination but can be ascertained using imaging procedures more sensitive to detecting urate deposition than plain radiography, such as ultrasonography (US), CT, magnetic resonance imaging (MRI), and dual-energy CT (DECT).[22] Therefore, the presence of apparent tophi is to be considered only the tip of the iceberg of MSUCs deposition in tissues and correlates with higher radiographic scores of structural damage[23] and poorer function.[24]

Palpable tophi are more commonly located in areas exposed to pressure or friction. Whereas in the skin, in tendons, and in superficial joints they tend to be consistent, those located in synovial bursae may frequently coexist with varying amounts of effusion, which may make clinical evaluation and measurement difficult.[25] If measurement of palpable tophi is to be used in clinical practice as an outcome measure for urate-lowering therapy,[26] this fact should be taken into consideration, because it may induce great variability.[27]

Although palpable tophi in the auricular helix have been academically considered to be a paradigm of macroscopic MSUC deposition, they are uncommonly found in clinical practice.

Joint Limitation

In absence of either swelling or deformity, the presence of joint limitation on physical examination suggests the presence of what is known, but yet to be defined, as gouty arthropathy. As mentioned earlier, a recent study[10] reported that only 52% of patients who were supposed to have gouty arthropathy had structural radiographic damage.

MSUC deposition in musculoskeletal structures is more frequently found with advanced imaging than with either clinical examination or radiographs, and even in the presence of normal radiographs.[28] Persistent joint limitation may be caused by masses of aggregates of MSUCs in either articular or periarticular structures, mostly ligaments and tendons, which limit normal biomechanics (see **Fig. 1**).[29]

In the clinical scenario of joint limitation, careful, clinically based evaluation of the best imaging technique to prescribe should be considered, bearing in mind that US evaluates soft tissue including the synovial membrane but does not evaluate but only the surface of accessible bone, and CT/DECT does not reliably evaluate soft tissues but may show impressive MSUC deposition.[30]

Persistent Joint Swelling

Persistent joint swelling is also referred to as chronic gouty arthritis. Inflammation may be observed to persist, subclinically, in asymptomatic joints of patients with gout using power Doppler US[31] or gadolinium-enhanced MRI.[32] Therefore, chronic arthritis is a clinical term that should apply to the presence of persistent clinical signs of inflammation: pain, swelling, and dysfunction.

Nevertheless, as with tophi, joint swelling may not be perceived by many patients, becoming apparent only during thorough rheumatologic physical examination, a practice that we strongly encourage not only for any chronic joint disease.

The presence of joint swelling is most commonly related to persistent effusion caused by granulomatous inflammation of the synovial membrane induced by MSUCs (**Fig. 4**). Nevertheless, patients with gout may also suffer from other causes of persistent joint effusion (eg, the presence of concomitant osteoarthritis or meniscal derangements).

Detection of even asymptomatic joint effusion in a joint in patients suspected to suffer from gout, and especially if the joint was involved in previous EAIs, is an outstanding opportunity to obtain a sample of synovial fluid for gold-standard diagnosis (MSUC observation under microscopic examination, as recommended by the

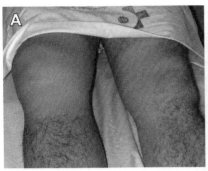
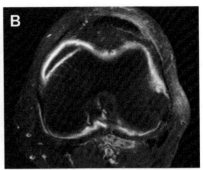

Fig. 4. (A) Patient referred because of persistent knee joint swelling; synovial fluid had <1000 leukocytes per microliter and MSUCs; (B) gadolinium-enhanced MRI showing intense uptake in thickened synovial membrane (*white* peripheral rim). (*Courtesy of* F. Perez-Ruiz, MD, PhD, Baracaldo, Spain; with permission.)

EULAR Task Force for Gout[33]) and also to ascertain the white cell count in the synovial fluid.

Deformity

Joint deformity develops most frequently late in the natural history of untreated gout, most often associated with extensive tophaceous deposition.[24] Structural damage of the joint structures leads to deformity and loss of function, especially if located in the joints of the hand (**Fig. 5**A).[24] In addition, extensive tendinous tophaceous deposition can induce deformities in the joints of the hands and feet that may mimic those found in patients with rheumatoid arthritis (see **Fig. 5**B).[34]

The natural course of untreated or neglected gout is progression to increasing frequency and intensity of EAIs and appearance of persistent clinical manifestations of gout, all of which are features of the disease that are preventable by proper and early diagnosis and treatment.

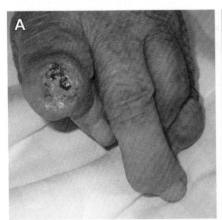
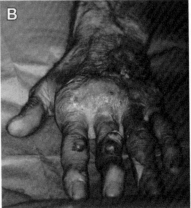

Fig. 5. (A) Severe structural damage of the joints of the hand, leading to complete loss of function. The huge, ulcerated tophus was believed to be a tumor; (B) extensive tendinous deposition, some of them ulcerated and draining, leading to pseudoswan-neck deformities. The patient was admitted with a previous diagnosis of rheumatoid arthritis. (*Courtesy of* F. Perez-Ruiz, MD, PhD, Baracaldo, Spain; with permission.)

NATURAL HISTORY OF UNTREATED (AND INEFFICIENTLY TREATED) DISEASE

The natural history of a disease is referred to as the evolution of untreated disease. If gout is to be considered as a deposition disease, undertreated or inefficiently treated hyperuricemia (not achieving target therapeutic[35] levels of serum urate lower than the threshold for saturation of urate, steadily, and in the long-term to completely dissolve MSUCs[36]) and untreated and undertreated gout could be considered as synonyms. A trend toward the most severe clinical involvement has been observed in the last 2 decades.[37]

Although it is not commonly believed that most patients with a first EAI (presumably) of gouty origin will not have further episodes, the natural history of the disease in the series reported by Gutman and Yü (whose studies of untreated primary gout and their conceptual approach to ULT are strongly recommended) showed that recurrence of EAIs was common in a relatively short period from clinical onset: in a series of 1266 male patients, "in about three fourths of these subjects a second attack developed within two years of the first."[19]

Also, in a report of 734 patients not treated with ULT, EAIs increased in frequency in 49% of the patients and in severity in 29% (**Fig. 6**),[38] considering that a ceiling effect for intensity may limit the possibility of increase in intensity of a typically excruciating pain.

An increase in the number of joints involved, or polyarticular gout, may be especially observed in untreated patients with the highest levels of serum urate. Heart transplant patients in the cyclosporine-A era (who were also on diuretics) may be illustrative: in a series of 178 patients without previous gout, with mean serum urate levels that increased from 10 to 14 mg/dL during follow-up, 22% developed gout at 4 years of follow-up and 43% of them developed polyarticular gout.[14]

Tophaceous deposits also increase with time in untreated gout. In a cohort of 392 patients with untreated gout[39] and showing no apparent signs of bone or joint involvement on plain radiography, the cumulative rate of development of radiographic abnormalities suggesting tophaceous deposition appeared to be linear, reaching 47% and 71% at 10 and 20 years of follow-up, respectively (**Fig. 7**). Development of tophi was associated with increasing serum urate levels in this cohort (**Fig. 8**).[39]

On the contrary, proper ULT to target serum urate levels has been associated not only with a reduction to zero in the number of EAIs[40] but also in the tophus burden,[25] body pain, and health-related quality-of-life outcomes.[41]

It should be considered that gout can be conceptually cured,[42] but structural[43] (and their associated functional) sequelae may not be reversible.

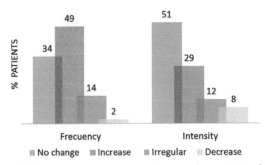

Fig. 6. In a cohort of 734 untreated patients with gout, the pattern of recurrence of EAIs showed an increase in frequency in half of the patients, but not in intensity, probably because of a ceiling effect. (*Courtesy of* F. Perez-Ruiz, MD, PhD, Baracaldo, Spain, with permission; and *Data from* Gutman AB. Treatment of primary gout: the present status. Arthritis Rheum 1965;8:911–20.)

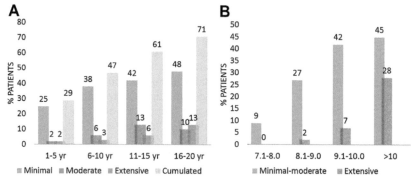

Fig. 7. (*A*) Data from 392 patients with untreated gout: tophi developed in 47% and 71% of the patients at 10-year and 20-year follow-up, respectively; (*B*) direct relationship between increasing serum urate levels and the development of tophi in a cohort of 12,989 patients with untreated gout. (*Courtesy of* F. Perez-Ruiz, MD, PhD, Baracaldo, Spain, with permission; and *Data from* Gutman AB. The past 4 decades of progress in the knowledge of gout, with an assessment of the present status. Arthritis Rheum 1973;16:431–45.)

Diagnosis of gout includes attaining the most accurate certainty of diagnosis, the evaluation of the burden of the disease, and consideration of the presence of other coexistent rheumatic diseases.

DIAGNOSIS OF GOUT

Diagnosis of gout comprises nosologic diagnosis (is it true gout?), evaluation of the burden of the deposition (how great and extensive is the deposition and how much is the structural damage induced?), and differential diagnosis. The evaluation of the mechanism of hyperuricemia is not discussed, because it is not within the scope of this article.

Nosologic Diagnosis

Nosologic diagnosis of gout is related to a simple and specific question: are the clinical manifestations related to MSUC deposition? The only reasonable answer is: certainly,

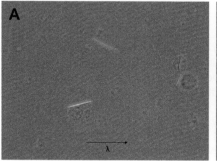

Fig. 8. MSUCs. (*A*) Polarized light microscopy 400×, with red compensator filter showing birefringent (shining) crystals yellow (negative elongation) when parallel to the polarizing axis (λ) and blue (positive elongation) when perpendicular; (*B*) easily identified large, square cholesterol crystals obtained from a persistent swelling of an olecranon bursa, which may lead one to oversee the urate crystal (*arrow*). Polarized, phase-contrast 400× microscopy. (*Courtesy of* F. Perez-Ruiz, MD, PhD, Baracaldo, Spain; with permission.)

if deposition of MSUCs is proved, especially considering that most patients are to be treated for the long-term, if not lifelong.

Evidence of the presence of MSUCs in a biological sample through microscopic examination remains the gold standard (see **Fig. 8**) as a definitive, inexpensive, accurate means of diagnosis of gout.[33] Nevertheless, in the face of a typical clinical presentation, a clinical diagnosis is reasonably accurate and acceptable when microscopy facilities or staff trained in tapping joints are not available,[44] although not definitive.[33] Use of new sophisticated imaging techniques such as US and DECT has increased as competitors to MSUC identification, because they have shown some specific findings[30]; however, their clinical usefulness has yet to be clarified. US may also be useful for guided puncture of joints or nodules in joint structures suspected to be tophi.[45] These topics are discussed elsewhere in this issue.

It is common clinical practice to use classification criteria[44,46] as a diagnostic tool in gout. This practice should be avoided, because classification criteria are not intended for diagnoses in clinical practice. The preliminary American Rheumatism Association 1977 criteria were limited to acute gouty arthritis; they have not been yet validated, and have limited applicability.[47,48] Other classification criteria have been recently proposed, but their extrinsic applicability is compromised because the population studied mostly had typical clinical manifestations of gout.[44] For example, patients presenting with a first EAI in the ankle, knee, or upper limb joints are not classified as having gout based on those criteria, particularly if serum urate levels are normal, a situation not infrequently encountered in clinical practice.[49]

Synovial fluid samples for examination of MSUCs may be obtained not only in close temporal proximity to EAIs but also in accessible joints previously inflamed.[33] These samples, if not immediately examined, may be preserved for some days if refrigerated or for months when frozen, although sample handling may have an impact on reliability.[50] In our practice, cryopreservation of synovial fluid samples is most easily performed using a 10% dilution with dimethylsulfoxide, a reliable procedure commonly used by hematologists, which retains viability of leukocytes for a short period after unfreezing.[51]

Samples for MSUC observation may also be obtained by puncturing nodules, preferably superficial but also deep if lesions suspicious for tophi are accessible by US examination.

Evaluation of the Burden of Deposition

The extent of deposition may be indirectly evaluated through a careful anamnesis and physical examination: the greater the number of EAIs, the number and location of joints ever involved by EAIs, the presence, size, and location of superficial tophi, persistence of pain, joint swelling, limitation of motion, and deformities denote the severity and extent of disease.

Imaging such as plain radiographs may be useful for patients with long duration of disease or to initially evaluate structural damage. In clinically selected patients in whom the clinical findings cannot be otherwise reasonably explained, advanced imaging procedures may be considered. Recently, a short 4-joint (including both knees and both first MTP joints) US screening has been proposed as a useful complement for clinical examination.[3]

A careful clinical evaluation may also be useful to ascertain the response of MSUC deposition to ULT. In selected patients, imaging may contribute to evaluating the expected reduction of the deposition.[26,52–54]

Differential Diagnosis

Misdiagnosis of gout is not infrequent.[55] As discussed earlier, oligoarticular or polyarticular presentation or the detection of tophi as the first clinical manifestations of gout are infrequent. Nevertheless, it seems that for diagnosis, the evaluation may be restricted to the present clinical grounds at medical visit. As a consequence, accuracy of diagnosis is higher for gout with monoarticular involvement compared with that involving an oligoarticular or polyarticular joint distribution.[56]

Polyarticular distribution, especially if the joints of the hands are affected, subcutaneous nodules are observed, or a positive rheumatoid factor is present, may be misdiagnosed as rheumatoid arthritis. Oligoarticular, lower limb, asymmetrical distribution of joint involvement may be considered to be a manifestation of spondyloarthropathies, especially when there is a familial or personal history of psoriasis or diarrhea has preceded the EAI of gout.

Monoarticular EAIs, especially in older patients with hyperuricemia, may be attributed to gout, acute pyrophosphate arthritis, and infectious arthritis. The presence of both hyperuricemia and chondrocalcinosis is frequent in the elderly and definite diagnosis may be difficult based on clinical grounds even with plain radiographic supportive findings. In these cases, obtaining synovial fluid samples is encouraged, although both MSUCs and calcium pyrophosphate crystals are not uncommonly found concomitantly.[57] Joint infection is not uncommon in patients with crystal-induced arthritis, and the presence of crystals in synovial fluid samples does not rule out infection.[58]

Monoarticular persistent effusion and inflammation of the knee joint is, in our practice, frequently misdiagnosed as pigmented villonodular synovitis, particularly because MRI of chronic granulomatous synovitis of gout may also show hypointense lesions on T1-weighted and T2-weighted sequences.[59]

Although the literature has considered the association between gout and other chronic inflammatory joint diseases to be infrequent, recent evidence has suggested that there is not a negative association: MSUCs may be retrieved from joints of patients with other rheumatic diseases,[57] and other diseases develop in patients with a correct previous diagnosis of gout, especially acute pyrophosphate arthritis in older patients, which may be difficult to differentiate in most instances.[60]

ACKNOWLEDGMENTS

This article is dedicated to all the patients with gout attending our gout clinic for the last 20 years, from whom we have learned as much as we have from reading the literature. They have been of great support to our amassing large databases for clinical investigation, and for giving permission for use of images. We also thank Mrs Rosario Lopez-Santamaria, Ms Inmaculada Iriondo, and Ms Begoña Balmaseda for their support during daily clinical practice at the office, and to Dr Alberto Alonso-Ruiz, Chief of Rheumatology Division at Hospital Universitario Cruces, for his encouraging attitude to our clinical investigations in gout.

REFERENCES

1. Pineda C, Amezcua-Guerra LM, Solano C, et al. Joint and tendon subclinical involvement suggestive of gouty arthritis in asymptomatic hyperuricemia: an ultrasound controlled study. Arthritis Res Ther 2011;13:R4.
2. De Miguel E, Puig JG, Castillo C, et al. Diagnosis of gout in patients with asymptomatic hyperuricaemia: a pilot ultrasound study. Ann Rheum Dis 2011;71:157–8.

3. Peiteado D, de ME, Villalba A, et al. Value of a short four-joint ultrasound test for gout diagnosis: a pilot study. Clin Exp Rheumatol 2012;30(6):830–7.

4. Perez Ruiz F, Herrero-Beites AM. Evaluation and treatment of gout as a chronic disease. Adv Ther 2012;29:935–46.

5. Campion EW, Glynn RJ, DeLabry LO. Asymptomatic hyperuricemia. Risks and consequences in the normative aging study. Am J Med 1987;82:421–6.

6. Perez-Ruiz F, Calabozo M, Alonso-Ruiz A. Gouty arthritis in the manubriosternal joint. Ann Rheum Dis 1997;56:571–2.

7. Konatalapalli RM, Lumezanu E, Jelinek JS, et al. Correlates of axial gout: a cross-sectional study. J Rheumatol 2012;39:1445–9.

8. Wendling D, Prati C, Hoen B, et al. When gout involves the spine: five patients including two inaugural cases. Joint Bone Spine 2013;80(6):656–9. http://dx.doi.org/10.1016/j.jbspin.2013.06.002.

9. Puig JG, Michán AD, Jimenez ML, et al. Female gout. Clinical spectrum and uric acid metabolism. Arch Intern Med 1991;151:726–32.

10. Lioté F, Lancrenon S, Lanz S, et al. GOSPEL: prospective survey of gout in France. Part I: design and patient characteristics (n = 1003). Joint Bone Spine 2012;79:464–70.

11. Rapado A, Castrillo JM. Gout disease. Its natural history based on 1,000 observations. Adv Exp Med Biol 1977;76B:223–30.

12. Simkin PA, Campbell PM, Larson EB. Gout in Heberden's nodes. Arthritis Rheum 1983;26:94–7.

13. Clive DM. Renal-transplant associated hyperuricemia and gout. J Am Soc Nephrol 2000;11:974–9.

14. Burack DA, Griffith BP, Thompson ME. Hyperuricemia and gout among heart transplant patients receiving cyclosporin. Am J Med 1992;92:141–4.

15. Hadler NM, Franck WA, Bress NM, et al. Acute polyarticular gout. Am J Med 1974;56:715–9.

16. Cohen H. Gout. In: Copeman WS, editor. Textbook of the rheumatic diseases. Edinburgh (United Kingdom): E&S Livingstone; 1948. p. 249–305.

17. Zhang Y, Chen C, Choi H, et al. Purine-rich foods intake and recurrent gout attacks. Ann Rheum Dis 2012;71:1448–53.

18. Schlesinger N. Response to application of ice may help differentiate between gouty arthritis and other inflammatory arthritides. J Clin Rheumatol 2006;12:275–6.

19. Yü TF, Gutman AB. Principles of current management of primary gout. Am J Med Sci 1967;254:893–907.

20. Vazquez-Mellado J, Cuan A, Magaña M, et al. Intradermal tophi in gout: a case-control study. J Rheumatol 1999;26:136–40.

21. Wernick R, Winkler C, Campbell S. Tophi as the initial manifestation of gout. Report of six cases and review of the literature. Arch Intern Med 1992;152:873–6.

22. Perez-Ruiz F, Naredo E. Imaging modalities and monitoring measures of gout. Curr Opin Rheumatol 2007;19:128–33.

23. Dalbeth N, Clark B, McQueen FM, et al. Validation of a radiographic damage index in chronic gout. Arthritis Rheum 2007;57:1067–73.

24. Dalbeth N, Collis J, Gregory K, et al. Tophaceous joint disease strongly predicts hand function in patients with gout. Rheumatology 2007;46:1804–7.

25. Perez-Ruiz F, Calabozo M, Pijoan JI, et al. Effect of urate-lowering therapy on the velocity of size reduction of tophi in chronic gout. Arthritis Rheum 2002;47:356–60.

26. Dalbeth N, Schauer C, MacDonald P, et al. Methods of tophus assessment in clinical trials of chronic gout: a systematic literature review and pictorial reference guide. Ann Rheum Dis 2011;70:597–604.
27. Schumacher HR, Becker MA, Palo WA, et al. Tophaceous gout: quantitative evaluation by direct physical measurement. J Rheumatol 2005;32:2368–72.
28. Carter JD, Kedar RP, Anderson SR, et al. An analysis of MRI and ultrasound imaging in patients with gout who have normal plain radiographs. Rheumatology (Oxford) 2009;48(11):1442–6.
29. Chen CK, Yeh LR, Pan HB, et al. Intra-articular gouty tophi of the knee: CT and MR imaging in 12 patients. Skeletal Radiol 1999;28:282–9.
30. Perez-Ruiz F, Schlesinger N, Dalbeth N, et al. Imaging of gout: findings and utility. Arthritis Res Ther 2009;11:232. http://dx.doi.org/10.1186/ar2687.
31. Thiele RG, Schlesinger N. Ultrasonography shows active inflammation in clinically unaffected joints in chronic tophaceous gout. Arthritis Rheum 2009;60:S565.
32. Perez-Ruiz F, Urresola A, Gorostiza D, et al. Validation of the measurement of tophi with magnetic resonance imaging as an outcome measure for chronic gout [abstract]. Arthritis Rheum 2011;63(Suppl 10):S77.
33. Zhang W, Doherty M, Pascual E, et al. EULAR evidence based recommendations for gout Part I. Diagnosis. Report of a Task Force of the EULAR Standing Committee for international clinical studies including therapeutics (ESCISIT). Ann Rheum Dis 2006;65:1301–11.
34. Schapira D, Stahl S, Izhak OB, et al. Chronic tophaceous gout mimicking rheumatoid arthritis. Semin Arthritis Rheum 1999;29:56–63.
35. Khanna D, Fitzgerald JD, Khanna PP, et al. 2012 American College of Rheumatology guidelines for management of gout. Part 1: systematic nonpharmacologic and pharmacologic therapeutic approaches to hyperuricemia. Arthritis Care Res (Hoboken) 2012;64:1431–46.
36. Perez-Ruiz F, Herrero-Beites AM, Carmona L. A two-stage approach to the treatment of hyperuricemia in gout: the "Dirty Dish" hypothesis. Arthritis Rheum 2011;63:4002–6.
37. Perez Ruiz F, Herrero Beites AM. Changes in gout patients' clinical profile in the last two decades. Arthritis Rheum 2012;64:S809–10.
38. Gutman AB. Treatment of primary gout: the present status. Arthritis Rheum 1965;8:911–20.
39. Gutman AB. The past four decades of progress in the knowledge of gout, with an assessment of the present status. Arthritis Rheum 1973;16:431–45.
40. Perez-Ruiz F, Calabozo M, Fernandez-Lopez MJ, et al. Treatment of chronic gout in patients with renal function impairment. An open, randomized, actively controlled. J Clin Rheumatol 1999;5:49–55.
41. Khanna PP, Perez-Ruiz F, Maranian P, et al. Long-term therapy for chronic gout results in clinically important improvements in the health-related quality of life: short form-36 is responsive to change in chronic gout. Rheumatology (Oxford) 2011;50:740–5.
42. Doherty M, Jansen TL, Nuki G, et al. Gout: why is this curable disease so seldom cured? Ann Rheum Dis 2012;71:1765–70.
43. Bloch C, Hermann G, Yü TF. A radiologic reevaluation of gout: a study of 2,000 patients. AJR Am J Roentgenol 1980;134:781–7.
44. Janssens HJ, Fransen J, van de Lisdonk EH, et al. A diagnostic rule for acute gouty arthritis in primary care without joint fluid analysis. Arch Intern Med 2010;170:1120–6.

45. Perez-Ruiz F, Martin I, Canteli B. Ultrasonographic measurement of tophi as an outcome measure for chronic gout. J Rheumatol 2007;34:1888–93.
46. Wallace SL, Robinson H, Masi AT, et al. Preliminary criteria for the classification of the acute arthritis of primary gout. Arthritis Rheum 1977;20:895–900.
47. Janssens HJ, Janssen M, Van de Lisdonk EH, et al. The limited validity of the criteria of the American College of Rheumatology for classifying gout patients in primary care. Ann Rheum Dis 2010;69(6):1255–6. http://dx.doi.org/10.1136/ard.2009.123687.
48. Malik A, Schumacher HR, Dinnella JE, et al. Clinical diagnostic criteria for gout: comparison with the gold standard of synovial fluid crystal analysis. J Clin Rheumatol 2009;15:22–4.
49. Logan JA, Morrison E, McGill PE. Serum uric acid in acute gout. Ann Rheum Dis 1997;56:696–7.
50. Graf SW, Buchbinder R, Zochling J, et al. The accuracy of methods for urate crystal detection in synovial fluid and the effect of sample handling: a systematic review. Clin Rheumatol 2013;32:225–32.
51. Stroncek DF, Xing L, Chau Q, et al. Stability of cryopreserved leukocytes preparations for donor leukocyte infusions. Transfusion 2011;51:2647–55.
52. Thiele RG, Schlesinger N. Ultrasonography shows disappearance of monosodium urate crystal deposition on hyaline cartilage after sustained normouricemia is achieved. Rheumatol Int 2010;30(4):495–503. http://dx.doi.org/10.1007/s00296-009-1002-8.
53. Dalbeth N, Aati O, Gao A, et al. Assessment of tophus size: a comparison between physical measurement methods and dual-energy computed tomography scanning. J Clin Rheumatol 2012;18:23–7.
54. Dalbeth N, Kalluru R, Aati O, et al. Tendon involvement in the feet of patients with gout: a dual-energy CT study. Ann Rheum Dis 2013;72(9):1545–8.
55. Wolfe F, Cathey MA. The misdiagnosis of gout and hyperuricemia. J Rheumatol 1991;18:1232–4.
56. Perez-Ruiz F, Ruiz Lopez J, Herrero Beites A. Influence of the natural history of disease on a previous diagnosis in patients with gout. Reumatol Clin 2009;5:248–51.
57. Oliviero F, Scanu A, Galozzi P, et al. Prevalence of calcium pyrophosphate and monosodium urate crystals in synovial fluid of patients with previously diagnosed joint diseases. Joint Bone Spine 2013;80(3):287–90. http://dx.doi.org/10.1016/j.jbspin.2012.08.006.
58. Shah K, Spear J, Nathanson LA, et al. Does the presence of crystal arthritis rule out septic arthritis? J Emerg Med 2007;32:23–6.
59. Narvaez JA, Narvaez J, Ortega R, et al. Hypointense synovial lesions on T2-weighted images: differential diagnosis with pathologic correlation. Am J Roentgenol 2003;181:761–9.
60. Perez-Ruiz F, Herrero-Beites AM. Prevalence of non-gout arthritis in patients with gout: not as sparing as previously thought. Arthritis Rheum 2012;64:S63.

Diagnosis and Clinical Manifestations of Calcium Pyrophosphate and Basic Calcium Phosphate Crystal Deposition Diseases

Hang-Korng Ea, MD, PhD[a,b,c], Frédéric Lioté, MD, PhD[a,b,c],*

KEYWORDS

- Calcium pyrophosphate • Basic calcium phosphate • Apatite • Calcification
- Calcific tendinitis • Chondrocalcinosis • Crowned dens syndrome • Ultrasonography

KEY POINTS

- Calcium pyrophosphate (CPP) and basic calcium phosphate (BCP) crystals are the 2 main families of calcium-containing crystals that can form simultaneously in all joint structures, ligament, tendon, muscle, and soft tissue.
- BCP and CPP crystal deposition are 2 common multifaceted diseases that can mimic alarming clinical manifestations.
- Ultrasonography seems to be an excellent imaging technique for CPP crystal detection but lacks efficacy for deep locations.
- Computed tomography remains the gold standard imaging modality for detection of calcification in the axial skeleton, especially at the cervical level.

INTRODUCTION

Calcium pyrophosphate (CPP) and basic calcium phosphate (BCP) crystals are the 2 main families of calcium-containing crystals that can form simultaneously in all joint structures, ligament, tendon, muscle, and soft tissue. Although these calcium crystal depositions are mostly asymptomatic, they can give rise to a wide range of clinical

This work is supported by ANR grant 2013-2017 (CAPYROSIS), "Association Rhumatisme et Travail," "Association ARPS."

[a] AP-HP, hôpital Lariboisière, Service de rhumatologie (centre Viggo Petersen), pôle appareil locomoteur, 2 Rue Ambroise Paré, Paris F-75010, France; [b] Sorbonne Paris Cité, University Paris Diderot (UFR de Médecine), 10 Avenue de Verdun, Paris F-75205, France; [c] INSERM, UMR-S 1132, Hopital Lariboisière, 2 Rue Ambroise Paré, Paris F-75010, France
* Corresponding author.
E-mail address: frederic.liote@lrb.aphp.fr

manifestations and syndromes, including acute inflammatory articular or periarticular attacks, chronic tendinitis, rapidly destructive arthropathies, or osteoarthritis (OA)-like lesions, as well as nervous compressions (**Table 1**). Some of these clinical symptoms have been referred to by a variety of names and confusing terms. Recently, a group of experts from the European League Against Rheumatism (EULAR) have elaborated 2 sets of recommendations for the terminology and diagnosis of CPP and its management.[1,2] Similar efforts should be made for BCP crystals.

Table 1
Summary of BCP and CPP crystal deposition-related manifestations

	CPP Crystals	BCP Crystals
Chemical composition	$Ca_2P_2O_7 \cdot 2H_2O$	$Ca_{10-x}(HPO_4)_x(PO_4)_{6-x}(OH)_{2-x}$
Ca^{2+}/P ratio	1.67	1.3
Members identified in human samples	Monoclinic Triclinic	Carbonated-apatite Octacalcium phosphate Whitlockite Tricalcium phosphate (?)
Intra-articular deposition	+++	+
Extra-articular deposition	+	+++
Clinical Manifestations		
Asymptomatic	++	++
Acute joint flare	++	?
Acute tendinitis	+	++
Acute bone erosion	+	+
Acute neck pain	++	+
Acute spinal pain	++	+
Chronic arthritis	++	+/−
OA associated	++	+++
Calcific tendinitis	+	+++
Milwaukee shoulder	?	++
Destructive arthropathies	+	+
Crowned dens syndrome	++	+
Spinal cord compression	+	+
Tumoral deposition	+	++
Synovial fluid detection	+++	+/−
Alizarin red staining	+	+
Radiographic pattern	Dense, linear	Dense, homogeneous without bone trabeculation
Ultrasonography	Hyperechoic deposits without posterior shadow	Hyperechoic with posterior acoustic shadowing
CT scan	+++	+++
Associated clinical conditions	Aging, OA, trauma Hemochromatosis hyperparathyroidism Hypomagnesemia Hypophosphatasia Wilson disease? Ochronosis?	Aging, OA Diabetes mellitus Chronic kidney disease Connective diseases Trauma, infection

CALCIFICATION FORMATION

Mechanisms of ectopic calcifications remain unresolved and have been reviewed recently.[3–8] Multiple factors contribute to this cellular driven process, including genetics, aging, imbalance between inhibitors and stimulators of calcification, alteration of calcium, phosphate and pyrophosphate metabolisms, extracellular matrix lesions, cellular differentiation state, and cell death.

Two types of CPP crystals have been identified in synovial fluid, hyaline cartilage, and fibrocartilage: monoclinic and triclinic CPP crystals.[9] BCP crystals encompass several types of crystals, including carbonated-apatite, octacalcium phosphate, and apatite-containing magnesium (whitlockite) crystals.[3]

The type of calcium-containing crystal depends on the levels of extracellular inorganic pyrophosphate (ePPi) and extracellular inorganic phosphate (ePi). High ePPi levels promote CPP crystal formation and inhibit BCP crystal nucleation. In contrast, high ePi concentration and low ePPi favor BCP crystal formation.[3,10] Several proteins regulate inorganic pyrophosphate (PPi) and inorganic phosphate (Pi) concentrations, including ANKH (ankylosis human), ENPP-1 (ectonucleotide pyrophosphate phosphodiesterase 1), or PC-1 (plasma-cell membrane glycoprotein 1), TNAP (tissue nonspecific alkaline phosphatase), PiT-1 (sodium-dependent phosphate transport protein 1), and CD73.[10–12] ANKH is a transmembrane protein that transports intracellular PPi across the cell membrane.[13] PC-1 converts extracellular nucleotide triphosphate into PPi and adenosine monophosphate (AMP). TNAP transforms PPi into orthophosphate. Pit-1 transports extracellular Pi into cell cytoplasm. CD73 converts AMP into adenosine and Pi. Adenosine inhibits TNAP activity (**Fig. 1**). Thus, ANKH, PC-1, and CD73 increase extracellular PPi concentration, which is decreased by TNAP. Mutations of these proteins have been associated with pathologic calcifications: gain-of-function mutations of *ANKH* or loss-of-function mutations of *TNAP* genes increase PPi concentration and lead to CPP crystal deposition (CPPD) disease[3,10]; loss-of-function mutations of *PC-1* and *NT5E* (gene encoding CD73 protein) genes decrease ePPi level and are associated with diffuse vascular calcifications and periarticular BCP crystal deposition.[11,14,15] Mutations of many other genes have been associated with vascular and joint calcification and are detailed in several reviews.[5,12,16]

According to EULAR recommendations, diagnosis of CPPD disease in young patients needs to be accompanied by ruling out of diseases such as hemochromatosis, primary hyperparathyroidism, chronic hypomagnesemia, and hypophosphatasemia.[1] There may also be an association between Wilson disease and CPPD (Marson L, Quemeneur AS, Trocello JM, et al, personal communication, 2013). A family history of CPPD disease suggests genetic disorder, especially a gain-of-function mutation of *ANKH* gene. This gene has been implicated in Spanish, Argentinean, and French families with CPPD disease.[17] Similarly, several clinical conditions favor BCP crystal deposition: chronic renal disease, diabetes mellitus, hyperparathyroidism, autoimmune diseases such as dermatomyositis, scleroderma, CREST syndrome, systemic lupus, trauma, and infection. Aging and OA are associated with CPPD and BCP crystal deposition in articular hyaline cartilages and fibocartilages.[18–21] BCP crystals are identified in 80% to 100% of OA cartilage according to different studies,[18,20,22,23] and CPPD prevalence is greater than 20% in people older than 80 years.[10,24] In the skeletal system, CPP crystals occur preferentially in articular tissues (synovial fluid, hyaline cartilage, fibrocartilage, intervertebral disk, ligament, joint synovium, and capsule), whereas BCP crystals are frequent in articular and extra-articular tissues involving especially tendons and soft tissue.

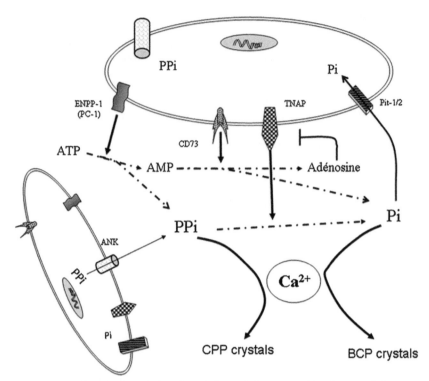

Fig. 1. Pyrophosphate (PPi) and phosphate balance (Pi). Increased local extracellular concentrations of PPi and Pi with local calcium concentration lead to CPP and BCP crystal formation, respectively. Ectoenzymes such as PC-1, membranous and extracellular nonspecific tissue alkaline phosphatase, and transmembrane channel ANK regulate these ionic concentrations. Regulatory components included local Mg concentrations, for example.

CLINICAL MANIFESTATIONS RELATED TO BCP AND CPPD

CPPD and BCP crystal deposition are often asymptomatic and identified as an incidental radiographic finding. However, both calcium crystals may be associated with several manifestations.[25] Intra-articular CPP crystals may cause acute and relapsing CPP crystal arthritis attacks, chronic CPP crystal inflammatory arthritis, and OA with CPP crystal.[1] Extra-articular CPP and BCP crystals can cause tenosynovitis, peripheral nerve and spinal cord compression, and pseudotumoral deposition.[25] Both CPPD and BCP crystal deposition around the odontoid process cause the crowned dens syndrome (CDS). Periarticular BCP crystal deposition may cause calcifying tendinitis, acute periarthritis, bursitis, and bone pain secondary to bone erosion.[26,27] Similarly, BCP crystals deposited in soft tissues may cause an acute inflammatory reaction, which is frequently associated with their resorption. Intra-articular BCP crystals may be responsible for severe destructive arthropathies known as the Milwaukee shoulder syndrome (MSS), as an example.[28–30]

Clinical Symptoms Related to BCP Crystals

Calcific periarthritis
Calcific tendinitis or calcific periarthritis most commonly involves the rotator cuff tendons of the shoulder joint and the medius gluteus tendon, but can occur at any tendon (**Fig. 2**).[31] Multiple localizations are common, occurring in 33%; bilateral calcification

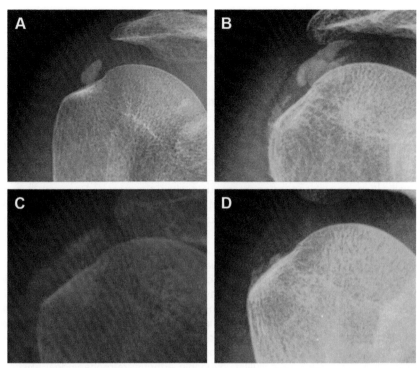

Fig. 2. Classification of calcific tendinitis of rotator cuff tendons. Different types of calcification of the supraspinatus tendon according to the system described by the French Society of Arthroscopy: type A, dense, well-defined, and circumscribed; type B, dense, well-defined, and segmented; type C, transparent and nonhomogeneous; and type D, dystrophic deposit at the origin of the tendon.

occurs in about half of shoulder cases, and deposits can be identified in other sites.[32] Calcium crystals are composed mainly of carbonated-apatite crystals.[33–35] Pathogenesis of periarticular calcification remains unresolved and involves systemic and local factors. Calcific periarthritis of the shoulder affects women more frequently in middle age and the dominant side (60%).[32,36] Boswoth[36] found a prevalence of 2.7% in 6061 asymptomatic office workers, with about 30% to 45% of individuals becoming symptomatic in a period of 3 years. In a prospective study, the prevalence of rotator cuff calcification was 7.3% in 1276 asymptomatic patients seen in the emergency department.[32] Calcifications occurred in 44% of patients between 40 and 50 years old. In painful shoulders, the prevalence was higher and varied between 7% and 50%.[37,38] The supraspinatus tendon (78%) is the most frequently involved tendon, followed by the infraspinatus (16%), the subscapularis (6%), and the long biceps tendons.[32,36] Calcific periarthritis may be associated with chronic pain and self-limited episodes of acute periarticular inflammation, which corresponds to the resorption phase of the crystals with migration in the subacromial bursae and acute bursitis. Persistent calcification can lead to local complications with joint tenderness, tendon tears, or adhesive capsulitis.

Cortical bone erosions
Cortical bone erosion and great tuberosity lysis are lesser known complications.[26,39] Flemming and colleagues[26] described in a retrospective series 50 cases of calcific

tendinitis with bone involvement. The humerus and femur were the 2 most frequent sites, with each representing 40% of cases (20 of 50 patients). Femoral involvement was posterior and subtrochanteric along the linea aspera in 95% of cases. Humeral involvement was located in the diaphysis at or near the insertion of the pectoralis major tendon (n = 9), in the lesser tuberosity (n = 6), and in the greater tuberosity (n = 5). The other sites included hand and wrist (n = 3), foot (n = 3), and cervical spine (n = 1). Calcification appeared solid in 50% of patients, stippled in 25%, and amorphous in 20%. Cortical erosion was evident in 78% of patients, periosteal reaction in 32%, and bone marrow involvement in 36%. Computed tomography (CT) is the key imaging tool, with a limitation between calcifications and the cortex of bone, whereas magnetic resonance imaging (MRI) can provide inflammatory figures and can mimic tumoral process.

Calcification may disappear spontaneously without symptom. Bosworth[36] found that radiographic resolution of calcification was around 6% per year, whereas Wölk and Wittenberg[40] reported an ultrasonographic (US) resolution rate of 82% within 8.6 years.

Acute calcific tendinitis and acute inflammatory reaction

BCP crystals like CPP crystals and urate crystals may induce self-limiting acute inflammatory attacks. Clinical symptoms may be impressive, with rapid onset of pain, important soft tissue swelling, and joint mobility reduction, inducing total or partial impotence. Fever may be present, and laboratory analysis may show increased inflammatory parameters and neutrophil count. Acute inflammatory attack related to uncommon BCP crystal localizations can be challenging and misdiagnosed with alarming conditions such as cellulitis, pyogenic arthritis, retropharyngeal abscess, infectious spondylitis, meningitides, or sarcoma.[26,41,42] This situation can lead to inappropriate management with invasive diagnostic procedures and therapies, including surgery and amputation. Diagnostic clues rely on awareness of this disease, history of a similar self-limiting flare, evidence of BCP crystal deposition by simple imaging procedures such as radiography, US, and mostly, CT scan examination.

Acute inflammatory flares may involve any tendons and commonly affects shoulder and hip joints followed by fingers, elbows, wrists, knees, ankles, and feet.[43] Acute attack of the longus colli muscle is rare but not infrequently reported. The longus colli muscle is a weak flexor of the neck, composed of 3 portions with superior, central, and inferior fibers. It extends from the level of the anterior tubercle of the atlas into the superior mediastinum to the level of the T3 vertebral body. Calcification involves mainly the superior fibers, which attach the tubercle of the atlas to the transverse processes of the C3-C5 vertebrae. Acute calcific tendinitis of the longus colli muscle was first described in 1964.[44,45] It usually affects patients who are between 30 and 60 years old, without gender predilection. Ring and colleagues[45] showed that this condition was caused by BCP crystal deposition with a foreign-body inflammatory response.[44] The most frequent presentation is neck pain with rapid onset, and stiffness, dysphagia, odynophagia, and headache. In some cases, there may be fever, with increased inflammatory markers. Clinical presentation can be confused with retropharyngeal abscess, infectious spondylitis, or meningitis pain and stiffness associated with odynophagia. The pathognomonic radiographic findings are prevertebral soft tissue swelling typically extending from C1 to C4 and the presence of amorphous calcification anterior to C2 at the insertion of the superior tendon of the muscle. However, these signs may be difficult to see on plain radiographs. CT is more sensitive than radiography for the detection of calcification and prevertebral soft tissue swelling (**Fig. 3**). It represents the method of choice, also allowing bone destruction or fracture to be ruled

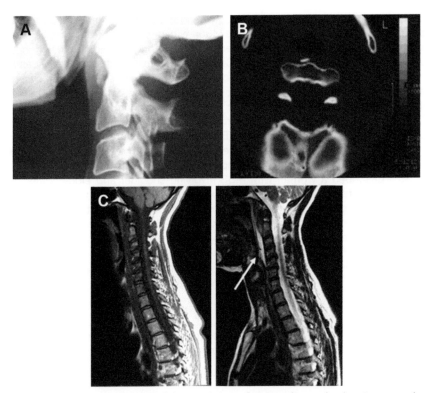

Fig. 3. Calcification of longus colli. (*A*) Lateral view of plain radiography showing amorphous calcification in front of C2 vertebral with a retropharyngeal soft tissue thickening. (*B*) Axial CT shows the calcification in front of the vertebral body. (*C*) Sagittal T1-weighted (*left*) and T2-weighted (*right*) MRI showing edema of prevertebral soft tissue (*arrow*).

out. Retropharyngeal soft tissue edema and muscle inflammation can be better visualized by MRI, which eliminates retropharyngeal abscess and cervical spondylitis. Thus, a correct diagnosis can be easily made by combining CT and MRI.[46] Treatment relies on a short course of antiinflammatory drugs and neck immobilization. Like other acute attacks secondary to BCP crystal deposition, symptoms usually spontaneously resolve within 1 to 2 weeks followed by calcification disappearence.

MSS, hemorrhagic shoulder of the elderly

MSS was described for the first time by McCarty and colleagues[30] in 1981. It has received several names, including hemorrhagic shoulder of the elderly, rapid destructive arthritis of the shoulder, and apatite-associated destructive arthritis. MSS is the prototypical BCP crystal–associated joint destructive arthropathy. It affects mainly elderly women (ratio of 4:1) and both shoulders in 60% to 80%.[28–30,47] The dominant side is involved in unilateral disease, and the disease is most severe in the dominant shoulder.[30] It is associated with rotator cuff defects and numerous aggregates of BCP crystals in the fluids of affected joints. Characteristically, shoulder pain is mild and intermittent and is exacerbated by motion and at night when lying in bed. Joint mobility is restricted or excessively mobile and instable (when the joint is completely destroyed). Large joint blood-stained effusions are common, with a low leukocyte count. Collagenase activity is increased in synovial fluids.[28–30] Usually, joint destruction occurs within months. Radiographs show initially superior subluxation of the humeral head from the glenoid fossa, secondary to widespread tear of the rotator cuff. Calcifications of periarticular soft tissues are frequent and noted in about 60% of affected shoulders. Bony sclerosis and cyst formation in the humeral head are common, as well as erosions of the greater tuberosity at the site of insertion of the rotator cuff.[30] Later, the glenohumeral joint is destroyed, with commonly, a large destruction of the humeral head and glenoid cavity. Diagnosis is helped by the identification of BCP crystals in synovial fluid using alizarin red staining. MSS can also affect the knee joint, involving more frequently the patellofemoral and lateral tibiofemoral compartments.[30,47] Recently, Ornetti and colleagues[48] described a woman with MSS involving shoulder and elbow joints. The natural history of the disease is unclear, but many cases seem to stabilize after a year or 2, with reduction of symptoms, joint effusions, and no further radiographic changes. MSS is also associated with OA in other joints. In their first description, MSS was associated with knee OA in more than 60% of cases.[30,47] Pons-Estel and colleagues[49] had reported kindred in which multiple members spanning several generations had features of MSS and OA in other joints. Genetic linkage was not identified.

Clinical Symptoms Related to CPPD

According to EULAR recommendations for terminology and diagnosis, 4 different clinical settings are associated with CPPD diseases:

1. Asymptomatic CPPD with no apparent clinical consequence
2. OA with CPPD
3. Acute CPP crystal arthritis (replacing the term pseudogout)
4. Chronic CPP crystal inflammatory arthritis[1]

Less commonly, atypical or periarticular CPP crystals may associate with tendinitis, bursitis, tumoral CPPD (especially in the temporomandibular joint and the foramen magnum), and acute spinal pain related to spine involvement.[1]

Asymptomatic CPPD

Asymptomatic CPPD is CPPD with no apparent clinical consequence. It may consist of isolated cartilage or fibrocartilage calcifications detected by plain radiographs (chondrocalcinosis [CC]), or OA with CPP crystals. Radiologic CC is not always caused by CPPD and is often an incidental finding. We and other investigators have shown that CPP and BCP crystals coexist in 20% of OA articular tibia cartilages harvested at the time of total joint arthroplasty.[18,20] The prevalence of CC varies from 3.7% in patients aged 55 to 59 years to 17.5% in patients aged 80 to 84 years.[24,50]

Acute CPP crystal arthritis

An acute joint attack caused by CPP crystals might mimic a gout flare and was formerly named pseudogout, which could give rise to confusion regarding the nature of the guilty crystals. The attack can be monoarticular, oligoarticular, or polyarticular. It is a common cause of monoarticular inflammation in elderly women. In a hospital series, CPP crystal inflammation was related to monoarthritis/oligoarthritis in 89% and to polyarthritis in 11%.[51] Knee, wrist, and metacarpophalangeal (MCP) joints are the most affected sites, but any joint can be involved, including uncommon ones such as acromion-clavicular, temporomandibular, sacroiliac, symphysis pubis, and spinal facet joints.[52–54] Characteristics of CPP crystal arthritis were highlighted by EULAR experts in 2 of 11 EULAR propositions[1]:

- EULAR proposition 2: "the rapid development of severe joint pain, swelling and tenderness that reaches its maximum within 6–24 h, especially with overlying erythema, is highly suggestive of acute crystal inflammation though not specific for acute CPP crystal arthritis."
- EULAR proposition 3: "presentation with features suggesting crystal inflammation involving the knee, wrist or shoulder of a patient over age 65 years is likely to be acute CPP crystal arthritis. The presence of radiographic CC and advanced age increases this likelihood, but definitive diagnosis needs to be crystal proven."

Thus, a rapid onset of acute synovitis with pain and marked soft tissue and joint swelling is highly characteristic of crystal inflammation without specificity for the type of crystal. Like microcrystal inflammation, CPP crystal attack is self-limited and lasts for 7 to 10 days. In a geriatric hospital series, acute CPP crystal arthritis resolved within 3 to 4 days.[1] Thus, a history of self-resolving flares is helpful for the diagnosis. However, because acute CPP crystal arthritis and infection may coexist, microbiological investigation should be performed even if CPP crystals are identified (EULAR proposition 10).[1] Laboratory tests show unspecific increase of C-reactive protein (CRP) and erythrocyte sedimentation rate (ESR). Acute CPP crystal inflammation, as observed in gout flares, can be favored by several stresses, including infection, surgery, cardiovascular events such as myocardial infarction or stroke, joint trauma, or surgery.[24] Joint lavage and meniscectomy are 2 classic factors inducing CPP crystal inflammation. The incidence of acute CPP crystal arthritis after arthroscopic lavage for knee OA with preexisting CC is estimated to be 26%.[55] A case-control study showed that patients with knee CC had 5 times more risk of acute CPP arthritis after meniscectomy than those without knee CC.[56] Other uncommon factors have been associated with acute CPP crystal arthritis: bisphosphonates, granulocyte colony-stimulating factor, and intra-articular injection of hyaluronan.[57,58]

Chronic CPP crystal arthritis

EULAR proposition 5 stipulated that "chronic CPP crystal inflammatory arthritis presents as chronic oligoarthritis or polyarthritis with inflammatory symptoms and signs and occasional systemic upset (with elevation of CRP and ESR); superimposed flares with characteristics of crystal inflammation support this diagnosis. It should be considered in the differential diagnosis of rheumatoid arthritis (RA) and other chronic inflammatory joint diseases in older adults. Radiographs may assist diagnosis, but the diagnosis should be 'crystal proven'."[1] However, physicians should pay attention to the addition of monoarthritis leading with time to bilateral asymmetrical polyarthritis involving both hands and wrists.

Chronic CPP crystal arthritis is not rare, occurring in 11% of CPP crystal inflammation.[51] It may be misdiagnosed as RA, or even as polymyalgia rheumatica when shoulders are affected. However, some clinicoradiologic features strongly suggest metabolic arthropathy and encourage searching for the GRAAL, which is the identification of CPP crystals; negativity of immunologic tests; involvement of the second and third MCP joints; presence of both spinal and peripheral articular symptoms; plain radiographs and US depicting characteristic abnormalities, including CC and the presence of hyperechoic deposits without posterior shadow within the cartilage (see diagnosis section).

OA with CPP and BCP crystals

The role of calcium-containing crystals in OA pathogenesis continues to be under debate.[59,60] Some investigators consider calcium crystals as bystanders of cartilage destruction, releasing bone mineral (eg, apatite crystals) into the joint cavity. However, recent clinical and research data[61] strongly suggest that calcium-containing crystals may induce a real crystal stress and contribute to cartilage destruction in OA. Crystal-associated OA is more severe and affects joints usually spared in primary OA. These features are highlighted by EULAR proposition 4: "OA with CPPD may associate with more inflammatory symptoms and signs, an atypical distribution (eg, radiocarpal or midcarpal, glenohumeral, hindfoot or midfoot involvement)...."[1]

BCP and CPP crystals are found frequently in OA femoral condyle, tibial, and femoral head cartilage, as well as OA knee joint fluid. Their presence is correlated with more severe radiographic scores.[18,20,23,62,63] Furthermore, BCP crystals appear with joint degeneration.[63] Calcium-containing crystal formation is a cell-driven process involving several factors, including aging, chondrocyte hypertrophy, apoptosis, and cartilage extracellular matrix alteration.[61] In vitro studies have shown that both BCP and CPP crystals induce inflammatory, catabolic, and apoptotic responses.[3] In vivo, intra-articular injection of CPP crystals worsens OA lesions induced by partial lateral meniscectomy and section of the fibular collateral and sesamoid ligaments in a rabbit model.[64] Similarly, intra-articular injection of BCP crystals into mouse knees induces synovial inflammation and cartilage degradation.[65]

The knee is a common target site for OA and the most common site for CPPD. BCP crystals are identified in 100% of femoral condyle and tibia plateau cartilages harvested at the time of joint replacement.[18,20] A strong association between OA and CPPD was noted in analysis conducted as part of the EULAR recommendations.[1] The pooled odds ratio (OR) is 2.66 (95% confidence interval [CI] 2.00–3.54) and is consistent between cross-sectional (2.52, 95% CI 1.86–3.44) and case-control (2.80, 95% CI 1.44–5.47) studies, suggesting that people with OA are more than twice as likely to have CPPD than not.[1] Compared with isolated OA, OA with CPPD may occur in less typical locations (eg, radiocarpal joints, elbows, shoulders, ankles) and have more patellofemoral and lateral tibiofemoral compartment involvement.[30,66–68] In hip OA, the presence of CPP crystals is associated with rapidly destructive OA.[24] A prospective observational study noted that the presence of CPP crystals in synovial fluids or CC is associated with radiographic progression, with an OR of 3.44 (95% CI 1.97–6.02).[69] However, in 2 longitudinal studies, the presence of knee CC at baseline was negatively associated with cartilage loss assessed by MRI.[70] These contradictory results keep the debate active. However, studies are heterogeneous, involving different joints and different populations. Calcium-containing crystals may have different properties according to the site where they deposit. In vitro, they induce different cellular responses according to cell type.[3]

Less common CPP crystal-related manifestations

Spine-related CPP crystals Although CPPD occurs preferentially in target areas such as second and third MCP joints, wrists (triangular ligament), knees (menisci) and symphysis pubis, these crystals have been identified in mostly all ligaments and musculoskeletal tissue. Resnick and Pineda[71] in a radiographic and pathologic analysis of more than 1000 cadaveric spinal specimens reported that CPPD occurs in practically all vertebral structures: intervertebral, apophyseal, and sacroiliac joints; median atlantoaxial articulations; intraspinal and extraspinal ligaments, including interspinous and supraspinous ligaments, ligamentun flavum, periodontoid ligaments, and posterior longitudinal ligament. These CPPDs can give rise to acute attacks and OA-like and destructive lesions. Massive CPPD may induce nervous compression with myelopathy, radicular pain, or cauda equine syndrome.[72–74]

Numerous vertebral abnormalities have been reported, including degenerative disk disease, vertebral destruction, scoliosis, spondylolisthesis, atlantoaxial subluxation, vertebral ankylosis, occipitoatlantoaxial joint collapse, and thickening of spinal ligaments.[71,72]

CDS The CDS is a clinical-radiologic entity, first described by Bouvet and colleagues,[75] characterized by acute neck pain caused by calcium deposition around the odontoid process. The calcium deposits are mostly CPP crystals, although BCP crystals have also been identified.[76–82] Clinical presentations may be asymptomatic or alarming, with acute febrile neck pain, cervical stiffness, and increased inflammatory markers. CDS, like acute tendinitis of the longus colli, can be misdiagnosed with meningitis, infectious spondylitis, temporal arteritis, polymyalgia rheumatica, metastatic bone disease, and spinal tumor.[77,83] Diagnosis is made by the identification of calcification deposition around the atlantoaxial joint by CT scan (**Fig. 4**). A characteristic pattern is the presence of calcification surrounding the top and sides of the odontoid process in a crownlike or horseshoelike deposition. Calcifications involve mainly the transverse ligament of the atlas, and 3 calcification patterns have been described: curvilinear, stippled, or mixed.[80] Calcifications can also occur in the other periodontoid structures, including synovial membrane, the articular capsule, alar ligaments, apical ligament, and longitudinal fiber of cruciate ligament. Recently, Kobayashi and colleagues[84] showed that acute neck pain in patients with transverse ligament calcification could be secondary to acute CPP arthritis of

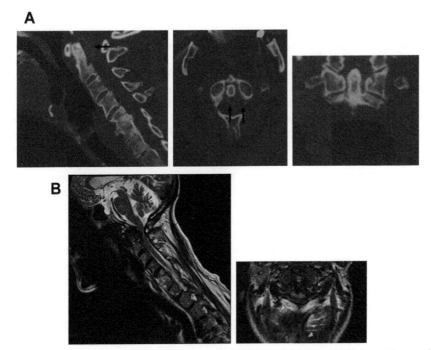

Fig. 4. Crowned dens syndrome. (*A*) CT scan with sagital, axial and coronal views. Linear calcifications are shown with *black arrows*. (*B*) MRI study with pseudo-tumor of the foramen magnum.

the lateral atlantoaxial joint. CT showed calcification of the transverse ligament in 22 of 27 (81.5%) patients and calcification of the longus colli muscle in 2 of 27 (7.5%) patients. Lateral atlantoaxial joint puncture allowed collecting synovial fluid in 16 patients (59.3%). CPP crystals were identified in 10 of 16 (62.5%) of the synovial fluid.[84] Thus, dramatic improvement was also observed after joint puncture in all patients. Pain decreased from 81.9 ± 16.3 mm before puncture to 35.6 ± 24.4 mm within 30 minutes of the procedure. Whether the improvement persisted was not mentioned.[84] Similarly, how atlantoaxial puncture improved pain secondary to longus colli tendinitis was not discussed. However, this study highlighted a possible association between CDS and acute CPP crystal arthritis of the atlantoaxial joint. Careful attention should be taken in MRI analysis to rule out this setting. Compared with CT, MRI is also more sensitive for soft tissue assessment and spinal cord compression (see Fig. 4B). Along with crystal deposition, CT can show subchondral cysts and erosion involving the odontoid process and atlantoaxoidal destructive arthropathy.[85] Prevalence of CDS varies from 6% in unselective patients undergoing CT to 71% in patients with articular CC.[80,85,86] A case-control study[87] found a prevalence of cervical calcifications in patients with proven articular CPP crystal disease in 24 of 35 patients (69%) compared with 4 of 35 (11%) in control patients. In a recent prospective study including 513 patients,[88] the overall prevalence of atlantoaxial CPPD shown by cervical spine CT was 12.5%. Prevalence increased with age, reaching 34% for patients aged 60 years and older and 49% for patients aged 80 years and older.[88]

Acute attacks of CPP crystals can occur in all spine structures, leading to numerous differential diagnoses, including infectious spondylitis and epidural abscess, leading to frequently reported misdiagnosis and inappropriate surgery.[89,90] Awareness of these conditions improves care.

Lumbar canal stenosis and compressive cervical myelopathy Lumbar canal stenosis and compressive cervical myelopathy are rare but well described and threatening complications of tumoral CPPD, leading to surgery decompression.[72,86,91–93] Cervical myelopathy compression can be anterior by periodontoid deposition of CPP crystals or posterior by ligamentum flavum deposition of CPP crystals or OA-like apophyseal lesions. Clinical symptoms include neck pain, neuralgia, numbness, and a varying degree of disabilities, such as lost of hand dexterity, weakness, gait impairment, and sphincter troubles. Fenoy and colleagues[92] reviewed in a retrospective study 21 patients with CPPD around the odontoid process. Mean age was 70.3 years and mean symptom duration 17.5 months. Patients had neck pain (85%), numbness, or paresthesias (61%). Calcification of the mass or transverse ligament was seen on CT in all patients. Overall, 19 of 21 patients underwent transoral-transpalatopharyngeal resection. Eighteen patients (86%) had improvement or resolution of symptoms after treatment. Mwaka and colleagues[93] retrospectively identified 26 of 465 patients (5.6%) who had been operated for cervical myelopathy compression caused by CPPD in ligamentun flavum. Ligamentum flavum calcification was observed mainly at C3-4 level (n = 13), C4-5 (n = 17), C5-6 (n = 12), and C6-7 (n = 5). Ten patients showed nodular calcification, whereas 16 showed a diffuse type of deposition.[93] CPP crystals analyzed by scanning electronic microscopy appeared as pinlike, rodlike, or rectangular crystals, and their characteristics were confirmed by x-ray diffraction. Histology and immunostaining analysis showed the presence of hypertrophic and apoptotic chondrocytes, suggesting a critical role of chondrocyte metaplasia in CPPD.[93] Spinal stenosis secondary to CPPD can occur at thoracic and lumbar levels. Markiewitz and colleagues[74] found that the incidence of CPPD in the ligamentum flavum was 24.5% in a retrospective study involving 102 patients undergoing lumbar spine decompression laminectomy.

Hemarthrosis related to CPP crystals Similar to BCP crystals, which can induce shoulder arthropathy with hemorrhagic effusion, spontaneous hemarthrosis may occur during the progression of articular CPPD. It affects mainly older women and involves also large joints, such as the knee and the shoulder joints. The disorder may recur in the same or in different joints. A study of 11 case histories suggests that bleeding occurs more readily in CC than in OA alone.[94] Cayla and colleagues[95] reported a series of 32 hemarthrosis (20 knees and 12 shoulders) associated with CPPD. Degenerative radiological changes with rupture of the rotator cuff are common. Three patients had joint destructions like neuropathic joint. Isotopic synoviorthesis seems effective in recurrent hemarthrosis. Mechanisms of hemarthrosis are unknown.

Destructive arthropathy with CPP crystals Joint destruction can mimic neuroarthropathy, with severe destruction leading frequently to complete lysis of the bone epiphysis. Knee, hip, shoulder, and wrist joints are the most affected sites.[96,97] Joint destruction has also been reported in the cervical spine, involving the atlantoaxial joint and intervertebral disks (**Fig. 5**). Destructive arthropathy secondary to CPP crystals occurs more frequently in patients with generalized OA.[96] Careful clinical examination rules out proprioceptive trouble and laboratory analysis rules out infection, syphilis, diabetes mellitus, and primary hyperparathyroidism. Analysis of synovial fluid can readily identify CPP crystals. Mostly, CPPD is widespread and plain radiographs of target areas show CC or radiographic features of CPPD disease.[97] The involvement of the femoropatellar joint shows characteristic signs in radiography: the patella wraps round the femoral condyle[97] and evolves to patella/femoral condyle indenting (see **Fig. 5**).

DIAGNOSIS

Diagnosis of BCP and CPP crystal–related diseases relies on clinical history, radiography, and synovial fluid analysis whenever possible. Although some radiographic and US characteristics (location of calcification, radiography patterns) may differentiate BCP crystal deposition from CPPD, only microscopic examination of synovial fluid permits correct identification of CPP crystals. Detection of BCP crystals by light microscopy is unusual, because these crystals are too small. Alizarin red staining of synovial fluid can identify the presence of calcium-containing crystals without distinguishing BCP from CPP crystals. To distinguish between the 2, spectrometry methods such as x-ray diffraction and infrared-transformed Fourier spectroscopy are necessary. Easier means of identifying BCP crystals are needed.

Radiographic and US Features Related to BCP Crystal Deposition

Radiographic features of BCP crystals show variable density and homogeneous calcium-containing deposits without trabeculation, which allow them to be differentiated from heterotopic ossifications or accessory ossicles. Calcification size varies between a few millimeters and centimeters. They are mostly ovoid but can also be linear and triangular. Their margins may be smooth and well defined or ill defined. Their density is variable. Calcifications can be classified according to the radiographic system described by Gärtner and Heyer (type I, dense with well-defined borders; type II, dense with indistinct borders or transparent with well-defined borders; type III, transparent with indistinct borders) or to the system described by the French Society of Arthroscopy (SFA) (type A, dense, well defined, and circumscribed; type B, dense, well defined, and segmented; type C, transparent and nonhomogeneous; and type

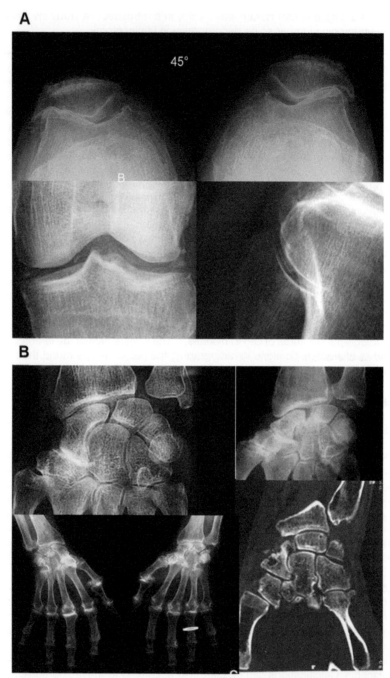

Fig. 5. Common and uncommon radiographic patterns of CPPD. (*A*) Knee joint with notched patella, common calcifications of the menisci and cartilages; calcification of the upper tibiofibular joint. (*B*) Calcifications of the triangular ligaments and intercarpal joints; scapholunar diastasis and ascension of the capitatum; CT scan showing calcifications and geodes.

D, dystrophic deposit at the origin of the tendon) (see **Fig. 2**).[98,99] However, the inter-observer and intraobserver agreements for both Gärtner and SFA classifications were poor, especially for differentiating type A and type B calcifications.[32] Type B is more frequent than type A and C, identified in 47%, 31%, and 22%, respectively.[32,100]

CT is superior to radiography for the detection of calcifications and bone lesions. It is helpful in acute flares involving the cervical spine (longus colli tendinitis, CDS, spondylitis) or bone with cortical bone erosion. CT permits identification of calcification and prevention of misdiagnosis.

US is an excellent tool to identify calcifications and to assess concurrently the status of the rotator cuff tendons, the subacromial-subdeltoid bursae, and presence of joint effusion. The calcifications appear as hyperechoic lesions within the tendon either as a single large focus or as multiple smaller foci. Calcifications show posterior acoustic shadowing, which varies in intensity depending on the size of the calcification, its location within the tendon, and its proximity to bone.[100] Performance of US is dependent on the experience of the practitioner.

CPPD Diagnosis

According to EULAR proposition 6: "Definitive diagnosis of CPPD is by identification of characteristic CPP crystals (parallelepipedic, predominantly intracellular crystals with absent or weak positive birefringence) in synovial fluid or occasionally biopsied tissue."[1] When synovial fluid analysis is not possible, characteristic CPP crystal signs observed by radiography of target areas and US can support the diagnosis.

Synovial fluid analysis

To increase sensitivity of microscopic synovial fluid examination, analysis should be performed on fresh synovial fluid after centrifugation to increase the concentration of crystals.[101] However, CPP crystals persist for up to 3 days if synovial fluid is stored at 4°C or even at stable room temperature (20°C).[102] CCP crystals are 1 to 20 μm long and appear as rhomboid, rectangular, acicular, and rod-shaped forms. CCP crystals are better identified under ordinary light microscopy. Under polarized microscopy, they may show positive birefringence with variable intensity, mostly weak or absent (**Fig. 6**). Because of this weak birefringence and their small size, CPP crystals may be missed if synovial fluid is examined only under polarized light microscopy. A study performed on 10 synovial fluids obtained from patients with acute knee arthritis with

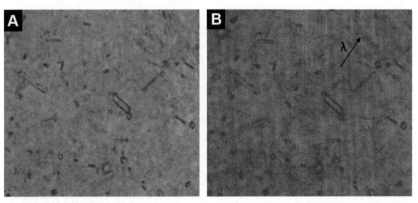

Fig. 6. CPP crystals observed under polarized microscopy. (*A*) Light microscopy, (*B*) Polarized microscopy.

CPP crystals showed that only about 20% of all CPP crystals identified were birefringent.[103] Numerous studies have shown a lack of consistency between different observers to identify CPP crystals. The sensitivity and specificity for CPP crystal detection vary between 12% and 83%, and 12% and 96%, respectively, according to laboratory expertise and CPP crystal concentration.[104–107] An observer's performance can be improved by training. After a 3-month course, 4 residents with no previous experience of synovial fluid analysis identified CPPD crystals with a sensitivity and specificity of 92.7% and 92.1%, respectively.[108] CPP crystals can be identified in uninflamed joints of patients with CPP crystal arthropathy. By analyzing 74 synovial fluid samples of patients with CPP crystal arthropathy, Martinez-Sanchis and Pascual[109] found that all samples contained CPP crystals. All samples contained CPP crystals inside the cells, and most of the intracellular crystals were inside mononuclear cells. The presence of intracellular crystals did not correlate with pain. Thus, synovial fluid analysis should be performed even in intercritical periods when CPP crystal disease is suspected.

When CPP crystals are not found by synovial fluid analysis, plain radiographs and US may help support the diagnosis, as proposed by EULAR recommendations 7 and 8.[1]

Radiographic features of CCPD
Radiographic CC is a useful imaging marker, often taken as a surrogate for CPP crystal disease. Detection of CC in proven cases of CPP crystal arthritis varies from 29% to 93%, depending on population and joint examined.[1,51,109] There are several possible reasons for discordance between CC and SF crystal positivity, including lack of specificity of CC for CPPD (BCP crystal deposits may also cause radiographic CC); low sensitivity of radiographs for detecting CC; and reduced ability to identify CC when there is significant cartilage loss.

CPPD in fibrocartilage can be visualized in target areas: menisci of the knee, triangular fibrocartilage of the wrist, labra of the acetabulum, symphysis pubis, and annulus fibrosus of the intervertebral disk. Less common sites are the sternoclavicular and acromioclavicular joints and glenoid labra,[110] or even the proximal tibiofibular joint. Hyaline cartilage calcification occurs commonly in the wrist, knee, elbow, and hip joints and is identified on radiographs as a thin dense line parallel to the subchondral bone. Synovial calcification is seen most often in the knee, MCP joints, and the radiocarpal and distal radioulnar joints of the wrist.

Besides calcification deposition, several characteristic radiographic features strongly suggest CPP crystal disease: subchondral sclerosis, scaphotrapezial arthropathy without trapezial-MCP OA, scapholunate collapse, ascension of the capitatum bone inducing scapholunate disjunction, inferior radioulnar arthropathy, and femoropatellar indentation (see **Fig. 5**).[67,97,111] Structural joint changes that are associated with CPPD are common and similar to those of OA, including joint space narrowing, subchondral sclerosis, and subchondral cyst formation. They are not always accompanied by calcifications discernible by radiographs and, in this case, it may be difficult to differentiate regular OA from OA associated with CPPD arthropathy.[112]

US features of CPPD
In the last decade, US has become an excellent technique for detecting CPPDs in joints and periarticular tissues. EULAR recommendations state, "ultrasonography can demonstrate CPPD in peripheral joints, appearing typically as thin hyperechoic bands within hyaline cartilage and hyperechoic sparkling spots in fibrocartilage.

Sensitivity and specificity appear excellent and possibly better than those of conventional x-rays."

Based on their experience, Frediani and colleagues proposed in 2005 US features for CPPD and considered as CPP calcifications all hyperechoic deposits that presented one of the following patterns:

i. Thin hyperechoic bands, parallel to the surface of the hyaline cartilage (frequently observed in the knee)
ii. A punctate pattern, composed of several thin hyperechoic spots, more common in fibrous cartilage and in tendons
iii. Homogeneous hyperechoic nodular or oval deposits localized in bursae and articular recesses (frequently mobile)[113]

With these patterns, US of the knee appears sensitive (0.87, 95% CI 0.69–1.04) and specific (0.96, 95% CI 0.90–1.03) for detection of synovial fluid CPP crystals.[114] Positive US findings may strongly suggest the diagnosis of CPPD (likelihood ratio = 24.2, 95% CI 3.51–168.01).[1] One direct comparison showed US to be more sensitive (100%) than radiographs (82%) in identifying CPPD.[113] This result is further confirmed by a recent study in which Barskova and colleagues[115] compared 3 imaging methods in 25 patients with crystal-proven CPPD disease. These investigators reported that US imaging detected CPP crystals in 100% of patients, CT in 15 of 18 (72%), and radiographs in only 11 of 25 (52%) patients. However, US remained insensitive for deep structures (eg, spine).

CT (and MRI) in BCP and CPP Crystal Diseases

CT can accurately show small intra-articular and periarticular calcifications because of its high spatial resolution. It is the gold standard imaging technique for detection of spinal calcification, as shown in CDS and acute tendinitis of the longus colli muscle. Its role in the assessment of peripheral joint involvement in crystal-induced arthropathies has been little explored. CT plays an important role in acute bone erosion induced by BCP crystal resorption as well. It permits accurate diagnosis and prevents inappropriate therapies. Clinical signs may be alarming, and differential diagnosis such as muscle sarcoma may even be considered. Showing calcification localized next to tendon insertion by CT is then helpful. CT imaging is highly accurate in predicting the consistency of BCP crystal deposits in relation to their mean attenuation value. The mean density for homogeneous and well-defined calcifications has a mean attenuation value of 476 HU (range 333–945 HU).[110] In addition, CT can depict cortical pseudocysts and irregularities in calcific tendinitis.[26]

The place of MRI in BCP and CPP crystal disease is limited. Its interest resides only in spinal involvement permitting assessment of neurologic complications and soft tissue edema. Calcific deposits are most typically associated with loss of signal intensity on MRI.

SUMMARY

BCP and CPPD are 2 common multifaceted diseases that can mimic alarming clinical manifestations. Awareness of less common presentations is helpful and prevents misdiagnosis. Diagnosis is based on direct and indirect identification of calcium-containing crystals and deposits. US seems to be an excellent imaging technique for CPP crystal detection but lacks efficacy for deep locations. CT remains the gold standard imaging modality for detection of calcification in the axial skeleton, especially at the cervical level.

REFERENCES

1. Zhang W, Doherty M, Bardin T, et al. European League Against Rheumatism recommendations for calcium pyrophosphate deposition. Part I: terminology and diagnosis. Ann Rheum Dis 2011;70(4):563–70.
2. Zhang W, Doherty M, Pascual E, et al. EULAR recommendations for calcium pyrophosphate deposition. Part II: management. Ann Rheum Dis 2011;70(4): 571–5.
3. Ea HK, Lioté F. Advances in understanding calcium-containing crystal disease. Curr Opin Rheumatol 2009;21(2):150–7.
4. Kirsch T. Biomineralization–an active or passive process? Connect Tissue Res 2012;53(6):438–45.
5. Nitschke Y, Rutsch F. Genetics in arterial calcification: lessons learned from rare diseases. Trends Cardiovasc Med 2012;22(6):145–9.
6. Sallam T, Cheng H, Demer LL, et al. Regulatory circuits controlling vascular cell calcification. Cell Mol Life Sci 2013;70(17):3187–97.
7. Schurgers LJ, Uitto J, Reutelingsperger CP. Vitamin K-dependent carboxylation of matrix Gla-protein: a crucial switch to control ectopic mineralization. Trends Mol Med 2013;19(4):217–26.
8. Taylor AM. Metabolic and endocrine diseases, cartilage calcification and arthritis. Curr Opin Rheumatol 2013;25(2):198–203.
9. Liu YZ, Jackson AP, Cosgrove SD. Contribution of calcium-containing crystals to cartilage degradation and synovial inflammation in osteoarthritis. Osteoarthritis Cartilage 2009;17(10):1333–40.
10. Abhishek A, Doherty M. Pathophysiology of articular chondrocalcinosis–role of ANKH. Nat Rev Rheumatol 2011;7(2):96–104.
11. St Hilaire C, Ziegler SG, Markello TC, et al. NT5E mutations and arterial calcifications. N Engl J Med 2011;364(5):432–42.
12. Markello TC, Pak LK, St Hilaire C, et al. Vascular pathology of medial arterial calcifications in NT5E deficiency: implications for the role of adenosine in pseudoxanthoma elasticum. Mol Genet Metab 2011;103(1):44–50.
13. Ho AM, Johnson MD, Kingsley DM. Role of the mouse ank gene in control of tissue calcification and arthritis. Science 2000;289(5477):265–70.
14. Rutsch F, Ruf N, Vaingankar S, et al. Mutations in ENPP1 are associated with 'idiopathic' infantile arterial calcification. Nat Genet 2003;34(4):379–81.
15. Rutsch F, Vaingankar S, Johnson K, et al. PC-1 nucleoside triphosphate pyrophosphohydrolase deficiency in idiopathic infantile arterial calcification. Am J Pathol 2001;158(2):543–54.
16. Sage AP, Tintut Y, Demer LL. Regulatory mechanisms in vascular calcification. Nat Rev Cardiol 2010;7(9):528–36.
17. Netter P, Bardin T, Bianchi A, et al. The ANKH gene and familial calcium pyrophosphate dihydrate deposition disease. Joint Bone Spine 2004;71(5): 365–8.
18. Fuerst M, Bertrand J, Lammers L, et al. Calcification of articular cartilage in human osteoarthritis. Arthritis Rheum 2009;60(9):2694–703.
19. Mitsuyama H, Healey RM, Terkeltaub RA, et al. Calcification of human articular knee cartilage is primarily an effect of aging rather than osteoarthritis. Osteoarthritis Cartilage 2007;15(5):559–65.
20. Nguyen C, Bazin D, Daudon M, et al. Revisiting spatial distribution and biochemical composition of calcium-containing crystals in human osteoarthritic articular cartilage. Arthritis Res Ther 2013;15(5):R103.

21. Sun Y, Mauerhan DR, Honeycutt PR, et al. Calcium deposition in osteoarthritic meniscus and meniscal cell culture. Arthritis Res Ther 2010;12(2):R56.
22. Fuerst M, Niggemeyer O, Lammers L, et al. Articular cartilage mineralization in osteoarthritis of the hip. BMC Musculoskelet Disord 2009;10:166.
23. Gordon GV, Villanueva T, Schumacher HR, et al. Autopsy study correlating degree of osteoarthritis, synovitis and evidence of articular calcification. J Rheumatol 1984;11(5):681–6.
24. Richette P, Bardin T, Doherty M. An update on the epidemiology of calcium pyrophosphate dihydrate crystal deposition disease. Rheumatology (Oxford) 2009; 48(7):711–5.
25. Molloy ES, McCarthy GM. Calcium crystal deposition diseases: update on pathogenesis and manifestations. Rheum Dis Clin North Am 2006;32(2):383–400, vii.
26. Flemming DJ, Murphey MD, Shekitka KM, et al. Osseous involvement in calcific tendinitis: a retrospective review of 50 cases. AJR Am J Roentgenol 2003; 181(4):965–72.
27. Fritz P, Bardin T, Laredo JD, et al. Paradiaphyseal calcific tendinitis with cortical bone erosion. Arthritis Rheum 1994;37(5):718–23.
28. Halverson PB, Cheung HS, McCarty DJ, et al. "Milwaukee shoulder"–association of microspheroids containing hydroxyapatite crystals, active collagenase, and neutral protease with rotator cuff defects. II. Synovial fluid studies. Arthritis Rheum 1981;24(3):474–83.
29. Halverson PB, Garancis JC, McCarty DJ. Histopathological and ultrastructural studies of synovium in Milwaukee shoulder syndrome–a basic calcium phosphate crystal arthropathy. Ann Rheum Dis 1984;43(5):734–41.
30. McCarty DJ, Halverson PB, Carrera GF, et al. "Milwaukee shoulder"–association of microspheroids containing hydroxyapatite crystals, active collagenase, and neutral protease with rotator cuff defects. I. Clinical aspects. Arthritis Rheum 1981;24(3):464–73.
31. Carcia CR, Scibek JS. Causation and management of calcific tendonitis and periarthritis. Curr Opin Rheumatol 2013;25(2):204–9.
32. Clavert P, Sirveaux F. Shoulder calcifying tendinitis. Rev Chir Orthop Réparatrice Appar Mot 2008;94(Suppl 8):336–55 [in French].
33. Chiou HJ, Hung SC, Lin SY, et al. Correlations among mineral components, progressive calcification process and clinical symptoms of calcific tendonitis. Rheumatology (Oxford) 2010;49(3):548–55.
34. Faure G, Daculsi G. Calcified tendinitis: a review. Ann Rheum Dis 1983; 42(Suppl 1):49–53.
35. Hamada J, Ono W, Tamai K, et al. Analysis of calcium deposits in calcific periarthritis. J Rheumatol 2001;28(4):809–13.
36. Bosworth BM. Calcium deposits in the shoulder and subacromial bursitis: a survey of 12,122 shoulders. JAMA 1941;116:2477–82.
37. Harmon PH. Methods and results in the treatment of 2,580 painful shoulders, with special reference to calcific tendinitis and the frozen shoulder. Am J Surg 1958;95(4):527–44.
38. Kachewar SG, Kulkarni DS. Calcific tendinitis of the rotator cuff: a review. J Clin Diagn Res 2013;7(7):1482–5.
39. Porcellini G, Paladini P, Campi F, et al. Osteolytic lesion of greater tuberosity in calcific tendinitis of the shoulder. J Shoulder Elbow Surg 2009;18(2):210–5.
40. Wolk T, Wittenberg RH. Calcifying subacromial syndrome–clinical and ultrasound outcome of non-surgical therapy. Z Orthop Ihre Grenzgeb 1997;135(5): 451–7 [in German].

41. Doumas C, Vazirani RM, Clifford PD, et al. Acute calcific periarthritis of the hand and wrist: a series and review of the literature. Emerg Radiol 2007;14(4):199–203.
42. Ellika SK, Payne SC, Patel SC, et al. Acute calcific tendinitis of the longus colli: an imaging diagnosis. Dentomaxillofac Radiol 2008;37(2):121–4.
43. Bonavita JA, Dalinka MK, Schumacher HR Jr. Hydroxyapatite deposition disease. Radiology 1980;134(3):621–5.
44. Gabra N, Belair M, Ayad T. Retropharyngeal calcific tendinitis mimicking a retropharyngeal phlegmon. Case Rep Otolaryngol 2013;2013:912628.
45. Ring D, Vaccaro AR, Scuderi G, et al. Acute calcific retropharyngeal tendinitis. Clinical presentation and pathological characterization. J Bone Joint Surg Am 1994;76(11):1636–42.
46. Offiah CE, Hall E. Acute calcific tendinitis of the longus colli muscle: spectrum of CT appearances and anatomical correlation. Br J Radiol 2009;82(978):e117–21.
47. Halverson PB, Carrera GF, McCarty DJ. Milwaukee shoulder syndrome. Fifteen additional cases and a description of contributing factors. Arch Intern Med 1990;150(3):677–82.
48. Ornetti P, Vernier N, Fortunet C. Milwaukee shoulder syndrome affecting the elbow. Arthritis Rheum 2013;65(2):538.
49. Pons-Estel BA, Gimenez C, Sacnun M, et al. Familial osteoarthritis and Milwaukee shoulder associated with calcium pyrophosphate and apatite crystal deposition. J Rheumatol 2000;27(2):471–80.
50. Neame RL, Carr AJ, Muir K, et al. UK community prevalence of knee chondrocalcinosis: evidence that correlation with osteoarthritis is through a shared association with osteophyte. Ann Rheum Dis 2003;62(6):513–8.
51. Louthrenoo W, Sukitawut W. Calcium pyrophosphate dihydrate crystal deposition: a clinical and laboratory analysis of 91 Thai patients. J Med Assoc Thai 1999;82(6):569–76.
52. el Maghraoui A, Lecoules S, Lechevalier D, et al. Acute sacroiliitis as a manifestation of calcium pyrophosphate dihydrate crystal deposition disease. Clin Exp Rheumatol 1999;17(4):477–8.
53. Hakozaki M, Kikuchi S, Otani K, et al. Pseudogout of the acromioclavicular joint: report of two cases and review of the literature. Mod Rheumatol 2011;21(4):440–3.
54. Yamakawa K, Iwasaki H, Ohjimi Y, et al. Tumoral calcium pyrophosphate dihydrate crystal deposition disease. A clinicopathologic analysis of five cases. Pathol Res Pract 2001;197(7):499–506.
55. Pasquetti P, Selvi E, Righeschi K, et al. Joint lavage and pseudogout. Ann Rheum Dis 2004;63(11):1529–30.
56. Doherty M, Watt I, Dieppe PA. Localised chondrocalcinosis in postmeniscectomy knees. Lancet 1982;1(8283):1207–10.
57. Ames PR, Rainey MG. Consecutive pseudogout attacks after repetitive granulocyte colony-stimulating factor administration for neutropenia. Mod Rheumatol 2007;17(5):445–6.
58. Wendling D, Tisserand G, Griffond V, et al. Acute pseudogout after pamidronate infusion. Clin Rheumatol 2008;27(9):1205–6.
59. McCarthy GM, Cheung HS. Point: hydroxyapatite crystal deposition is intimately involved in the pathogenesis and progression of human osteoarthritis. Curr Rheumatol Rep 2009;11(2):141–7.
60. Pritzker KP. Counterpoint: hydroxyapatite crystal deposition is not intimately involved in the pathogenesis and progression of human osteoarthritis. Curr Rheumatol Rep 2009;11(2):148–53.

61. Ea HK, Nguyen C, Bazin D, et al. Articular cartilage calcification in osteoarthritis: insights into crystal-induced stress. Arthritis Rheum 2011;63(1):10–8.
62. Derfus BA, Kurian JB, Butler JJ, et al. The high prevalence of pathologic calcium crystals in pre-operative knees. J Rheumatol 2002;29(3):570–4.
63. Nalbant S, Martinez JA, Kitumnuaypong T, et al. Synovial fluid features and their relations to osteoarthritis severity: new findings from sequential studies. Osteoarthritis Cartilage 2003;11(1):50–4.
64. Fam AG, Morava-Protzner I, Purcell C, et al. Acceleration of experimental lapine osteoarthritis by calcium pyrophosphate microcrystalline synovitis. Arthritis Rheum 1995;38(2):201–10.
65. Ea HK, Chobaz V, Nguyen C, et al. Pathogenic role of basic calcium phosphate crystals in destructive arthropathies. PLoS One 2013;8(2):e57352.
66. Muehleman C, Li J, Aigner T, et al. Association between crystals and cartilage degeneration in the ankle. J Rheumatol 2008;35(6):1108–17.
67. Resnick D, Niwayama G, Goergen TG, et al. Clinical, radiographic and pathologic abnormalities in calcium pyrophosphate dihydrate deposition disease (CPPD): pseudogout. Radiology 1977;122(1):1–15.
68. Yang BY, Sartoris DJ, Djukic S, et al. Distribution of calcification in the triangular fibrocartilage region in 181 patients with calcium pyrophosphate dihydrate crystal deposition disease. Radiology 1995;196(2):547–50.
69. Ledingham J, Regan M, Jones A, et al. Factors affecting radiographic progression of knee osteoarthritis. Ann Rheum Dis 1995;54(1):53–8.
70. Neogi T, Nevitt M, Niu J, et al. Lack of association between chondrocalcinosis and increased risk of cartilage loss in knees with osteoarthritis: results of two prospective longitudinal magnetic resonance imaging studies. Arthritis Rheum 2006;54(6):1822–8.
71. Resnick D, Pineda C. Vertebral involvement in calcium pyrophosphate dihydrate crystal deposition disease. Radiographic-pathological correlation. Radiology 1984;153(1):55–60.
72. Baba H, Maezawa Y, Kawahara N, et al. Calcium crystal deposition in the ligamentum flavum of the cervical spine. Spine (Phila Pa 1976) 1993;18(15):2174–81.
73. Doita M, Shimomura T, Maeno K, et al. Calcium pyrophosphate dihydrate deposition in the transverse ligament of the atlas: an unusual cause of cervical myelopathy. Skeletal Radiol 2007;36(7):699–702.
74. Markiewitz AD, Boumphrey FR, Bauer TW, et al. Calcium pyrophosphate dihydrate crystal deposition disease as a cause of lumbar canal stenosis. Spine (Phila Pa 1976) 1996;21(4):506–11.
75. Bouvet JP, Le Parc JM, Michalski B, et al. Acute neck pain due to calcifications surrounding the odontoid process: the crowned dens syndrome. Arthritis Rheum 1985;28(12):1417–20.
76. Ali S, Hoch M, Dadhania V, et al. CPPD crowned dens syndrome with clivus destruction: a case report. J Radiol Case Rep 2011;5(8):30–7.
77. Aouba A, Vuillemin-Bodaghi V, Mutschler C, et al. Crowned dens syndrome misdiagnosed as polymyalgia rheumatica, giant cell arteritis, meningitis or spondylitis: an analysis of eight cases. Rheumatology (Oxford) 2004;43(12):1508–12.
78. Godfrin-Valnet M, Godfrin G, Godard J, et al. Eighteen cases of crowned dens syndrome: presentation and diagnosis. Neurochirurgie 2013;59(3):115–20.
79. Malca SA, Roche PH, Pellet W, et al. Crowned dens syndrome: a manifestation of hydroxy-apatite rheumatism. Acta Neurochir (Wien) 1995;135(3–4):126–30.

80. Roverano S, Ortiz AC, Ceccato F, et al. Calcification of the transverse ligament of the atlas in chondrocalcinosis. J Clin Rheumatol 2010;16(1):7–9.
81. Scutellari PN, Galeotti R, Leprotti S, et al. The crowned dens syndrome. Evaluation with CT imaging. Radiol Med 2007;112(2):195–207.
82. Sekijima Y, Yoshida T, Ikeda S. CPPD crystal deposition disease of the cervical spine: a common cause of acute neck pain encountered in the neurology department. J Neurol Sci 2010;296(1–2):79–82.
83. Wu DW, Reginato AJ, Torriani M, et al. The crowned dens syndrome as a cause of neck pain: report of two new cases and review of the literature. Arthritis Rheum 2005;53(1):133–7.
84. Kobayashi T, Miyakoshi N, Konno N, et al. Acute neck pain caused by arthritis of the lateral atlanto-axial joint. Spine J 2013. http://dx.doi.org/10.1016/j.spinee.2013.10.054.
85. Kakitsubata Y, Boutin RD, Theodorou DJ, et al. Calcium pyrophosphate dihydrate crystal deposition in and around the atlantoaxial joint: association with type 2 odontoid fractures in nine patients. Radiology 2000;216(1):213–9.
86. Constantin A, Marin F, Bon E, et al. Calcification of the transverse ligament of the atlas in chondrocalcinosis: computed tomography study. Ann Rheum Dis 1996; 55(2):137–9.
87. Finckh A, Van Linthoudt D, Duvoisin B, et al. The cervical spine in calcium pyrophosphate dihydrate deposition disease. A prevalent case-control study. J Rheumatol 2004;31(3):545–9.
88. Chang EY, Lim WY, Wolfson T, et al. Frequency of atlantoaxial calcium pyrophosphate dihydrate deposition at CT. Radiology 2013;269(2):519–24.
89. Bartlett CS 3rd, Casden AM, Abdelwahab IF. Calcium pyrophosphate deposition disease mimicking infection in the lumbar spine. Orthopedics 1999;22(1): 79–81.
90. Mikhael MM, Chioffe MA, Shapiro GS. Calcium pyrophosphate dihydrate crystal deposition disease (pseudogout) of lumbar spine mimicking osteomyelitis-discitis with epidural phlegmon. Am J Orthop (Belle Mead NJ) 2013;42(8): E64–7.
91. Assaker R, Louis E, Boutry N, et al. Foramen magnum syndrome secondary to calcium pyrophosphate crystal deposition in the transverse ligament of the atlas. Spine (Phila Pa 1976) 2001;26(12):1396–400.
92. Fenoy AJ, Menezes AH, Donovan KA, et al. Calcium pyrophosphate dihydrate crystal deposition in the craniovertebral junction. J Neurosurg Spine 2008; 8(1):22–9.
93. Mwaka ES, Yayama T, Uchida K, et al. Calcium pyrophosphate dehydrate crystal deposition in the ligamentum flavum of the cervical spine: histopathological and immunohistochemical findings. Clin Exp Rheumatol 2009;27(3):430–8.
94. Phelip X, Verdier JM, Gras JP, et al. The hemarthroses of articular chondrocalcinosis. Rev Rhum Mal Osteoartic 1976;43(4):259–66 [in French].
95. Cayla J, Huchet B, Rondier J, et al. Hemarthrosis of articular chondrocalcinosis. A propos of 28 cases. Importance of treatment by isotopic synoviorthesis. Rev Rhum Mal Osteoartic 1982;49(4):281–5 [in French].
96. Gerster JC, Vischer TL, Fallet GH. Destructive arthropathy in generalized osteoarthritis with articular chondrocalcinosis. J Rheumatol 1975;2(3):265–9.
97. Richards AJ, Hamilton EB. Destructive arthropathy in chondrocalcinosis articularis. Ann Rheum Dis 1974;33(3):196–203.
98. Gartner J, Simons B. Analysis of calcific deposits in calcifying tendinitis. Clin Orthop Relat Res 1990;(254):111–20.

99. Mole D, Kempf JF, Gleyze P, et al. Results of endoscopic treatment of non-broken tendinopathies of the rotator cuff. 2. Calcifications of the rotator cuff. Rev Chir Orthop Réparatrice Appar Mot 1993;79(7):532–41 [in French].
100. Saboeiro GR. Sonography in the treatment of calcific tendinitis of the rotator cuff. J Ultrasound Med 2012;31(10):1513–8.
101. Robier C, Quehenberger F, Neubauer M, et al. The cytospin technique improves the detection of calcium pyrophosphate crystals in synovial fluid samples with a low leukocyte count. Rheumatol Int 2013. [Epub ahead of print].
102. Tausche AK, Gehrisch S, Panzner I, et al. A 3-day delay in synovial fluid crystal identification did not hinder the reliable detection of monosodium urate and calcium pyrophosphate crystals. J Clin Rheumatol 2013;19(5):241–5.
103. Ivorra J, Rosas J, Pascual E. Most calcium pyrophosphate crystals appear as non-birefringent. Ann Rheum Dis 1999;58(9):582–4.
104. Hasselbacher P. Variation in synovial fluid analysis by hospital laboratories. Arthritis Rheum 1987;30(6):637–42.
105. Schumacher HR, Sieck M, Clayburne G. Development and evaluation of a method for preservation of synovial fluid wet preparations for quality control testing of crystal identification. J Rheumatol 1990;17(10):1369–74.
106. Swan A, Amer H, Dieppe P. The value of synovial fluid assays in the diagnosis of joint disease: a literature survey. Ann Rheum Dis 2002;61(6):493–8.
107. von Essen R, Holtta AM, Pikkarainen R. Quality control of synovial fluid crystal identification. Ann Rheum Dis 1998;57(2):107–9.
108. Lumbreras B, Pascual E, Frasquet J, et al. Analysis for crystals in synovial fluid: training of the analysts results in high consistency. Ann Rheum Dis 2005;64(4):612–5.
109. Martinez Sanchis A, Pascual E. Intracellular and extracellular CPPD crystals are a regular feature in synovial fluid from uninflamed joints of patients with CPPD related arthropathy. Ann Rheum Dis 2005;64(12):1769–72.
110. Paparo F, Fabbro E, Ferrero G, et al. Imaging studies of crystalline arthritides. Reumatismo 2011;63(4):263–75.
111. Doherty W, Lovallo JL. Scapholunate advanced collapse pattern of arthritis in calcium pyrophosphate deposition disease of the wrist. J Hand Surg Am 1993;18(6):1095–8.
112. Steinbach LS. Calcium pyrophosphate dihydrate and calcium hydroxyapatite crystal deposition diseases: imaging perspectives. Radiol Clin North Am 2004;42(1):185–205, vii.
113. Frediani B, Filippou G, Falsetti P, et al. Diagnosis of calcium pyrophosphate dihydrate crystal deposition disease: ultrasonographic criteria proposed. Ann Rheum Dis 2005;64(4):638–40.
114. Filippou G, Frediani B, Gallo A, et al. A "new" technique for the diagnosis of chondrocalcinosis of the knee: sensitivity and specificity of high-frequency ultra-sonography. Ann Rheum Dis 2007;66(8):1126–8.
115. Barskova VG, Kudaeva FM, Bozhieva LA, et al. Comparison of three imaging techniques in diagnosis of chondrocalcinosis of the knees in calcium pyrophosphate deposition disease. Rheumatology (Oxford) 2013;52(6):1090–4.

Imaging in the Crystal Arthropathies

Fiona M. McQueen, MBChB, MD, FRACP[a,b,]*,
Anthony Doyle, MBChB, FRANZCR, ABR[c,d],
Nicola Dalbeth, MBChB, MD, FRACP[b,e]

KEYWORDS

- Imaging • Gout • Crystal arthropathies • Magnetic resonance imaging
- Ultrasonography • Computed tomography

KEY POINTS

- Advanced imaging in gout using computed tomography (CT) scanning, dual-energy CT (DECT), and magnetic resonance imaging (MRI) has revealed the close association between erosions and tophi suggesting a mechanistic link.
- The ultrasound double-contour sign in gout is likely to represent monosodium urate crystals deposited over hyaline cartilage, and often appears adjacent to tophi.
- Some imaging techniques, especially ultrasonography, CT, and DECT, may be useful to reveal tophus resolution during trials of urate-lowering therapy in gout.
- Plain radiography remains the imaging investigation of choice for the diagnosis of calcium pyrophosphate dihydrate (CPPD) arthropathy, as it reveals the typical pattern and distribution of crystal deposits.
- CT is important in the investigation of neck pain, as it can reveal CPPD deposition adjacent to C1/C2 that leads to the crowned dens syndrome, or retropharyngeal tendinitis, resulting from deposition of calcium hydroxyapatite crystals within fibers of the longus colli muscle.

The authors confirm that they have not received any financial support or benefits from commercial sources for the work reported in this article. The authors have no financial interests that would create a conflict of interest with regard to this work.
[a] Department of Molecular Medicine and Pathology, University of Auckland, 85 Park Road, Grafton, Auckland 1023, New Zealand; [b] Auckland District Health Board, Department of Rheumatology, Greenlane Clinical Centre, 214 Green Lane West, Auckland 1051, New Zealand; [c] Department of Anatomy and Radiology, University of Auckland, 85 Park Road, Grafton, Auckland 1023, New Zealand; [d] Auckland District Health Board, Department of Radiology, Auckland City Hospital, 2 Park Road, Grafton, Auckland 1023, New Zealand; [e] Bone & Joint Research Group, Department of Medicine, University of Auckland, 85 Park Road, Grafton, Auckland 1023, New Zealand
* Corresponding author. Department of Molecular Medicine and Pathology, Faculty of Medical and Health Sciences, University of Auckland, 85 Park Road, Grafton, Auckland, New Zealand.
E-mail address: f.mcqueen@auckland.ac.nz

INTRODUCTION

Over the last decade there have been important advances in imaging of the crystal arthropathies. Although plain radiography remains the cornerstone modality in this setting and is most familiar to rheumatologists and radiologists, it is now possible with advanced techniques to visualize not only joint damage but also soft-tissue inflammation, including synovitis and tenosynovitis, crystal deposition, and cartilage change. Three-dimensional (3D) multislice imaging via computed tomography (CT), dual-energy computed tomography (DECT), and magnetic resonance imaging (MRI) provide an opportunity to identify abnormalities in complex regions such as the midfoot, a common site of gouty involvement,[1] and the upper cervical spine, where calcium pyrophosphate dihydrate (CPPD) and hydroxyapatite (HA) arthropathies may contribute to significant pathologic features.[2] Ultrasonography (US) is also contributing to the understanding of these conditions, in particular by revealing crystal deposition within cartilage with variable patterns that have diagnostic implications.[3] The opportunity provided by CT and DECT scanning to visualize tophi in extraordinary detail has helped to elucidate the pathologic links between deposition of monosodium urate (MSU) crystals and the development of bone erosion in gout.[4] Advanced imaging is also increasingly being used in the setting of clinical trials, as digitized formats allow comparison of data, such as tophus volume, over time. In the clinical arena diagnostic applications are expanding, especially regarding gout, whereby imaging now sometimes offers the opportunity to identify MSU crystals without invasive joint aspiration. This article reviews the use of imaging techniques in the crystal arthropathies, with an emphasis on recent advances in this field and evolving clinical applications.

GOUT
Radiography

Most often the radiographic appearance of acute gout, especially at the time of the first attack, is nonspecific. Plain radiographs (XRs) are frequently normal apart from soft-tissue swelling in the affected region, and typical gouty erosions can take up to 10 years to develop as timed from the first attack.[5,6] However, plain radiography is part of the workup of acute gout not only to look for erosions but also to help exclude other differential diagnoses and investigate for possible complicating factors such as septic arthritis or osteomyelitis (typically associated with the rapid development of erosion and bone lysis on both sides of the joint). In addition, an XR will give some information about other forms of arthropathy such as osteoarthritis, which frequently coexists with gout.[7]

The typical radiographic appearance of chronic gout is of an asymmetric erosive arthropathy, most prominent at the feet (especially involving the first metatarsophalangeal [MTP] joint), but potentially affecting any joint in the peripheral skeleton including the hands, as shown in **Fig. 1**. Axial involvement may also occur but is rare.[8] Tophi appear as soft-tissue opacities, which often (but not invariably) overlie erosions. Erosions have a characteristic well-corticated appearance, often with overhanging margins, and they may be sited away from the margins of the joint (extramarginal) or within the joint, and/or sometimes be fully enclosed within periarticular bone without a breach of the cortex (intraosseous). In contrast to the XR appearances of rheumatoid arthritis (RA), there is typically no periarticular osteopenia in gout and, indeed, adjacent bone tends to be sclerotic. The bone beneath the joint margin may appear cystic or be subject to subchondral collapse. Hence the 2006 European League Against Rheumatism (EULAR) task force included the finding of "asymmetric joint swelling" and "subcortical cysts without erosion" in their list of 10 key diagnostic features of gout,[9] consistent

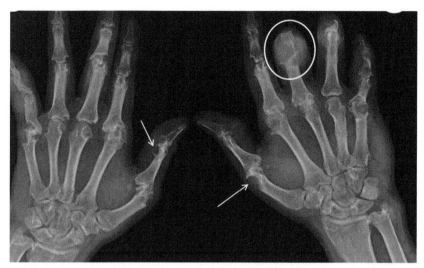

Fig. 1. Advanced tophaceous gout in a 44-year-old man of Samoan ethnicity. Multiple well-corticated erosions are seen, many with typical overhanging margins (*arrows*). At some sites of extensive tophus deposition there has been complete bone lysis (*circle*). Bone density is well preserved.

with the 1977 American Rheumatism Association preliminary gout classification criteria.[10] However, the EULAR guidelines development group acknowledged that plain radiography usually plays only a minor role in diagnosis, especially when gout is early or acute, when XRs are frequently normal. Rettenbacher and colleagues[11] formally examined the sensitivity and specificity of plain radiography for a gout diagnosis, in comparison with a clinical gold standard, and found a sensitivity of 31% and specificity of 93%. An XR scoring system for evaluating damage in gouty arthropathy has been developed,[12] based on a modified Sharp/van der Heijde scoring method[13] with inclusion of the distal interphalangeal joints. This aspect is of particular importance now that potent disease-modifying urate-lowering therapies (ULTs) have become available that may actually modify structural damage. A recent pilot study revealed that use of pegloticase over a 12-month period in patients with erosive tophaceous gout could actually lead to a reduction in erosion scores, with regression of soft-tissue masses and increased sclerosis at the time of the follow-up plain radiographic assessment.[14]

In addition to bone erosion in gout, there has been recent interest in new bone formation (NBF). A study of paired XRs and CT scans found that NBF in gout can appear in the form of bone sclerosis, osteophytes, bony spurs and, rarely, periosteal deposition and ankylosis.[15] NBF was more likely to occur when erosions were present, and there was also a strong association with tophi, as determined from CT scans. Results suggested a link between tophus, bone erosion, and NBF during joint remodeling in gout; interestingly, a somewhat similar association has been observed in some patients with the mutilans form of psoriatic arthritis.[16]

Advanced Imaging in Gout

CT scanning

Multislice helical CT scanning is useful for imaging bone and tophi in gout, as the very thin slices (0.5 mm) and potential for 3D reconstruction allow excellent resolution to be achieved. **Fig. 2** shows a CT 3D reconstruction of the wrist in a patient with long-standing tophaceous gout, revealing multiple tophi (typically with a density of density

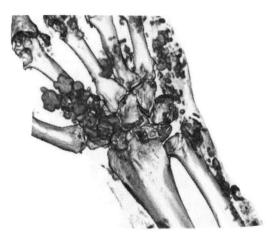

Fig. 2. Computed tomography (CT) scan of the right wrist taken from the patient shown in **Fig. 1** shows extensive tophus deposition overlying the dorsal aspect of the base of the second metacarpal, and scattered tophus throughout the carpus (Philips Brilliance 16-slice scanner, Philips Medical Systems, Best, The Netherlands; reconstruction using a soft-tissue algorithm, 512-pixel matrix, also to 0.8-mm slices with a 0.4-mm increment).

of 160–170 Hounsfield units) adjacent to erosions and also extending into soft tissues. 3D imaging with CT is particularly successful for revealing bone erosions and their relationship with tophi, as shown in **Fig. 3**. This relationship was also illustrated in the study by Dalbeth and colleagues,[4] where CT scans from 20 patients with gout were assessed for tophi and erosions. Of those joints where CT erosions were detected, 82% were separately scored as positive for the presence of tophi. When CT erosions of greater than 5 mm diameter were considered, this figure increased to 95%. These data suggest that erosions are likely to represent regions of bone that have been mined by tophus deposition, via several mechanisms including cytokine-mediated osteoclast activation.[17,18] The Auckland group also used CT to examine surface tophi and compared results with those of a physical examination. Of those tophi identified clinically, 89% were scored on CT scanning, and there was a very strong correlation between the 2 methods in terms of measured size of lesions.[19] Thus, CT has potential both as a diagnostic tool in gout and as an instrument with which to measure progressive erosive damage and, indeed, tophus growth or resolution. Its metrics demonstrate excellent reader reliability, and a scoring system for use in the feet has recently been developed.[20]

DECT
DECT is a recent arrival on the imaging scene in rheumatology, but has been used in other medical settings for some years. In urology, DECT has been used to determine the composition of renal calculi[21] and has been used in cardiology for imaging coronary anatomy, characterizing atherosclerotic plaque, and, more recently, evaluating myocardial perfusion.[22] This technique uses 2 x-ray tubes with different voltages, aligned at 90° to each other. Data are acquired simultaneously at 2 different energy levels (80 kV and 140 kV), creating 2 different data sets, which are then processed by specialized software and analyzed using an image-based 2-material decomposition algorithm to separate calcium from monosodium urate, using soft tissue as a baseline.[23] Calcium, which has a high atomic number, causes a greater change in attenuation of X-rays than MSU, which has low atomic number

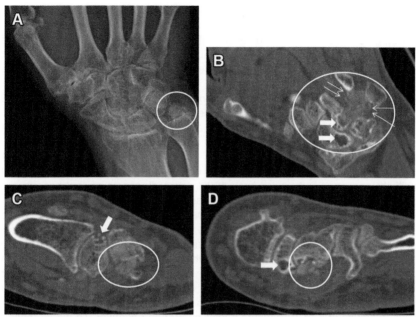

Fig. 3. Imaging from a 50-year-old New Zealand–European man with an 18-year history of gout. (*A*) Radiograph of the right wrist shows calcification within the triangular fibrocartilage (*circle*). (*B*) CT scan (coronal) of the same region shows large, well-corticated erosions (*wide arrows*) and an area of partially calcified tophus within the carpus (*fine arrows*). (*C*) Sagittal image with cut at second-metacarpophalangeal level showing erosion at the trapezoid (*wide arrow*) and tophus within capitate erosion (*circle*). (*D*) Sagittal image with a more medial cut shows corticated erosion (*wide arrow*) and tophus within capitate (*circle*).

components. These materials are then given different color coding, which allows them to be differentiated on the resultant CT scan (**Fig. 4**). The detection of MSU does depend on the computer software settings and in particular the parameter ratio, which dictates the slope of the line that is used to help differentiate MSU from

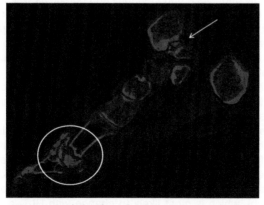

Fig. 4. Dual-energy CT image of the foot from a patient with tophaceous gout (lateral view), showing monosodium urate (MSU) crystals deposited within and overlying a large erosion at the first metacarpophalangeal joint (*circle*). Further MSU crystals are shown within the subtalar joint (*arrow*).

calcium.[23] Although this work by Nicolaou and colleagues[23] suggests using a parameter ratio of 1.28, a recent comparative study with 3T MRI indicated that a ratio of 1.55 had greater sensitivity.[24] However, higher ratios frequently lead to nonspecific artifact. Further investigation into the operating characteristics of DECT in gout may be necessary to optimize the scanning procedure and minimize the potential for false positives or negatives.

There is an unmet clinical need for an imaging procedure that will detect MSU deposits and help diagnose gout in those patients for whom joint aspiration is not possible. The idea that this could be achieved using DECT is very attractive to patients and physicians alike. Choi and colleagues[25] reported the first study of DECT in gout in 2009, and described its ability to reveal multiple intra-articular and extra-articular urate deposits, many of which were undetectable clinically. Sensitivity and specificity were both 100% for a diagnosis of tophaceous gout, as all 20 patients studied were DECT-positive and the regions where deposits were detected were aspirate-positive for MSU crystals, whereas all 10 controls were DECT-negative. Another retrospective DECT study examining a larger group used 2 separate readers and found interreader agreement to be very high for scoring DECT deposits (κ value 0.87). In their hands DECT scans were positive for urate deposits in all 12 patients with clinically suspected gout, where the same joints were MSU-aspirate–positive (100% sensitivity).[26] Specificity was 89% for reader 1 (false-positive DECT scans in 2 of 19 patients) and 79% for reader 2 (false positives in 4 of 19 patients if joint-aspiration negative). To clarify these issues, a larger prospective study was performed by Choi and colleagues.[27] Forty crystal-proven gout patients and 40 patients with other arthritic conditions acting as controls underwent DECT scanning of all peripheral joints. The specificity and sensitivity of DECT in this setting were 93% and 78%, indicating that both were very high, but diagnostic accuracy was not 100%. Glazebrook and colleagues[28] have provided further evidence of this recently with their report of a false-negative DECT scan in a patient with acute aspirate-proven gout affecting the third metacarpophalangeal (MCP) joint. Thus, DECT may be a useful diagnostic tool but is not infallible, and more information is needed about its sensitivity and specificity in acute or nontophaceous gout for which the clinical diagnosis remains in doubt.

DECT has also provided new insights into gout pathology, including the finding that urate very commonly deposits around tendons and bursae as well as joints. In a prospective DECT study of 92 patients with tophaceous gout where scans of the feet were obtained, 39% of all Achilles tendons imaged showed MSU deposition, followed in terms of frequency by 18% of peroneal tendons and 10% of extensor hallucis longus tendons.[29] Much of this tophus was observed in the region of the enthesis, raising the possibility that biomechanical strain may influence patterns of urate deposition. Thus, gout is definitely more than a joint disease, and the deposition of tophaceous material in soft tissues has clinical implications ranging from nerve compression syndromes[30] to tendon rupture.[31]

DECT also has the potential to be useful in a randomized clinical trial (RCT) setting to follow the reduction in urate burden achieved with effective ULT, because DECT can quantify urate using automated, computerized volume assessment software, providing reproducible data that may be stored digitally and compared with subsequent measurements over time. It also enables measurement of the crystal component of tophi, which is most likely to change with ULT, as opposed to the soft-tissue granulomatous response that makes up the bulk of the tophus.[1] Only one longitudinal study has been published to date reporting the relationship between DECT urate volumes and serum urate (SU) measurements in 73 patients observed over 12 months.[32] Although higher SU levels were observed in patients with increased DECT urate volumes, there was no consistent relationship between these parameters in terms of change over time, and it is possible that DECT may not be as useful as hoped in this context. Clearly, however, further studies are warranted.

Ultrasonography
US has an emerging role in gout, to both facilitate joint aspiration for confirmation of the presence of MSU crystals and assist in making a diagnosis in its own right because of certain US-specific imaging features. US can detect joint inflammation in terms of synovitis and tenosynovitis by revealing synovial thickening using gray-scale US, often with additional vascular signal detected using power Doppler US. There may be an associated signal-free region, representing a synovial effusion. These features are nonspecific and common to all inflammatory arthropathies.[33] A recent systematic review by Chowalloor and Keen[34] examined the literature related to US-detected pathologic features in gout,[34] and found that tophi have been well studied using this technique. It should be recalled that not all sites of possible tophus deposition are accessible to US (including regions of the tarsus and carpus), and also that intraosseous tophi cannot be detected by this modality. Where tophi are accessible to US, they are typically ovoid in shape, with a hypoechoic border and an internal stippled signal, as shown in **Fig. 5**.[35] Validation of US tophi has been performed against MRI and histology as gold standards.[36,37] Perez-Ruiz and colleagues[36] reported that MSU crystals could be aspirated from 83% of US-defined tophi. In some cases, floating hyperechoic foci have been described within synovial fluid, likely representing microtophi, resulting in a snowstorm appearance.[11] A longitudinal study has shown

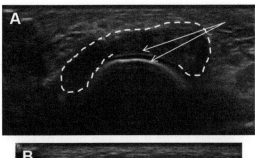

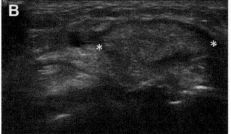

Fig. 5. Ultrasonography images of tophi from the patient shown in **Fig. 3**. (*A*) Transverse view of tophaceous deposit overlying the second metacarpal head, which appears hypoechoic (*dotted line*). The double-contour sign is shown (*double arrow*). (*B*) Another tophus from the same patient overlying the distal radius is shown between asterisks (longitudinal view). Typical features include ovoid shape, hypoechoic border, stippled center, and lack of vascularity.

that the US measurement of tophi is reliable and responsive to change, suggesting a possible role for RCTs to monitor the efficacy of ULT.[38] Of note, patients with asymptomatic hyperuricemia have also been found to have evidence of US tophi within joints, tendons, and soft tissues.[39] However, different studies have designated tophi in different ways, and more standardized definitions are required.[34,40] Estimation of reliability also needs further work, as most US studies in gout have assessed this by rereading stored images. Given the potential variability in technique used when performing a US scan, future studies need to incorporate a true test of interreader reliability by reimaging patients on 2 consecutive occasions and employing 2 separate readers.

US erosions have also been well studied and compared with radiographic and MRI erosions.[37,41,42] Wright and colleagues[41] compared high-resolution US (HRUS) with XR at the first MTP joints of 39 male gout patients and 22 matched controls. Poor agreement was found between HRUS and XR for erosion detection (κ = 0.2), and the investigators concluded that there were a large number of false-negative XRs. Ten erosions were detected by HRUS, compared with 3 using XR, in 22 MTP joints that had never been clinically affected by gout, and it was concluded that US is a much more sensitive modality than XR for erosion detection. Rettenbacher and colleagues[11] compared US with XR in a larger prospective study of 105 patients with a clinical suspicion of gout. XR findings suggested gout with sensitivity of 31% and specificity of 93% (compared with the final clinical diagnosis), whereas US had sensitivity of 96% and specificity of 73%. It is instructive to balance these very positive reports with that of Carter and colleagues,[37] who studied an "index joint," which had been affected by clinical gout but remained free of XR erosions, using US and MRI. Of 27 subjects, 15 (56%) had erosions on MRI of their index joint, whereas only 1 (4%) had erosions identified by US. Therefore US would seem to be much less sensitive than MRI, but further comparative studies are needed.

The double-contour sign was described by Thiele and Schlesinger[43] in 2010. One hyperechoic line is due to a US signal bouncing off cortical bone, for example at the head of an MCP or MTP joint, while a second outer line is thought to represent the deposition of MSU crystals in a fine layer over hyaline cartilage, forming a new reflective barrier. Sandwiched between these lines is the articular hyaline cartilage, which is not echogenic (see **Fig. 5**). This sign has been described as being relatively common in gout, detected in symptomatic and asymptomatic joints, and also in asymptomatic hyperuricemia.[42,44,45] It has also been detected (uncommonly) in controls.[41] Naredo and colleagues[40] recently reported an ultrasound-guided aspiration study of intra-articular hyperechoic aggregates from joints or tendons from 49 gout patients and 8 control patients. Aspirated material was positive for MSU crystals in 78% of gout patients and none of the controls, and negative for crystals in 20% of gout patients. Calcium pyrophosphate crystals were found in 1 gout patient and 1 control. This study is the closest approximation to comparative imaging/histologic verification that is available. A cadaveric study of gout cartilage from the 1950s described cartilage surfaces as being "diffusely dusted with white crystal deposits" in 11 gout patients.[46] A more recent arthroscopic study of the wrist described "diffuse synovitis and crystalline deposits throughout the radiocarpal joint with focal crystalline precipitates on the scapholunate and lunotriquetral ligaments,"[47] but there was no imaging comparator. The sensitivity and specificity of the double-contour sign in diagnosing gout have been estimated by one group as 44% and 99%, respectively.[48] Ottaviani and colleagues[49] found in their MSU-aspirate–positive gout patients that all those with urate levels greater than 600 μM

(10 mg/dL) had a double-contour sign in at least 1 assessed joint. Disappearance of this sign has been observed in response to ULT.[43] However, pitfalls certainly exist in interpreting this feature, particularly when echogenicity at the interface between synovial fluid and cartilage can be variable. Therefore it cannot yet be recommended as a reliable diagnostic feature that might replace the necessity for joint aspiration.

MRI

MRI has not been as widely studied in gout as the other imaging modalities already mentioned, but is quite frequently used clinically for diagnostic reasons.[50] Like US, it allows joint inflammation to be assessed as well as joint damage, and has some advantages over the latter in terms of greater accessibility for certain joint regions and less operator dependence. Tophi have particular characteristics when imaged using MRI. Tophi are visible as discrete masses or nodules with low signal on T1-weighted (T1w) images, whereas T2-weighted (T2w) signal intensity ranges from low to high, and there may be variable contrast enhancement related to vascularity (**Fig. 6**).[51] Comparative US and MRI studies are few, but Perez-Ruiz and colleagues[36] validated the measurement of tophi by US against MRI as a gold standard, and found a good correlation between the 2 methods for tophus detection but only moderate agreement for measurement of tophus dimensions. Digitized MRI data have the potential to be useful for longitudinal review, and Schumacher and colleagues[52] suggested MRI tophus volume could be a useful outcome measure in clinical trials of ULT. However, this would involve a time-consuming manual outlining procedure for computation of volume, and thus far there are no reports of this application. A recent study comparing MRI with DECT for detection of tophi at the wrist found a good correlation between the 2 modalities, with MRI having a specificity of 0.98 and a sensitivity of 0.63 for detecting tophi, using DECT as a gold standard.[24] Thus MRI could have a place in assisting in gout diagnosis, especially in situations where DECT scanning is not available.

Some new insights into the pathophysiology of gout are also emerging from MRI studies. Poh and colleagues[53] described a 10-year retrospective study from New Zealand, involving predominantly Pacific and Maori patients with gout. The investigators made the interesting observation that whereas features of synovitis and bone erosion were frequently detected and often florid, MRI bone edema was relatively

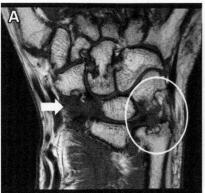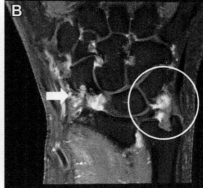

Fig. 6. Magnetic resonance imaging scans of the wrist in a 68-year-old Samoan man with tophaceous gout. (A) T1-weighted coronal image showing multiple erosions and adjacent amorphous tophaceous material (*circle* and *arrow*). (B) Postcontrast T1-weighted fat-saturated (FS) coronal image. These regions show variable enhancement post contrast.

uncommon and mild in gout. However, in those cases where there was concomitant osteomyelitis, bone edema was usually severe. In RA, osteitis has been found to be the histopathologic correlate of MRI bone edema on imaging/histologic studies,[54] but in gout no such characterization of the bone edema lesion has been possible, owing to difficulty obtaining bone samples. Recently, a prospective MRI study of the wrist in 40 gout patients confirmed MRI bone edema to be relatively rare and mild in uncomplicated gout, being scored at 1% of wrist sites in 5 of 40 patients.[55] This study examined associations between the various MRI features of gout including tophi, synovitis, bone erosions, and bone edema, and found erosions to be strongly associated with tophi (as already observed from CT studies[4]) but not with synovitis or bone edema. These findings highlight the unique nature of the osteopathology of gout, which contrasts with that of immune-mediated arthropathies such as RA.

CPPD ARTHROPATHY
Radiography

CPPD crystal deposition disease is a common form of crystalline arthropathy characterized clinically by a variety of patterns including the most common asymptomatic state (radiographic chondrocalcinosis, **Fig. 7**), acute monoarthritis (pseudogout), and a symmetric polyarticular destructive arthropathy that mimics RA.[56] A formal diagnosis of CPPD crystal deposition disease requires synovial fluid analysis and the finding of typical rhomboidal crystals with specific birefringence characteristics. However, in many patients the diagnosis is suggested through typical features on XR, which remains the investigation of choice for several reasons. First, multiple joints can be imaged so that typical appearances at specific locations, such as the wrist or knee, can be identified. Second, the typical appearances of CPPD arthropathy rely on the deposition of calcium and the formation of erosions, both well seen by all forms of radiography. Lastly, associated conditions including osteoarthritis, hyperparathyroidism, or hemochromatosis also have characteristic radiographic features, so that useful additional diagnostic data may be captured by this modality.

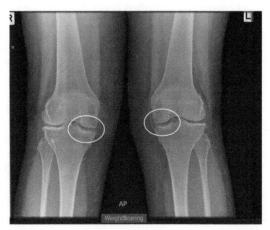

Fig. 7. Weight-bearing radiograph of the knees in an elderly male who was asymptomatic. Typical linear CPPD deposits are seen within hyaline cartilage at the medial compartments of both knee joints (*circles*) with concomitant osteoarthritic features including joint space narrowing, sclerosis and osteophyte formation.

In 1977, Resnick and colleagues[57] described the typical radiographic and pathologic abnormalities of CPPD arthropathy in 85 patients, with concomitant analysis of cadaveric or surgical tissue when this was available. Calcification of cartilage (hyaline and fibrocartilage), synovium, joint capsule, tendons, ligaments, and soft tissues was the primary finding, often associated with an arthropathy that superficially resembled osteoarthritis but was more destructive, with "extensive collapse and fragmentation of subchondral bone." Where surgical material was available, cartilaginous and osseous material were found embedded within synovial membrane, associated with marked cellular proliferation. Favored sites for calcification included the triangular fibrocartilage of the wrist and the menisci of the knee. Other radiographic signs associated with CPPD arthropathy include the wrap-around patella, describing marked loss of joint space at the patellofemoral joint with exuberant osteophytosis,[58] and typical changes at the radiocarpal joint where loss of cartilage space may occur with scapholunate advanced collapse (SLAC wrist).[59] Within the spine, CPPD deposits may be located within the intervertebral discs, ligamentum flavum, apophyseal joints, and surrounding the odontoid peg, resulting in the so-called crowned dens sign.[60] This region is even more accurately imaged using CT (see next section), and soft-tissue masses that may cause cord compression may be identified with MRI.

CT Scanning

CT scanning is the gold standard for identifying the crowned dens syndrome. Scutellari and colleagues[61] used CT to evaluate 38 patients with neck pain, and found calcific deposits around the dens in 12. Compression of the cervical cord was associated in a minority of cases, and additional MRI scanning was used to investigate for myelopathic change within the cord. Another group described a strong association between cervical CPPD arthropathy of this type and type 2 odontoid fractures with obvious potential clinical sequelae.[62]

Ultrasonography

There has been recent interest in identifying calcium pyrophosphate crystal deposition in cartilage using US.[63] The sonographic findings described include a thin hyperechoic band parallel to the bone cortex but separated from it by a hypoechoic region (representing cartilage) in a similar way to the double-contour sign of gout as described by Thiele and Schlesinger.[42] However, these investigators noted a more "punctate pattern" in CPPD arthropathy which appeared to differ from the "smoother" line typical of gout. Others have described hyperechoic rounded amorphous shaped regions within for example the triangular fibrocartilage at the wrist and the menisci of the knee.[3] However, to date there have been no rigorous comparative studies of this form of imaging compared with histopathology as a gold standard and the sensitivity and specificity of US for detecting CPPD arthropathy (for example when radiography is negative) remains speculative.

HYDROXYAPATITE ARTHROPATHY
Radiography and CT Scanning

Calcium hydroxyapatite is the largest mineral component of bone. HA crystals are small (70–300 nm in diameter) and may be difficult to identify from synovial fluid, but have been characterized as having a "shiny coin" appearance on phase-contrast light microscopy, with distinctive morphology on transmission and scanning electron microscopy.[64,65] HA deposition disease may occur in patients with renal failure in the form of tumoral calcinosis.[65] A more common presentation is in older patients with normal renal function who develop the acutely painful condition of calcific periarthritis at the shoulder.[66] HA deposits appear to form where ischemic conditions in the region of the rotator cuff favor crystal deposition.[67] The much more severe and uncommon erosive arthropathy, christened "Milwaukee shoulder" by Halverson and colleagues,[68] is also an HA-associated arthropathy. Plain radiography remains the cornerstone imaging investigation for HA arthropathy. Early HA deposits often appear as cloudy, poorly defined opacities in the periarticular region adjacent to the acromion. Older lesions are denser and more defined, with a smooth border and an ovoid shape, as shown in **Fig. 8**. These lesions are frequently seen at the greater tuberosity of the humerus within the distal supraspinatus tendon insertion.[69] Erosion of adjacent bone may also sometimes be apparent. Where anatomy is complex, CT is the optimal radiographic modality, as in the syndrome of acute retropharyngeal tendinitis resulting from deposition of calcium hydroxyapatite crystals in the superior oblique fibers of the longus colli muscle.[70] These patients present with neck pain exacerbated on swallowing, and an axial CT scan of cervical spine at odontoid level typically shows calcification in the tendon of the longus colli muscle anterior to odontoid process (**Fig. 9**).

MRI and US

On MRI, the calcific deposits of HA arthropathy are of low signal on T1w and T2w images.[71] When crystals in the rotator cuff rupture they cause synovitis, leading to the clinical presentation, which is dominated by severe pain caused by adjacent tenosynovitis and subacromial bursitis. These inflammatory features are well seen on MRI using postcontrast T1w and T2w or proton-density sequences. The shoulder is not the only site to be involved, and MRI is a useful modality for identifying HA arthropathy at the hip, where it commonly involves the gluteus medius tendon.[72] Calcific periarthritis of the longus colli muscle may have typical MRI features as shown in **Fig. 9**, with associated inflammation and free fluid in the retropharyngeal space (appearing as a bright signal). There is very little literature on the specific US characteristics of HA

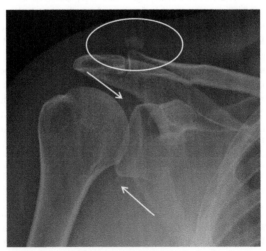

Fig. 8. Large calcified deposit adjacent to the acromioclavicular joint (*ellipse*) in a 68-year-old woman with hydroxyapatite arthropathy. Tiny deposits are also seen at the upper and lower margins of the glenoid within the triceps origins (*arrows*).

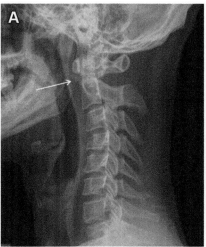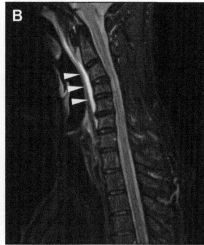

Fig. 9. Acute calcific prevertebral tendonitis of the longus colli muscle caused by calcium hydroxyapatite deposition in the superior oblique fibers (extending from the anterior arch of C1 to the T3 vertebral body). (*A*) Plain radiograph of the cervical spine (lateral view) showing calcific deposit below the arch of the atlas (*arrow*). (*B*) T2-weighted FS magnetic resonance image shows retropharyngeal fluid as a bright signal (*arrowheads*).

arthropathy, although US-assisted joint aspiration may have diagnostic applications. US will also identify the features of bursitis and tendonitis associated with calcific tendonitis at the shoulder.[3]

SUMMARY

There have been recent exciting advances in imaging that are directly relevant to the diagnosis and management of the crystal arthropathies. CT and DECT are important additions in gout diagnosis, revealing the volume and distribution of tophi in vastly better detail than could be gleaned previously from XRs. However, these modalities entail exposure to ionizing radiation and are not as widely available as plain radiography. As in other forms of arthritis, MRI and US inform about the inflammatory response affecting soft tissues, synovium, and tenosynovium, as well as revealing joint damage in terms of erosion, cartilage change, and tendon rupture. MRI offers some advantages with its potential to image all tissues at all sites (although scans are generally confined to one anatomic region), in addition to a lack of radiation exposure. However, it has drawbacks including expense and inability to accurately detect MSU deposition in gout. US has been heralded as an important new addition to the imaging armamentarium in gout because of its ability to show crystal deposition in cartilage, but its reliability as a diagnostic tool and where it will fit as a management aid to the clinician remain to be defined. Which form of imaging to use depends, as always, on the clinical setting, and in many instances radiography remains the most suitable, especially in CPPD and HA arthropathies. **Table 1** provides a summary of the utility of these imaging modalities in the 3 crystal arthritides discussed. Often multiple forms of imaging are used in complex patients, but this may represent a waste of resources. Finding the most appropriate form of imaging to answer the relevant clinical question remains a challenge for rheumatologists and radiologists alike, but many more imaging options are now open, offering the potential for better disease outcomes in patients with crystal arthropathies.

Table 1
Summary of clinical applications of imaging modalities in the crystal arthropathies

Type of Crystal Arthropathy	Imaging Modality				
	Plain Radiography	CT Scanning	DECT Imaging	MRI	US
Gout	Good coverage: multiple areas imaged at low cost. Erosions and joint space change best seen in long-standing gout. Tophi seen as soft-tissue opacities and may be calcified. Sensitivity of 31% and specificity of 93% for gout diagnosis vs clinical gold standard[11] Limited exposure to ionizing radiation Widely available	Excellent imaging of erosions and tophi: better detection than radiography because of 3-dimensional multiplanar modality. Area scanned is more limited than that in radiography. Exposure to ionizing radiation Cost	Excellent imaging of tophi (color coded according to decomposition algorithm to reveal MSU crystals). Area scanned is more limited than that in radiography. Sensitivity of 78%–100% and specificity of 79%–93% vs MSU aspiration for gout diagnosis[26,27] Exposure to ionizing radiation. Cost. Available only in specialist centers	Useful clinical tool for complex presentations (eg, if concomitant osteomyelitis suspected). Reveals synovitis, tenosynovitis, soft-tissue inflammation, bone erosion, and tophi. 3-T MRI has specificity of 98% and sensitivity of 63% for detecting tophi vs DECT gold standard[24] No exposure to ionizing radiation	Convenient hands-on tool for trained rheumatologist. Assists joint aspiration for crystal identification. Very good for detecting tophi (but not all areas accessible). Images synovitis, tenosynovitis, effusions, and soft-tissue inflammation. Double-contour sign indicates MSU deposition in cartilage. Sensitivity 96% and specificity 73% for diagnosing gout vs a clinical gold standard[11]

CPPD arthropathy	Ideal for revealing CPPD crystal deposition in a wide range of locations. Typical radiographic appearance (located in hyaline and fibrocartilage) Can show associated erosion and joint disorganization in destructive CPPD arthropathy	Most useful application in regions where anatomy is complex (eg, cervical spine). Helpful for diagnosis of crowned dens syndrome.[61]	Not applicable	Useful for imaging detailed anatomy at shoulder or hip girdle. Calcific deposits well seen. Can reveal associated synovitis and tenosynovitis as well as tendon attrition and rupture	May be used to assist joint aspiration to obtain CPPD crystals for diagnosis. Images calcific deposits, erosions, synovitis, tenosynovitis, and joint effusion. May reveal crystal deposition in cartilage[3]
HA arthropathy	Most useful imaging modality for diagnosis: typical radiographic patterns such as calcific periarthritis at the shoulder[69]	Specific application where anatomy is complex such as the cervical spine (acute calcific prevertebral tendonitis)[70] or hip periarthritis[72]	Not applicable	As for CPPD	As for CPPD Few data on US

Abbreviations: CPPD, calcium pyrophosphate dihydrate; CT, computed tomography; DECT, dual-energy computed tomography; HA, calcium hydroxyapatite; MRI, magnetic resonance imaging; MSU, monosodium urate; US, ultrasonography.

REFERENCES

1. Dalbeth N, Aati O, Gao A, et al. Assessment of tophus size: a comparison between physical measurement methods and dual-energy computed tomography scanning. J Clin Rheumatol 2012;18(1):23–7.
2. Feydy A, Liote F, Carlier R, et al. Cervical spine and crystal-associated diseases: imaging findings. Eur Radiol 2006;16(2):459–68.
3. Delle Sedie A, Riente L, Iagnocco A, et al. Ultrasound imaging for the rheumatologist X. Ultrasound imaging in crystal-related arthropathies. Clin Exp Rheumatol 2007;25(4):513–7.
4. Dalbeth N, Clark B, Gregory K, et al. Mechanisms of bone erosion in gout; a quantitative analysis using plain radiography and computed tomography. Ann Rheum Dis 2009;68(8):1290–5. http://dx.doi.org/10.1136/ard.2008.094201.
5. Watt I, Middlemiss H. The radiology of gout. Review article. Clin Radiol 1975; 26(1):27–36.
6. Barthelemy CR, Nakayama DA, Carrera GF, et al. Gouty arthritis: a prospective radiographic evaluation of sixty patients. Skeletal Radiol 1984;11(1):1–8.
7. Roddy E, Zhang W, Doherty M. Are joints affected by gout also affected by osteoarthritis? Ann Rheum Dis 2007;66(10):1374–7. http://dx.doi.org/10.1136/ard. 2006.063768.
8. Nygaard HB, Shenoi S, Shukla S. Lower back pain caused by tophaceous gout of the spine. Neurology 2009;73(5):404.
9. Zhang W, Doherty M, Pascual E, et al. EULAR evidence based recommendations for gout. Part I: diagnosis. Report of a task force of the Standing Committee for International Clinical Studies Including Therapeutics (ESCISIT). Ann Rheum Dis 2006;65(10):1301–11.
10. Wallace SL, Robinson H, Masi AT, et al. Preliminary criteria for the classification of the acute arthritis of primary gout. Arthritis Rheum 1977;20(3):895–900.
11. Rettenbacher T, Ennemoser S, Weirich H, et al. Diagnostic imaging of gout: comparison of high-resolution US versus conventional X-ray. Eur Radiol 2008; 18(3):621–30.
12. Dalbeth N, Clark B, McQueen F, et al. Validation of a radiographic damage index in chronic gout. Arthritis Rheum 2007;57(6):1067–73.
13. van der Heijde DM, van Riel PL, Nuver-Zwart IH, et al. Effects of hydroxychloroquine and sulphasalazine on progression of joint damage in rheumatoid arthritis. Lancet 1989;1(8646):1036–8.
14. Dalbeth N, Doyle AJ, McQueen FM, et al. Exploratory study of radiographic change in patients with tophaceous gout treated with intensive urate-lowering therapy. Arthritis Care Res 2013;66(1):82–5.
15. Dalbeth N, Milligan A, Doyle AJ, et al. Characterization of new bone formation in gout: a quantitative site-by-site analysis using plain radiography and computed tomography. Arthritis Res Ther 2012;14:R165.
16. Ly J, Pinto C, Doyle A, et al. Axial bone proliferation causing cervical myelopathy in the mutilans form of psoriatic arthritis despite peripheral bone erosion. Ann Rheum Dis 2009;68(3):443–4.
17. McQueen FM, Chhana A, Dalbeth N. Mechanisms of joint damage in gout: evidence from cellular and imaging studies. Nat Rev Rheumatol 2012;8(3):173–81. Available at: http://dx.doi.org/10.1038/nrrheum.2011.207.
18. Dalbeth N, Smith T, Nicolson B, et al. Enhanced osteoclastogenesis in patients with tophaceous gout: urate crystals promote osteoclast development through interactions with stromal cells. Arthritis Rheum 2008;58(6):1854–65.

19. Dalbeth N, Clark B, Gregory K, et al. Computed tomography measurement of tophus volume: comparison with physical measurement. Arthritis Rheum 2007;57(3):461–5.
20. Dalbeth N, Doyle A, Boyer L, et al. Development of a computed tomography method of scoring bone erosion in patients with gout: validation and clinical implications. Rheumatology 2011;50(2):410–6.
21. Primak AN, Fletcher JG, Vrtiska TJ, et al. Noninvasive differentiation of uric acid versus non-uric acid kidney stones using dual-energy CT. Acad Radiol 2007; 14(12):1441–7.
22. Pontone G, Grancini L, Andreini D, et al. Myocardial perfusion imaging using dual-energy computed tomography: a clinical case. Eur Heart J Cardiovasc Imaging 2013;14(8):835.
23. Nicolaou S, Yong-Hing CJ, Galea-Soler S, et al. Dual-energy CT as a potential new diagnostic tool in the management of gout in the acute setting. AJR Am J Roentgenol 2010;194(4):1072–8.
24. McQueen F, Doyle A, Dalbeth N. DECT urate deposits: now you see them now you don't. Ann Rheum Dis 2013;72(3):458–9. http://dx.doi.org/10.1136/annrheumdis-2012-202452.
25. Choi HK, Al-Arfaj AM, Eftekhari A, et al. Dual energy computed tomography in tophaceous gout. Ann Rheum Dis 2009;68(10):1609–12.
26. Glazebrook KN, Guimaraes LS, Murthy NS, et al. Identification of intraarticular and periarticular uric acid crystals with dual-energy CT: initial evaluation. Radiology 2011;261(2):516–24.
27. Choi HK, Burns LC, Shojania K, et al. Dual energy CT in gout: a prospective validation study. Ann Rheum Dis 2012;71(9):1466–71.
28. Glazebrook KN, Kakar S, Ida CM, et al. False-negative dual-energy computed tomography in a patient with acute gout. J Clin Rheumatol 2012;18(3):138–41. Available at: http://dx.doi.org/10.1097/RHU.0b013e318253aa5e.
29. Dalbeth N, Kalluru R, Aati O, et al. Tendon and ligament involvement in gout: a dual energy computed tomography study. Ann Rheum Dis 2013;72(9): 1545–8.
30. Chen CK, Chung CB, Yeh L, et al. Carpal tunnel syndrome caused by tophaceous gout: CT and MR imaging features in 20 patients. AJR Am J Roentgenol 2000;175(3):655–9.
31. Iwamoto T, Toki H, Ikari K, et al. Multiple extensor tendon ruptures caused by tophaceous gout. Mod Rheumatol 2010;20(2):210–2. http://dx.doi.org/10.1007/s10165-009-0258-x.
32. Rajan A, Aati O, Kalluru R, et al. Lack of change in urate deposition by dual-energy computed tomography among clinically stable patients with long-standing tophaceous gout: a prospective longitudinal study. Arthritis Res Ther 2013; 15(5):R160.
33. Joshua F. Ultrasound applications for the practicing rheumatologist. Best Pract Res Clin Rheumatol 2012;26(6):853–67. Available at: http://dx.doi.org/10.1016/j.berh.2012.10.002.
34. Chowalloor PV, Keen HI. A systematic review of ultrasonography in gout and asymptomatic hyperuricaemia. Ann Rheum Dis 2013;72(5):638–45. Available at: http://dx.doi.org/10.1136/annrheumdis-2012-202301.
35. Fernandes EA, Lopes MG, Mitraud SA, et al. Ultrasound characteristics of gouty tophi in the olecranon bursa and evaluation of their reproducibility. Eur J Radiol 2012;81(2):317–23. Available at: http://dx.doi.org/10.1016/j.ejrad.2010.12.051.

36. Perez-Ruiz F, Martin I, Canteli B. Ultrasonographic measurement of tophi as an outcome measure for chronic gout. J Rheumatol 2007;34(9):1888–93.
37. Carter JD, Kedar RP, Anderson SR, et al. An analysis of MRI and ultrasound imaging in patients with gout who have normal plain radiographs. Rheumatology 2009;48(11):1442–6.
38. Perez-Ruiz F, Calabozo M, Pijoan JI, et al. Effect of urate-lowering therapy on the velocity of size reduction of tophi in chronic gout. Arthritis Rheum 2002;47(4): 356–60. http://dx.doi.org/10.1002/art.10511.
39. Pineda C, Amezcua-Guerra LM, Solano C, et al. Joint and tendon subclinical involvement suggestive of gouty arthritis in asymptomatic hyperuricemia: an ultrasound controlled study. Arthritis Res Ther 2011;13(1):R4.
40. Naredo E, Uson J, Jiménez-Palop M, et al. Ultrasound-detected musculoskeletal urate crystal deposition: which joints and what findings should be assessed for diagnosing gout? Ann Rheum Dis 2013. http://dx.doi.org/10.1136/annrheumdis-2013-203487.
41. Wright SA, Filippucci E, McVeigh C, et al. High-resolution ultrasonography of the first metatarsal phalangeal joint in gout: a controlled study. Ann Rheum Dis 2007;66(7):859–64.
42. Thiele RG, Schlesinger N. Diagnosis of gout by ultrasound. Rheumatology 2007; 46(7):1116–21.
43. Thiele RG, Schlesinger N. Ultrasonography shows disappearance of monosodium urate crystal deposition on hyaline cartilage after sustained normouricemia is achieved. Rheumatol Int 2010;30(4):495–503.
44. Howard RG, Pillinger MH, Gyftopoulos S, et al. Reproducibility of musculoskeletal ultrasound for determining monosodium urate deposition: concordance between readers. Arthritis Care Res 2011;63(10):1456–62. Available at: http://dx.doi.org/10.1002/acr.20527.
45. De Miguel E, Puig J, Castillo C, et al. Diagnosis of gout in patients with asymptomatic hyperuricaemia: a pilot ultrasound study. Ann Rheum Dis 2012;71(1): 157–8. http://dx.doi.org/10.1136/ard.2011.154997.
46. Levin MH, Lichtenstein L, Scott HW. Pathologic changes in gout; survey of eleven necropsied cases. Am J Pathol 1956;32(5):871–95.
47. Wilczynski MC, Gelberman RH, Adams A, et al. Arthroscopic findings in gout of the wrist. J Hand Surg Am 2009;34(2):244–50. Available at: http://dx.doi.org/10.1016/j.jhsa.2008.10.022.
48. Filippucci E, Riveros MG, Georgescu D, et al. Hyaline cartilage involvement in patients with gout and calcium pyrophosphate deposition disease. An ultrasound study. Osteoarthritis Cartilage 2009;17(2):178–81.
49. Ottaviani S, Allard A, Bardin T, et al. An exploratory ultrasound study of early gout. Clin Exp Rheumatol 2011;29(5):816–21.
50. McQueen FM, Doyle A, Dalbeth N. Imaging in gout—what can we learn from MRI, CT, DECT and US? Arthritis Res Ther 2011;13(6):246.
51. Gentili A. The advanced imaging of gouty tophi. Curr Rheumatol Rep 2006;8(3): 231–5.
52. Schumacher HR Jr, Becker MA, Edwards NL, et al. Magnetic resonance imaging in the quantitative assessment of gouty tophi. Int J Clin Pract 2006;60(4):408–14. http://dx.doi.org/10.1111/j.1368-5031.2006.00853.x pii: IJCP853.
53. Poh YJ, Dalbeth N, Doyle A, et al. MRI bone oedema is not a major feature of gout unless there is concomitant osteomyelitis: ten year findings from a high prevalence population. J Rheumatol 2011;38(11):2475–81.

54. McQueen FM, Gao A, Østergaard M, et al. High grade MRI bone oedema is common within the surgical field in rheumatoid arthritis patients undergoing joint replacement and is associated with osteitis in subchondral bone. Ann Rheum Dis 2007;66:1581–7. http://dx.doi.org/10.1136/ard.2007.070326.
55. McQueen FM, Doyle A, Reeves Q, et al. Bone erosions in patients with chronic gouty arthropathy are associated with tophi but not bone oedema or synovitis: new insights from a 3T MRI study. Rheumatology 2014;53(1):95–103.
56. McCarty DJ. Crystals and arthritis. Dis Mon 1994;40(6):255–99.
57. Resnick D, Niwayama G, Goergen TG, et al. Clinical, radiographic and pathologic abnormalities in calcium pyrophosphate dihydrate deposition disease (CPPD): pseudogout. Radiology 1977;122(1):1–15.
58. Reginato AJ, Tamesis E, Netter P. Familial and clinical aspects of calcium pyrophosphate deposition disease. Curr Rheumatol Rep 1999;1(2):112–20.
59. Chen C, Chandnani VP, Kang HS, et al. Scapholunate advanced collapse: a common wrist abnormality in calcium pyrophosphate dihydrate crystal deposition disease. Radiology 1990;177(2):459–61.
60. Bouvet JP, le Parc JM, Michalski B, et al. Acute neck pain due to calcifications surrounding the odontoid process: the crowned dens syndrome. Arthritis Rheum 1985;28(12):1417–20.
61. Scutellari PN, Galeotti R, Leprotti S, et al. The crowned dens syndrome. Evaluation with CT imaging. Radiol Med 2007;112(2):195–207.
62. Kakitsubata Y, Boutin RD, Theodorou DJ, et al. Calcium pyrophosphate dihydrate crystal deposition in and around the atlantoaxial joint: association with type 2 odontoid fractures in nine patients. Radiology 2000;216(1):213–9.
63. Filippucci E, Scire CA, Delle Sedie A, et al. Ultrasound imaging for the rheumatologist. XXV. Sonographic assessment of the knee in patients with gout and calcium pyrophosphate deposition disease. Clin Exp Rheumatol 2010;28(1):2–5 pii:945.
64. Schumacher HR, Smolyo AP, Tse RL, et al. Arthritis associated with apatite crystals. Ann Intern Med 1977;87(4):411–6.
65. Grinlinton FM, Vuletic JC, Gow PJ. Rapidly progressive calcific periarthritis occurring in a patient with lupus nephritis receiving chronic ambulatory peritoneal dialysis. J Rheumatol 1990;17(8):1100–3.
66. Carcia CR, Scibek JS. Causation and management of calcific tendonitis and periarthritis. Curr Opin Rheumatol 2013;25(2):204–9. Available at: http://dx.doi.org/10.1097/BOR.0b013e32835d4e85.
67. Giachelli CM. Inducers and inhibitors of biomineralization: lessons from pathological calcification. Orthod Craniofac Res 2005;8(4):229–31.
68. Halverson PB, McCarty DJ, Cheung HS, et al. Milwaukee shoulder syndrome: eleven additional cases with involvement of the knee in seven (basic calcium phosphate crystal deposition disease). Semin Arthritis Rheum 1984;14(1):36–44.
69. Hayes CW, Conway WF. Calcium hydroxyapatite deposition disease. Radiographics 1990;10(6):1031–48.
70. Wakabayashi Y, Hori Y, Kondoh Y, et al. Acute calcific prevertebral tendonitis mimicking tension-type headache. Neurol Med Chir (Tokyo) 2012;52(9):631–3.
71. Zubler C, Mengiardi B, Schmid MR, et al. MR arthrography in calcific tendinitis of the shoulder: diagnostic performance and pitfalls. Eur Radiol 2007;17(6):1603–10.
72. Sakai T, Shimaoka Y, Sugimoto M, et al. Acute calcific tendinitis of the gluteus medius: a case report with serial magnetic resonance imaging findings. J Orthop Sci 2004;9(4):404–7.

Comorbidities in Patients with Crystal Diseases and Hyperuricemia

Sebastian E. Sattui, MD[a], Jasvinder A. Singh, MBBS, MPH[b,c,d],
Angelo L. Gaffo, MD, MSPH[e,f,*]

KEYWORDS

- Crystal arthropathies • Comorbidities • Gout • Hyperuricemia
- Cardiovascular disease • Metabolic syndrome • Renal disease
- Calcium pyrophosphate arthropathy

KEY POINTS

- Recent evidence has shown that asymptomatic hyperuricemia, as well as hyperuricemia in patients with gout, plays a significant role in the development of cardiovascular comorbidities.
- In addition to an already proven association between hypertension and hyperuricemia, interventional trials are showing a positive effect of urate-lowering therapy in early stages of hypertension in young individuals.
- An association between hyperuricemia and other cardiovascular diseases such as coronary heart disease, congestive heart failure, and stroke is still not clear.

Continued

S.E. Sattui and A.L. Gaffo have no conflict of interest. J.A. Singh has received research grants from Takeda and Savient and consultant fees from Savient, Takeda, Allergan, and Regeneron. J.A. Singh is supported by grants from the Agency for Health Quality and Research Center for Education and Research on Therapeutics (CERTs), National Institute of Arthritis, Musculoskeletal and Skin Diseases (NIAMS), National Institute of Aging (NIA), and National Cancer Institute (NCI) and the resources and use of facilities at the Birmingham VA Medical Center, AL.
[a] Division of Clinical Immunology and Rheumatology, Department of Medicine, School of Medicine, University of Alabama, Faculty Office Tower 813, 510 20th Street South, Birmingham, AL 35294, USA; [b] Medicine Service, Center for Surgical Medical Acute Care Research and Transitions (C-SMART), 700 19th Street South, Birmingham VA Medical Center, Birmingham, AL 35233, USA; [c] Division of Clinical Immunology and Rheumatology, Department of Medicine, School of Medicine, University of Alabama, Faculty Office Tower 805B, 200 First Street South West, Rochester, MN 55905, USA; [d] Department of Orthopedic Surgery, Mayo Clinic College of Medicine, Rochester, MN, USA; [e] Section of Rheumatology, Veterans Affairs Medical Center, 700 19th Street South, Birmingham, AL 35233, USA; [f] Division of Clinical Immunology and Rheumatology, Department of Medicine, School of Medicine, University of Alabama, Shelby Building 201, 1825 University Boulevard, Birmingham, AL 35294, USA
* Corresponding author. Department of Medicine, University of Alabama School of Medicine, 1720 2nd Avenue South, FOT 1203, Birmingham, AL 35294-3412.
E-mail address: agaffo@uab.edu

Rheum Dis Clin N Am 40 (2014) 251–278
http://dx.doi.org/10.1016/j.rdc.2014.01.005
0889-857X/14/$ – see front matter
© 2014 Elsevier Inc. All rights reserved.

Continued

- A link between hyperuricemia, insulin resistance, and the metabolic syndrome has been shown by fructose-fed animal models and may explain the association between 2 overlapping and increasing diseases.
- Hyperuricemia is associated with an increased risk of chronic kidney disease, but the use of urate-lowering therapy in these patients is still not clear.
- Evidence regarding calcium pyrophosphate arthropathy and associated comorbidities is still scarce and not conclusive.

Crystal arthropathies are among the most common cause of arthritis worldwide. Of these arthropathies, gout represents the highest known burden of crystal-induced arthritis and is likely the most common type of inflammatory arthritis in adults in the United States.[1,2] Calcium pyrophosphate arthropathies, initially described as pseudogout,[3] and other calcium crystal arthropathies are less commonly recognized than gout. Although initially observed only as a painful inflammatory arthropathy, in recent years, more evidence has been building up the case for an association between gout and hyperuricemia and important cardiovascular-metabolic conditions.[4–8] This article presents an updated review of the evidence for these associations, as well as comorbidities associated with calcium crystal arthropathies.

COMORBIDITIES ASSOCIATED WITH HYPERURICEMIA AND GOUT

Hyperuricemia, defined as a serum urate (SU) concentration higher than the point of saturation of 6.8 mg/dL or more,[9] is the most common biochemical abnormality associated with the development of gout, but it is not a sufficient causative factor. Individuals in whom SU concentrations are increased above saturation levels but have not developed clinical manifestations of gout are considered to have asymptomatic hyperuricemia. Data from the US National Health and Nutrition Examination Survey (NHANES) 2007–2008 study estimated a gout prevalence of 3.9% (5.9% for men; 2.0% for women), but a higher hyperuricemia prevalence of 21.4% (21.2% for men; 21.6% for women).[5] In the following sections, the experimental and epidemiologic evidence linking gout and various comorbidities and their complex interrelationships is summarized.

Cardiovascular Disease

Urate and the endothelium: laboratory and animal studies
In vitro studies that used urate concentrations similar to in vivo levels have shown several potential vascular effects. These effects include suppression of nitric oxide (NO) levels,[10,11] increased platelet-derived growth factor expression, local thromboxane production, and cyclooxygenase 2 stimulation, as well as induction of endothelial proliferation, angiotensin II production, and increased markers of oxidative stress.[12–14] The key role of the renin-angiotensin system (RAS) was proved by the reversibility of these effects by adding captopril or losartan.[13] Other significant in vitro observations include the increased production of endothelin 1, a powerful vasoconstrictor, on human aortic smooth muscle cells and cardiac fibroblasts under different urate concentrations.[15,16] All of these effects are facilitated by the entry of urate to vascular smooth muscle cells via the urate anion transporter 1 (URAT-1), an integral membrane protein that serves as a urate transporter and was initially described in afferent renal arterioles.[17]

In vivo animal models have also supported data from in vitro studies. Hyperuricemia was induced in rats through the administration of oxonic acid, a uricase inhibitor, which led to renal vascular disease characterized by cortical vasoconstriction, afferent arteriolar swelling, and glomerular hypertension.[18,19] Partial attenuation of these abnormalities was obtained through the administration of the nonreversible xanthine oxidase inhibitor, febuxostat.[20,21] Other animal models supported these observations and have also shown that although early hypertension can be corrected with SU reduction, after prolonged hyperuricemia, urate reduction does not translate into control of blood pressure and avoidance of arteriolar thickening. Prolonged hyperuricemia results in an irreversible sodium-sensitive urate-insensitive hypertension.[14,22] These observations have pointed to a 2-stage model, with an early hypertension mediated by increased renal renin activity and reduction of circulating plasma nitrates, and a later irreversible phase secondary to an altered intrarenal vascular architecture (**Fig. 1**).[23]

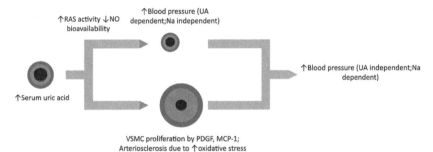

Fig. 1. Proposed 2-stage urate-mediated hypertension. An initial stage of urate-dependent vasoreactive hypertension is induced. Later, when anatomic changes that include wall thickening and smooth muscle proliferation have occurred, a second and definitive sodium-dependent hypertension is established. MCP-1, monocyte chemotactic protein 1; Na, sodium; PDGF, platelet-derived growth factor; UA, urate; VSMC, vascular smooth muscle cell. (*Adapted from* Feig DI. The role of uric acid in the pathogenesis of hypertension in the young. J Clin Hypertens (Greenwich) 2012;14(6):346–52; with permission.)

Hypertension

In 1999, a study of the Framingham cohort reported an association between hyperuricemia and hypertension, which has been confirmed by other epidemiologic studies in different populations.[24–31] Recently, NHANES 2007–2008 analyzed the prevalence of gout, hyperuricemia, and comorbidities in noninstitutionalized adults. Hypertension was present in 74% with gout, and in 47% with hyperuricemia (defined as an SU >7.0 mg/dL for men and >5.7 mg/dL for women) but no history of gout, compared with a population-estimated prevalence of 24% among normouricemic patients. Prevalence among the population with gout with and without hyperuricemia was 77.7% and 70.8%, respectively, higher compared with individuals with asymptomatic hyperuricemia. The prevalence of hypertension was significantly higher among individuals in the highest SU category (SU $\geq$10 mg/dL) compared with those in the lowest SU category (SU <4 md/dL).[5]

A meta-analysis that pooled 11 studies showed a significantly increased risk ratio for incident hypertension of 1.41 (95% confidence interval [CI] 1.23–1.58) among individuals with hyperuricemia, after adjusting for traditional risk factors, including age, body mass index (BMI), and alcohol and tobacco use. This risk appeared more pronounced in younger individuals and women. An increased pooled relative risk (RR) for incident hypertension of 1.13 (95% CI 1.06–1.20) per each mg/dL increase in SU was calculated from 6 studies.[32] Another meta-analysis including 8 prospective studies also reported an increased risk, pooled RR 1.55 (95% CI 1.32–1.82), for hypertension when comparing the highest quartile with the lowest one of SU. However, the analysis presented showed significant heterogeneity ($P<.05$).[33]

Most interventional studies come from the adolescent or pediatric population. A relationship between primary hypertension and high SU levels has been observed even at concentrations less than the supersaturation level of 6.8 mg/dL, and 1 study reported increased SU levels (>5.5 mg/dL) in up to 90% in children with primary hypertension.[34–36] A small randomized, controlled, crossover trial of 30 treatment-naive adolescents (11–17 years old) with stage I hypertension and hyperuricemia randomized individuals to receive oral allopurinol 200 mg daily versus placebo followed by a washout period and then the crossover intervention. After treatment, 20 of 30 participants achieved normal blood pressures compared with 1 participant taking placebo.[37] A randomized, double-blind, placebo-controlled study[38] compared allopurinol with probenecid in prehypertensive obese adolescents. Both treatment arms had a significant decrease in SU and led to a reduction in systolic and diastolic blood pressure of 10.2 and 9.0 mm Hg, respectively. These results suggested that reduction in blood pressure was related to the urate-lowering effect and not to decreased xanthine oxidase activity. A similar study with a small sample of hyperuricemic adults receiving allopurinol 300 mg daily also supported the blood pressure reduction effects of urate-lowering therapy (ULT).[39] Despite these encouraging results, a recent Cochrane review on pharmacotherapy for hyperuricemia and the reduction of blood pressure concluded that evidence is still insufficient to recommend ULT.[40]

Atherosclerosis, coronary heart disease, and peripheral arterial disease

Several mechanisms such as maintenance of a proinflammatory state, promoting a proliferative response in vascular smooth muscle cells, and alterations in the RAS and promotion of hypertensive state may explain the link between urate concentrations and cardiovascular disease. Contributing to this association, increased levels of monosodium urate have also been observed in atherosclerotic plaques.[41] Carotid intima-media thickness (IMT), regarded as a surrogate marker for atherosclerosis, has been shown to have a significant association with SU levels in cohort of healthy postmenopausal women, and also in a different cohort of hypertensive individuals with and without hyperuricemia.[42,43] Another study[44] also reported a dose response relation between SU and carotid atherosclerotic plaques in men with and without cardiovascular risk factors. However, the same group did not find any association between the levels of SU and coronary artery calcification (CAC).[45] The associations between SU, CAC, and IMT were reevaluated in an analysis of 5115 young adults aged 18 to 30 years and followed for 25 years. Using CAC and carotid IMT as markers of subclinical atherosclerosis, the investigators reported increased risks for CAC progression from years 15 to 25 with respect to baseline SU. For carotid IMT, SU at year 15 significantly predicted greater IMT at year 20, but this association remained significant in men only after adjusting for BMI. Greater increments in SU concentrations from years 0 to 15 were associated with higher risks of CAC progression and IMT.[46] These findings supported a role for SU as a potential biomarker of subclinical atherosclerosis in young adults.

Urate-induced endothelial dysfunction secondary to reduced NO production precedes plaque formation[47] and may play a more direct role (**Fig. 2**). A recent review and meta-analysis of the use of xanthine oxidase inhibitors for the treatment of cardiovascular disease[48] evaluated 3 outcome parameters (brachial artery flow–mediated

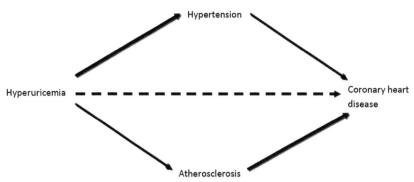

Fig. 2. Association and causality between hyperuricemia and coronary heart disease. Hyperuricemia has an indirect effect in the development of coronary heart disease through the development of hypertension and atherosclerosis. However, evidence on a direct and independent effect (*dashed arrow*) on the development of coronary heart disease is still not conclusive. (*Adapted from* Gaffo AL, Edwards NL, Saag KG. Gout. Hyperuricemia and cardiovascular disease: how strong is the evidence for a causal link? Arthritis Res Ther 2009;11(4):240.)

dilation, forearm blood flow responses to acetylcholine infusion, and circulating markers of oxidative stress) and showed a significant improvement in each of them in patients with, or at risk of, cardiovascular disease. However, data on this aspect are still not conclusive.

Since the Framingham Heart Study in 1999 failed to identify a significant association between SU, cardiovascular disease, and cardiovascular death,[49] several other population studies have presented contradictory evidence. An NHANES 2007–2008 analysis reported a 14% prevalence of myocardial infarction among individuals with gout, with an age-adjusted and sex-adjusted odds ratio (OR) of 2.68 (1.45 for men; 6.86 for women) compared with individuals who did not have gout. Prevalence of myocardial infarction in individuals with hyperuricemia was 5.7%, with an OR of 1.21 compared with normouricemic individuals. Prevalence of myocardial infarction was significantly higher in hyperuricemic or normouricemic individuals with gout (11.6% and 14.1%, respectively) compared with hyperuricemic individuals with no diagnosis of gout (5.7%).[5] Other studies also support an increased risk of coronary heart disease (CHD) in women with gout.[50] Recently, a population-based study of a Taiwanese cohort[51] also reported gout as an independent risk factor for myocardial infarction and stated that this risk was greater in younger individuals without cardiovascular risk factors.

An initial meta-analysis on the subject[52] reported a 13% increased risk (RR 1.13; 95% CI 1.07–1.20) of CHD among those in the top tertile of SU levels compared with those in the lowest tertile. A more recent meta-analysis of 26 studies with 402,997 adults[53] reported a modest but significant increased risk of CHD incidence and mortality on hyperuricemic individuals, 1.09 (95% CI 1.03–1.16) and 1.16 (95% CI 1.05–1.19), respectively, even after adjusting for traditional risk factors. A nonsignificant increased CHD mortality RR of 1.12 was reported for each 1-mg/dL SU increase, with only the women subgroup analysis having a statistically significant but modest increase. So, although statistically significant, evidence so far has shown a small increase in risk of both incidence and mortality in CHD with hyperuricemia.

Peripheral arterial disease (PAD) is another manifestation of atherosclerosis, and scarce evidence regarding an association with SU has been published. A cross-sectional study among 3987 participants in NHANES 1999–2009[54] found that higher

SU levels were significantly associated with PAD, independently from traditional cardiovascular risk factors. Another study analyzing data from the Multiple Risk Factor Intervention Trial[55] showed an increased, although nonsignificant, odds of having PAD in association with hyperuricemia with an OR of 1.23 (95% CI 0.98–1.54). However, a history of gout was associated with an OR of 1.33 (95% CI 1.07–1.66), even after adjustment of underlying hyperuricemia. These findings are regarded as insufficient to assume a possible therapeutic approach.[56,57]

Congestive heart failure

Increasing SU levels and hyperuricemia have been associated with increased incidence of congestive heart failure (CHF)[58,59] and increased mortality in patients with established CHF.[60–64] Data from NHANES 2007–2008 estimated increased point prevalences for CHF in hyperuricemic individuals compared with normouricemic individuals, with an OR of 2.52 (95% CI 1.58–4.04), and in individuals with gout compared with nongout, with an OR of 2.68 (95% CI 1.88–3.83).[5] An analysis of the Framingham offspring cohort of 4989 adults, with no clinical CHF at baseline, showed that individuals with gout had a 2 to 3 times higher incidence of CHF and echocardiographic measures of systolic dysfunction. Median follow-up time was 15.9 years. Mortality was increased in participants with gout, with an adjusted hazard ratio (HR) of 1.58 (95% CI 1.40–1.78), compared with people without gout, and this effect was also observed in subgroup analysis comparing individuals with gout and CHF compared with those with heart failure but without gout.[65]

However, evidence suggests that increased xanthine oxidase activity in damaged myocardial tissue results in the production of urate precursors and radical oxygen species, which are responsible for cardiac hypertrophy, myocardial fibrosis, left ventricular remodeling, and contractility impairment.[66] This finding poses urate as a marker of increased xanthine oxidase activity rather than a cause. Support for this hypothesis was provided by an analysis on CHF outcomes in patients with and without chronic kidney disease (CKD), which concluded that hyperuricemia is associated with a poor outcome in CHF without CKD but not in patients with CHF and CKD. In the former case, hyperuricemia would be secondary to increased xanthine oxidase activity, rather than impaired excretion like in CKD.[63] Although there are few therapeutic trials, data are suggestive of improvements in myocardial function and ejection fraction being secondary to xanthine oxidase inhibition rather than decreasing SU levels.[67–71]

Cerebrovascular disease

New evidence has emerged regarding an association between SU and cerebrovascular disease. A study using brain magnetic resonance imaging (MRI)[72] evaluated the aggregate volume of white matter hyperintense signals in a sample of 177 adults. High-normal SU (SU >5.75 mg/dL for men; >4.8 mg/dL for women) concentrations were associated with a significant increase in white matter hyperintense signals compared with participants with low to moderate SU levels. This association was still significant after adjusting for traditional risk factors. SU has also been postulated as a predictor of poor prognosis and recurrent events in stroke survivors.[73,74]

Results from NHANES 2007–2008[5] showed an increased incidence of stroke in individuals with gout, with an OR of 2.02 (95% CI 0.98–4.19) and hyperuricemia 1.74 (95% CI 1.16–2.59), compared with the control population. Although the risk was increased in women, this difference was not significant. A systematic review and meta-analysis[75] pooled a total of 16 studies including 238,449 adults and after adjusting for known risk factors, hyperuricemia was associated with a 47% (95% CI

1.19–1.76) increased risk of stroke and a 26% (95% CI 1.12–1.39) increased mortality. In this analysis, no significant difference by sex was observed. The intervention trials with ULT have had conflicting results on subclinical parameters,[76–78] and no evidence supporting use of ULT in stroke patients is available.

An association between SU concentrations and cardiovascular disease is becoming firmly established for hypertension and is an evolving field, with still insufficient evidence for atherosclerosis, coronary artery disease, stroke, and CHF. The first attempts at a leap to causality are being made by the development of interventional clinical trials aimed at decreasing SU levels and affecting cardiovascular outcomes.

Renal Disease

Urate and renal disease: laboratory and animal models
Almost 90% of the filtered urate is reabsorbed at the proximal tubule by the urate anion exchanger URAT-1, located at the apical membrane of tubular cells.[17,79] Urate regulation at the tubular level is a complex process that involves several other transporters, and conditions such as Lesch-Nyhan syndrome and tumor lysis syndrome, in which SU levels increase more than 10 mg/dL, cause renal damage through urate deposition in the tubuli.[79–81] Deposition of crystals within the tubuli has also been mentioned as an initial phase of the translocation of urate crystals to the interstitium and medulla, a component of the crystal-related nephropathy. This mechanism, which leads to tubular atrophy and vascular degeneration, used to be considered as the explanation for renal damage in patients with gout. However, with the decrease in incidence and severity of crystal nephropathy, this diagnosis is now considered only for specific subgroups, which include lead intoxication or genetic defeats leading to increased urate production.[79]

However, animal models have shown significant evidence of renal injury and disease in absence of crystal deposition. Systemic and glomerular hypertension with increased vascular resistance and reduced renal blood flow secondary to increased oxidative stress and endothelial dysfunction was observed in rats with oxonic acid–induced hyperuricemia. In 2 of these models, changes were reversed by using tempol (a superoxide scavenger) and L-arginine (a substrate for endothelial NO synthase).[18,82,83] Activation of the RAS also contributes to the development of vascular disease of the afferent arteriolar system and glomerular hypertrophy.[22,84] The development of arteriolopathy leads to glomerular hypoxia and ineffective autoregulation mechanisms, which further increases the damage to the glomerulus.[14,19] These changes result from specific mechanisms that involve stimulation of nicotinamide adenine dinucleotide phosphate (NADPH) oxidases with mitochondrial dysfunction,[85] production of reactive oxygen species,[86] activation of the RAS,[13] smooth muscle cell proliferation,[13] and induction of proinflammatory cytokines.[87] Recent data have also shown a direct effect of urate in tubular cells, promoting a phenotypic transition of renal tubular cells such as epithelial-to-mesenchymal transition by decreasing expression of E-cadherin synthesis.[88] Epithelial-to-mesenchymal transition is considered one of the initial phenomena in renal fibrosis.[89]

Hyperuricemia-induced renal damage has been shown to have a significant effect in animal models with preexisting renal disease. This effect has been proved in nephrectomy injury models, in which ULT was shown to improve blood pressure and renal function and decrease histologic changes.[21,90] In a model of cyclosporine nephropathy, increasing urate worsened renal disease and ULT ameliorated renal damage.[91,92] An animal model of diabetic mice also showed that reducing SU improved diabetic nephropathy by reducing tubulointerstitial injury, with no effect on glomerular damage.[93]

CKD

An association between hyperuricemia, including gout, and CKD has been frequently described in the literature and population studies. Data from NHANES 2007–2008 described a prevalence of CKD stage 3 or more in 19.9% of individuals with gout, associated with an OR of 2.32 (95% CI 1.65–3.26) when compared with individuals without gout. Prevalence in a hyperuricemic population was also significantly increased compared with a normouricemic population (14.8% vs 3.3%, respectively), with an OR of 3.96 (95% CI 2.63–5.97). Increased prevalence was observed with increasing values for SU.[5] Although the causality of these observations has been difficult to confirm, because of the increasing SU with declining renal function, evidence from experimental data explained a possible role of SU in the incidence and progression of CKD.

The largest epidemiologic study to date, which included 177,570 adults from the US Renal Data System for 25 years, reported an independent association between SU and risk for end-stage renal disease with an HR of 2.14 (1.65–2.77) when comparing the highest with the lowest quartile.[94] Another large cohort study evaluating 21,547 adults of the Vienna Health Screening project reported an almost double (OR 1.74; 95% CI 1.45–2.09) increased risk of kidney disease in individuals with SU levels between 7.0 and 8.9 mg/dL and a triple risk in individuals with levels more than 9.0 mg/dL (OR 3.12; 95% CI 2.29–4.25).[95] A pooled study from the Atherosclerosis Risks in Communities and the Cardiovascular Health Study cohorts and 2 analyses from the Okinawa General Health Maintenance Association Study cohort also support an association between SU and the development of end-stage renal disease.[96–98]

In IgA nephropathy, increased SU levels have also been reported as an independent predictor for the development of CKD.[99–101] In diabetic patients, increased SU levels have been described as an independent predictor of the development of diabetic nephropathy,[102] microalbuminuria and macroalbuminuria,[103] and declining renal function[104] in patients with type 1 diabetes. Hyperuricemia has also been associated, after adjusting for possible confounders, with an increased risk of incident CKD (OR 2.10; 95% CI 1.16–3.76) among patients with type 2 diabetes with normal kidney function.[105] However, data analyzing the association between progression of CKD and SU are still not conclusive. A recent study of middle-aged and elderly Taiwanese adults with stage 3 to 5 CKD concluded that increased urate levels increased the risk of renal disease only in stage 3 CKD but not in more advanced stages.[106] SU has also been reported as an independent risk factor for progression of kidney disease by other studies,[107,108] although no association has been reported.[109,110] This information may point to urate as a stronger risk factor for incidence rather than progression of CKD.[111]

Treatment with allopurinol in hyperuricemic individuals with normal renal function has shown a beneficial effect on estimated glomerular filtration rate (eGFR).[39,112] Interventional trials on patients with CKD, although scarce and small, have also shown supporting results. A randomized study of allopurinol and placebo in 54 patients with stage 3 to 4 CKD[113] showed a slowing in disease progression in the treatment arm compared with placebo. Another study[114] that included 113 patients with eGFR <60 mL/min/1.73 m^2 randomized patients either to allopurinol 100 mg/d or placebo for 24 months. After 24 months, there was no significant change in eGFR in the allopurinol group, whereas a significant decrease in eGFR was noticed in the control group. Allopurinol treatment slowed renal disease progression, estimating an HR reduction of 0.53 (95% CI 0.28–0.99). A beneficial effect on cardiovascular end points was also observed. A study using a different approach[115] randomized 50 patients with CKD 3 to 4 already on allopurinol for treatment of mild hyperuricemia, to either continuation or withdrawal of allopurinol. After allopurinol withdrawal, there was a significant acceleration in the decline of renal function as well as worsening hypertension. In a post hoc analysis of the RENAAAL (Reduction of Endpoints in NIDDM with the Angiotensin II Antagonist Losartan) trial, in which the intervention was treatment with the antihypertensive losartan, a reduction of 6% of renal events was observed for every 0.5-mg/dL reduction of SU. The impact of SU reduction over time on the renoprotective effect of losartan was estimated by adjusting for the residual SU in the analysis of renal events, and after observing a mild reduction on the effect of losartan (from 22% to 17%), the investigators concluded that one-fifth of the observed renoprotective effect of losartan was attributed to its uricosuric effect.[116] In diabetic patients with diabetic nephropathy, a small randomized placebo-controlled trial of 40 patients showed a reduction of proteinuria in patients treated with allopurinol.[117]

Acute kidney injury
Hyperuricemia and acute kidney injury (AKI), via crystal-dependent mechanisms, have usually been associated in the context of tumor lysis syndrome. However, based on the observations of experimental models on crystal-independent renal injury, a possible association of SU and AKI has been described. In a small trial evaluating the incidence of postoperative AKI in patients undergoing high-risk cardiovascular surgery,[118] SU greater than 6 mg/dL was associated with a 4-fold increase for AKI (OR 3.98; 95% CI 1.10–14.33). Poor survival after coronary artery bypass grafting has also been associated with increasing SU levels.[119] A more recent study of 190 patients who underwent cardiovascular surgery[120] reported increasing incidences of AKI (defined as absolute increase in serum creatinine level ≥ 0.3 mg/dL from baseline within 48 hours after surgery) with increasing levels of SU. In the multivariate analysis, SU levels starting from equal to or more than 5.5 mg/dL were associated with an increased risk, ascending up to a 35-fold (OR 35.4; 95% CI 9.7–128.7) with SU equal to or more than 7 mg/dL. A double-blind, placebo-controlled, randomized interventional trial using preoperative rasburicase in hyperuricemic patients undergoing high-risk cardiovascular surgery showed no benefit on postoperative serum creatinine levels. However, a decrease in the urine neutrophil–associated lipocalin (a predictive marker of AKI in cardiovascular surgery patients) was reported in the rasburicase-treated patients.[121] Information on this subject is still scarce and inconclusive.

Urolithiasis
Urate nephrolithiasis represents 7% to 10% of all nephrolithiases in the United States.[122] Most individuals suffering from urate kidney stones are neither hyperuricemic nor suffer from gout, because the usual abnormality observed in these individuals is consistently acidic urine (pH <5.5).[123,124] However, a large population study did report an association between the diagnosis of gout and an increased risk of incident kidney stones (RR 2.12; 95% CI 1.22–3.68).[125] Hyperuricosuria, decreased urinary pH, and low urinary volume are considered the 3 main factors involved in the development of urate nephrolithiasis.[80] The role of hyperuricemia and gout as risk factors may still not be clear, especially because studies have shown that most patients with gout are urate underexcretors.[124,126] A stronger association between urate nephrolithiasis with type 2 diabetes mellitus and obesity has been described and explained in the basis of predisposition to an acidic urinary environment.[80,122]

Evidence for urate crystal–independent mechanisms of renal injury, coupled to epidemiologic data, show a role for urate in the development of CKD. However, its importance in the progression of the disease and the potential use of ULT in patients with CKD is still unclear. Further clinical trials in patients with CKD are needed, as well as further information on the possible role of SU as a risk factor for AKI.

Metabolic Disease

Urate pathways and fructose: laboratory and animal models

The increased renal reabsorption of SU at the proximal tubules secondary to hyperinsulinemia has been regarded as the main hypothesis for the association between hyperuricemia and the metabolic syndrome (MS).[127,128] However, models incorporating fructose metabolism are uncovering the contributory role of urate in the MS. Fructose consumption, either in the forms of table sugar or high-fructose corn syrup (in beverage and food sweetening), has increased in the last 30 years, and epidemiologic data have shown similar increments in obesity and associations with certain components of the MS.[129–133] Fructose is phosphorylated by the enzyme fructokinase, which by having no negative feedback mechanism works uninterruptedly, causing intracellular phosphate and adenosine triphosphate depletion and increased activity by the adenosine monophosphate deaminase, leading to increased levels of urate.[134,135] An overlap of the increasing consumption of fructose and a corresponding trend of SU has been recognized.[136] Fructose-induced hyperuricemia has been proved to result in the development of insulin resistance (IR), hypertension, and renal injury in several animal models.[137–140] This process has also been reversed by the administration of xanthine oxidase inhibitors (allopurinol and febuxostat) and uricosuric drugs (benzodiarone), suggesting a dependency on SU concentrations and not xanthine oxidase activity.[139,140] Recent data on a trial using oxonic acid on rats fed with physiologic concentrations of fructose showed that although hyperuricemia did not increase body weight, blood pressure, or triglyceride levels, it did cause structural renal damage and significant increase in plasma insulin levels.[141] Increased plasma insulin level, through development of IR, is regarded as the potential central promoter of the MS.[142–144]

Based on findings and observations from experimental data, 2 different mechanisms that could explain the induction of IR, and hence hyperinsulinemia, have been proposed (**Fig. 3**).[111] First, hyperuricemia reduces endothelial NO bioavailabilty.[10,11] Because NO is necessary for glucose uptake in skeletal muscle, alterations in carbohydrate metabolism occur secondary to this deficiency.[145] Hypertension, another result of reduced NO bioavailability and damage to the endothelium has also been pointed as a possible mediator of the MS.[146] A second important mechanism results from the inflammatory and oxidative changes in adipose tissue secondary to exposure to increased concentrations of urate. Intracellular urate in adipocytes, probably after translocation by URAT-1 transporters, increases oxidative stress by an increase in the enzymatic activity of the reduced form of the NADPH oxidase, giving rise to

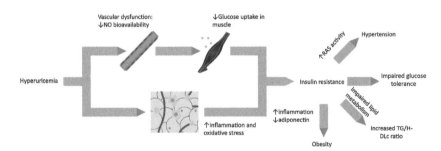

Fig. 3. Hyperuricemia, IR, and the MS. Experimental models have shown that hyperuricemia-induced vascular dysfunction, inflammation, and increased oxidative stress lead to IR, which leads to impaired glucose tolerance and predisposes to the other components of the MS. HDLc, high-density lipoprotein cholesterol; TG, triglycerides.

reactive oxygen species, which lead to protein nitrosylation, lipid peroxidation, and further NO reduction.[86] This process also induces macrophage infiltration, liberation of other inflammatory molecules such as monocyte chemotactic protein 1, and reduction of adiponectin.[146,147] These inflammatory and oxidative changes in adipocytes have been shown to cause MS in obese mice.[148] A study with obese hyperuricemic mice[147] showed that after decreasing urate levels with allopurinol, the proinflammatory endocrine imbalance was improved, with reduction of macrophage infiltration in adipose tissue, increase in adiponectin levels and reduction in IR.

IR and diabetes

As already seen in animal models, human studies have also shown an inverse correlation between high urate levels and insulin sensitivity.[149,150] A large population study of 53,477 Korean adults showed that SU levels were independently correlated with IR and that this risk, as for the MS, was maintained when patients were within the normal range.[151] Although a causal association is still in debate, a recent 15-year follow-up study of 5012 US nondiabetic adults has supported the contribution of SU to IR. After using regression models, it showed that individuals with hyperuricemia (defined as >7.0 mg/dL) were more likely to develop IR and prediabetes (HR 1.36 [95% CI 1.23–1.51] and 1.25 [95% CI 1.04–1.52], respectively).[152] Another study also supported a higher risk of developing hyperinsulinemia with increased baseline urate levels in nondiabetic patients.[153] Although interventional studies are still missing, a clinical trial of ULT with benzbromarone in patients with CHF and decreasing SU showed an improvement in IR.[71]

Type 2 diabetes mellitus, the final expression of IR, has also been associated with increasing SU concentrations in epidemiologic studies. A 15-year follow-up study reported an increased risk for the development of diabetes in individuals with hyperuricemia (HR 1.87; 95% CI 1.33–2.62).[152] An increased risk has also been reported by different cohorts.[29,154–158] Data from NHANES 2007–2008 showed that individuals with hyperuricemia presented an increased risk for diabetes (OR 1.63; 95% CI 1.13–2.34) and that this risk had a dose-dependent association with SU levels. Diabetes prevalence among individuals with gout was also increased compared with individuals without gout (25.7% and 7.8%, respectively), reflecting an increased risk for diabetes among individuals with gout.[5] However, data on this relation are still not conclusive, with several studies indicating either no association between SU and diabetes,[159] or even an inverse relationship between both.[160–162] Although results are based on epidemiologic data, causality is still controversial; use of SU as a predictor of all-cause mortality in type 2 diabetic patients was recommended in a study carried out on a cohort of 535 diabetic adults. This association remained significant after adjusting for other covariables.[163]

MS

The MS represents a cluster of physiologic and anthropometric abnormalities (IR, increased blood pressure, truncal obesity, hypertriglyceridemia, and low high-density lipoprotein cholesterol [HDLc]) and is regarded as a risk factor for the development of diabetes and cardiovascular diseases. An association between MS and hyperuricemia has been already been well described. An analysis of NHANES III data showed an increasing prevalence of the MS with increasing levels of SU, equal to or more than 10 mg/dL compared with individuals with levels less than 6.0 mg/dL (70.7% and 18.9%, respectively). A significant difference in prevalence between individuals with and without gout was also shown (62.8% and 25.4%, respectively).[164] The increasing risk of MS in individuals with higher SU levels has also been reported in other studies,[165,166] and the increased SU levels have also been observed to be significantly increased by the number of components of MS.[165,167,168] An increased risk has even been described in individuals with high-normal SU levels in a Korean cohort.[169]

Besides IR and hypertension, associations between SU and other individual components of the MS have also been described. In a study of 11,182 subjects older than 65 years old,[170] triglyceride levels and waist circumference showed a positive correlation with urate levels, whereas HDLc showed a negative correlation. These observations had been previously reported on patients with high cardiovascular risk in a population-based study in Spain.[171,172] A strong relationship between hyperuricemia, gout, and obesity has been well documented, and data from an analysis of NHANES 1988–1994 and 2007–2010 have shown a progressively greater prevalence of gout in higher BMI categories.[173] However, direct causality is still not clear, and it may involve leptin, adiponectin, and inflammation on adipocytes (see **Fig. 3**).[174] A study analyzing data from individuals with and without hyperuricemia in Taiwan[175] identified obesity and hypertriglyceridemia as possible potentiating factors on SU for the development of gout.

Neurologic Disorders

Antioxidants effects of urate

Compared with other mammals, higher levels of urate are secondary to the evolutionary loss of urate oxidase.[176,177] This mutation was seen as beneficial and part of adaptation by several investigators, who postulated the presence of urate as a stimulant with positive effects on cognition, alertness, and motivation,[178] or an antiaging effect through its ability to prevent oxidative damage.[179] Although the theories of the antioxidant capacity of urate were ignored because of the association of high urate levels and cardiovascular risk, evidence for its neuroprotective effects and association with neurodegenerative disorders have resurfaced.

Urate can act as a powerful scavenger for peroxynitrite,[180] peroxyl and hydroxyl radicals[181] and has been shown to reduce oxidative damage in DNA molecules.[182] In studies using cellular models of neurodegeneration, reduced oxidative stress and cell death have been associated with urate, and 1 study using a mouse model of Parkinson disease showed suppressed oxidative stress and death of dopaminergic cells.[183,184] In 1994, the first study reporting an association of SU and Parkinson disease in postmortem human tissue samples[185] showed that urate was significantly reduced in the substantia nigra of patients with Parkinson disease, and its addition decreased oxidation of dopamine in the caudate nucleus and substantia nigra.

Parkinson disease and other neurodegenerative conditions

The largest prospective study evaluating the relationship between hyperuricemia and the risk of developing Parkinson disease analyzed data from 18,018 men from the Health Professional Follow-up Study. During the observation period, 84 individuals were diagnosed with Parkinson disease, and after adjusting for other variables, the rate ratio for the highest quartile of uricemia compared with the lowest was 0.43 (95% CI 0.18–1.02).[186] Data from a more recent study, the Atherosclerosis Risk in Communities (ARIC) study,[187] reported a similar OR (0.4 [95% CI 0.2–10]), when comparing extreme quartiles of plasma urate. Data regarding risk of Parkinson disease on individuals with gout have also been reported by 2 studies. An analysis of the General Practice Research Database, which includes more than 3 million adults in the United Kingdom, reported that individuals with a previous history of gout had a lower risk, (OR 0.69; 95% CI 0.48–0.99) of developing Parkinson disease. This association was seen only in men.[188] Another study[189] based on an 8-year median follow-up of a Canadian cohort reported an adjusted RR of 0.70 (95% CI 0.59–0.83) among those with gout. A recent review on this subject[176] suggested, although still not at a clinical level, the feasibility of using SU as a risk, diagnostic, and prognostic marker for Parkinson disease.

Data supporting this association have also been observed in other neurodegenerative diseases. In multiple sclerosis, a study showed that lower urate levels correlated with a worse prognosis, which manifested as relapses.[190] A study of Huntington disease[191] showed that higher SU levels correlated with a slower disease progression and identified a trend of decreased worsening of motor function with increasing urate. Although evidence from interventional trials is lacking, a small trial with 11 patients with multiple sclerosis treated with inosine (aimed at increasing SU levels) showed clinical improvement in 3 of the patients, and no disease progression in the rest.[192] Evidence of this association is lacking, and further studies are needed to determine the nature of these observations.

COMORBIDITIES ASSOCIATED WITH CALCIUM PYROPHOSPHATE DIHYDRATE CRYSTAL DEPOSITION DISEASE

Pseudogout is just part of the spectrum of calcium pyrophosphate dihydrate crystal deposition (CPPD) disease, which also includes pyrophosphate arthropathy, asymptomatic chondrocalcinosis, and unusual presentations such as pseudorheumatoid arthritis or crowned dens syndrome.[193,194] Population studies using radiologic evidence of chondrocalcinosis have estimated prevalence ranging between 7% and 10%, usually in the population older than 60 years, and have proved a positive association with age.[195–198] However, prevalence can vary depending on the method of identification. Studies examining synovial fluid of osteoarthritic joints at the time of joint replacement have reported a 25% to 43% prevalence of CPPD crystals.[3] Data on CPPD, as well as on the associations with other comorbidities, are scarce. Most relevant evidence for these associations is presented in the following sections.

Osteoarthritis

An association between CPPD disease and osteoarthritis (OA) has been discussed and suggested for years; however, the precise nature of this relationship is still unclear, and the existence of common risk factors (eg, aging and joint injury), makes studying the relationship complex and challenging.[199,200] CPPD and other calcium crystals, such as basic calcium phosphate crystals, have been shown to generate calcium oscillations in articular chondrocytes[201] and a prolonged inflammatory response, which can contribute or amplify articular degeneration and joint damage.[202,203] Increased transcription of the progressive ankylosis homolog gene (ANKH), the mutations of which have been described in familial forms of CPPD disease,[204] has been reported in OA meniscal cells.[205]

The European League Against Rheumatism (EULAR) recommendations on CPPD disease analyzed the association with OA, taking into account 4 cross-sectional and 5 case-control studies. It estimated that people with OA were almost 3 times more likely to have CPPD (OR 2.66; 95% CI 2.00–3.54).[199] A study including 2 cohorts of people with knee OA and radiographic Kellgren scores of greater than or equal to 2 used MRI to explore the relation between radiographic chondrocalcinosis and OA progression. After 30 months of imaging and follow-up, cartilage loss, used as a proxy for progressive OA, showed no correlation with the presence of chondrocalcinosis.[206]

Table 1 Comorbidities and their association with hyperuricemia and gout		
Comorbidity	Evidence on Association and Causality	Evidence for Impact of Urate Therapies
Hypertension	Several population studies have proved an independent association between SU and development of hypertension[32,33] SU plays a key role in the initial stages of the development of hypertension[217]	Small-sampled controlled studies have shown reduction in blood pressure with ULT in young individuals[37,38] and adults[39]; however, evidence to recommend use of ULT is still not conclusive[40]
CHD	Although still not conclusive, evidence shows a small but significant increased risk of CHD in individuals with hyperuricemia[52,53] and patients with gout[51]	Trials on the use of allopurinol and angina exist, although evidence for CHD incidence and prognosis is still lacking
CHF	Although a constant association with increased incidence[58,59,65] and mortality,[60,61] causality is still under debate, because hyperuricemia may reflect only increased xanthine oxidase activity[63,66]	Small trials showing improvement in myocardial function and ejection fraction with allopurinol suggest benefits secondary to xanthine oxidase inhibition rather than SU decrease[69–71]
Stroke	Associations with cerebral ischemia,[72] increased incidence of stroke,[75] and poorer prognosis in patients with stroke have been reported[73,74]; however, causality is still not clear	Trials using ULT have shown conflicting results in subclinical parameters[76–78]
CKD	Experimental evidence on crystal-independent renal injury models[82–84] has supported epidemiologic evidence for a causative role of hyperuricemia on CKD[95–97]; however, data on effects of disease progression are still not conclusive[106,110]	Interventional studies with allopurinol have shown improvement in eGFR in normal individuals[39,112] and a decrease in renal function deterioration in patients with CKD[113–115]; data are still scarce to generalize recommendations for use of ULT
IR and MS	Experimental data have shown a causative role for urate in the development of IR, and an association with the development of IR[151,152] and the MS has been established[165,166,169]; associations with dyslipidemia[170] and obesity have been reported[173]	A role for ULT in animal models with MS has been shown,[140,147] and improvement in IR was seen in 1 trial with patients with CHF[71]; further trials are needed

(continued on next page)

Table 1
(continued)

Comorbidity	Evidence on Association and Causality	Evidence for Impact of Urate Therapies
Type 2 diabetes mellitus	Increasing incidence in individuals with hyperuricemia has been shown.[152,154,155] Studies of an association between gout and diabetes are still not conclusive, with some studies even showing an inverse relation between both[159,160,162]	Data on this subject are still lacking to consider further recommendations
Neurodegenerative disorders	An association between hyperuricemia and a decreased incidence with Parkinson disease[186–188] as a slower development of multiples sclerosis[190] and Huntington disease has been reported; data on the subject are scarce[191]	A small trial in patients with multiple sclerosis showed clinical improvements in 3 of the patients while increasing SU with inosine[192]; further trials are needed

Evidence about this subject is still not conclusive, and although calcium crystals may be involved in the process of OA, more studies are needed.

Metabolic and Endocrine Disorders

A relationship between hemochromatosis and CPPD disease has been described. A study of 178 patients diagnosed with hereditary hemochromatosis and not yet treated with phlebotomy[207] showed a 30% prevalence of chondrocalcinosis and a positive correlation between the number of joints involved with age, ferritin level, and PTH 44–68. An older case series of 54 patients with hemochromatosis reported a significant association (OR 6.81; 95% CI 2.02–22.95) with chondrocalcinosis.[208] Although still under debate, the significance of this association may be relatively small. This observation was shown by a study that carried out systematic genetic testing of 128 patients with chondrocalcinosis and pseudogout, which reported a low prevalence of C282Y homozygotes and C282Y/H63D compound heterozygotes (1.6% and 3.1%, respectively).[209]

The 2011 EULAR report on CPPD disease, which pooled data from 5 studies, described an association between CPPD disease and hyperparathyroidism, showing that patients with hyperparathyroidism were 3 times more likely to have CPPD than controls (OR 3.03; 95% CI 1.15–8.02).[199] Triggering of pseudogout attacks by parathyroidectomy has also been reported by some studies.[210,211] However, data on this association are still scarce.

A cross-sectional study of 72 patients with intestinal failure and in parenteral nutrition showed a significant association between hypomagnesemia and chondrocalcinosis. Compared with healthy controls, these patients with chronic hypomagnesemia presented a higher prevalence of chondrocalcinosis (16.6% vs 2.7% in controls), and prevalence of chondrocalcinosis was significantly higher (OR 13.5; 95% CI 2.76–127.3) in patients with lower serum magnesium levels.[212] Reports on Gitelman syndrome and chondrocalcinosis support this association.[213,214] CPPD arthropathy or pseudogout can be the onset of presentation of Gitelman syndrome, and this disease should be considered in the differential of younger patients presenting with CPPD disease.[215]

Hypophosphatasia, gout, ochronosis, familial hypocalciuric hypercalcemia, X-linked hypophostatemic rickets, Wilson disease, and acromegaly are additional diseases that have been linked to CPPD disease. However, data on these associations are based only on case reports.[216]

SUMMARY

The clinical significance of asymptomatic hyperuricemia and gout as risk factors for various comorbidities has been supported recently by the emergence of new data from experimental, epidemiologic, and clinical intervention trials (**Table 1**). Evidence available is supportive of a causal role of hyperuricemia on hypertension, leaving SU as a possible therapeutic target, especially on early stages. Although interventional data from small trials are available and do suggest a benefit, larger trials are needed to collect enough evidence to support indication of ULT. Evidence for CHD and stroke, although suggested, is still not clear and further studies are required. The association between CHF and urate is probably indirect and related to an increased activity by xanthine oxidase, and benefit of xanthine oxidase inhibition is still not conclusive. Cardiovascular comorbidities are an important consideration in the management of gout patients.

Although SU was initially not considered to be a cause for the development of the MS, fructose-fed animal models have shown evidence of involvement of urate in the pathologic process of IR. This association requires further studies but suggests a connection between the overlapping increases of their respective prevalences. However, an association between hyperuricemia, gout, and diabetes is still not clear. The relationship between hyperuricemia and CKD incidence is also becoming clearer in the light of new experimental and epidemiologic evidence; however, the relation to effects on CKD progression is still not conclusive. Recent data on AKI deserve further attention. The associations between SU and neurodegenerative diseases are still not clear, and further evidence is needed to show if this represents only an observation or a potential therapeutic strategy.

Calcium deposition diseases, such as CPPD, represent a low proportion of crystal arthropathies, and studies on the subject are still scarce. Although interest in the role of calcium crystals in the development of OA is increasing, data are still lacking for conclusions to be drawn. The association between CPPD disease and several metabolic and endocrine disorders has been established based on several small studies; however, the association is too small to consider an active search for these disorders in patients with CPPD disease.

REFERENCES

1. Lawrence RC, Felson DT, Helmick CG, et al. Estimates of the prevalence of arthritis and other rheumatic conditions in the United States. Part II. Arthritis Rheum 2008;58:26–35.
2. Zhu Y, Pandya BJ, Choi HK. Prevalence of gout and hyperuricemia in the US general population: the National Health and Nutrition Examination Survey 2007-2008. Arthritis Rheum 2011;63:3136–41.
3. Richette P, Bardin T, Doherty M. An update on the epidemiology of calcium pyrophosphate dihydrate crystal deposition disease. Rheumatology (Oxford) 2009;48:711–5.

4. Singh JA, Strand V. Gout is associated with more comorbidities, poorer health-related quality of life and higher healthcare utilisation in US veterans. Ann Rheum Dis 2008;67:1310–6.

5. Zhu Y, Pandya BJ, Choi HK. Comorbidities of gout and hyperuricemia in the US general population: NHANES 2007-2008. Am J Med 2012;125:679–87.e1.

6. Annemans L, Spaepen E, Gaskin M, et al. Gout in the UK and Germany: prevalence, comorbidities and management in general practice 2000-2005. Ann Rheum Dis 2008;67:960–6.

7. Robinson PC, Merriman TR, Herbison P, et al. Hospital admissions associated with gout and their comorbidities in New Zealand and England 1999-2009. Rheumatology (Oxford) 2013;52:118–26.

8. Sari I, Akar S, Pakoz B, et al. Hyperuricemia and its related factors in an urban population, Izmir, Turkey. Rheumatol Int 2009;29:869–74.

9. Loeb JN. The influence of temperature on the solubility of monosodium urate. Arthritis Rheum 1972;15:189–92.

10. Zharikov S, Krotova K, Hu H, et al. Uric acid decreases NO production and increases arginase activity in cultured pulmonary artery endothelial cells. Am J Physiol Cell Physiol 2008;295:C1183–90.

11. Khosla UM, Zharikov S, Finch JL, et al. Hyperuricemia induces endothelial dysfunction. Kidney Int 2005;67:1739–42.

12. Rao GN, Corson MA, Berk BC. Uric acid stimulates vascular smooth muscle cell proliferation by increasing platelet-derived growth factor A-chain expression. J Biol Chem 1991;266:8604–8.

13. Corry DB, Eslami P, Yamamoto K, et al. Uric acid stimulates vascular smooth muscle cell proliferation and oxidative stress via the vascular renin-angiotensin system. J Hypertens 2008;26:269–75.

14. Mazzali M, Kanellis J, Han L, et al. Hyperuricemia induces a primary renal arteriolopathy in rats by a blood pressure-independent mechanism. Am J Physiol Renal Physiol 2002;282:F991–7.

15. Chao HH, Liu JC, Lin JW, et al. Uric acid stimulates endothelin-1 gene expression associated with NADPH oxidase in human aortic smooth muscle cells. Acta Pharmacol Sin 2008;29:1301–12.

16. Cheng TH, Lin JW, Chao HH, et al. Uric acid activates extracellular signal-regulated kinases and thereafter endothelin-1 expression in rat cardiac fibroblasts. Int J Cardiol 2010;139:42–9.

17. Enomoto A, Kimura H, Chairoungdua A, et al. Molecular identification of a renal urate anion exchanger that regulates blood urate levels. Nature 2002;417:447–52.

18. Sanchez-Lozada LG, Tapia E, Santamaria J, et al. Mild hyperuricemia induces vasoconstriction and maintains glomerular hypertension in normal and remnant kidney rats. Kidney Int 2005;67:237–47.

19. Sanchez-Lozada LG, Tapia E, Avila-Casado C, et al. Mild hyperuricemia induces glomerular hypertension in normal rats. Am J Physiol Renal Physiol 2002;283:F1105–10.

20. Sanchez-Lozada LG, Tapia E, Soto V, et al. Treatment with the xanthine oxidase inhibitor febuxostat lowers uric acid and alleviates systemic and glomerular hypertension in experimental hyperuricaemia. Nephrol Dial Transplant 2008;23:1179–85.

21. Sanchez-Lozada LG, Tapia E, Soto V, et al. Effect of febuxostat on the progression of renal disease in 5/6 nephrectomy rats with and without hyperuricemia. Nephron Physiol 2008;108:69–78.

22. Mazzali M, Hughes J, Kim YG, et al. Elevated uric acid increases blood pressure in the rat by a novel crystal-independent mechanism. Hypertension 2001;38: 1101–6.
23. Feig DI. The role of uric acid in the pathogenesis of hypertension in the young. J Clin Hypertens (Greenwich) 2012;14:346–52.
24. Sundstrom J, Sullivan L, D'Agostino RB, et al. Relations of serum uric acid to longitudinal blood pressure tracking and hypertension incidence. Hypertension 2005;45:28–33.
25. Krishnan E, Kwoh CK, Schumacher HR, et al. Hyperuricemia and incidence of hypertension among men without metabolic syndrome. Hypertension 2007;49: 298–303.
26. Masuo K, Kawaguchi H, Mikami H, et al. Serum uric acid and plasma norepinephrine concentrations predict subsequent weight gain and blood pressure elevation. Hypertension 2003;42:474–80.
27. Mellen PB, Bleyer AJ, Erlinger TP, et al. Serum uric acid predicts incident hypertension in a biethnic cohort: the atherosclerosis risk in communities study. Hypertension 2006;48:1037–42.
28. Nagahama K, Inoue T, Iseki K, et al. Hyperuricemia as a predictor of hypertension in a screened cohort in Okinawa, Japan. Hypertens Res 2004;27:835–41.
29. Nakanishi N, Okamoto M, Yoshida H, et al. Serum uric acid and risk for development of hypertension and impaired fasting glucose or Type II diabetes in Japanese male office workers. Eur J Epidemiol 2003;18:523–30.
30. Gaffo AL, Jacobs DR Jr, Sijtsma F, et al. Serum urate association with hypertension in young adults: analysis from the Coronary Artery Risk Development in Young Adults cohort. Ann Rheum Dis 2013;72(8):1321–7.
31. Perlstein TS, Gumieniak O, Williams GH, et al. Uric acid and the development of hypertension: the normative aging study. Hypertension 2006;48:1031–6.
32. Grayson PC, Kim SY, LaValley M, et al. Hyperuricemia and incident hypertension: a systematic review and meta-analysis. Arthritis Care Res 2011;63:102–10.
33. Zhang W, Sun K, Yang Y, et al. Plasma uric acid and hypertension in a Chinese community: prospective study and metaanalysis. Clin Chem 2009;55:2026–34.
34. Feig DI, Johnson RJ. Hyperuricemia in childhood primary hypertension. Hypertension 2003;42:247–52.
35. Viazzi F, Antolini L, Giussani M, et al. Serum uric acid and blood pressure in children at cardiovascular risk. Pediatrics 2013;132:e93–9.
36. Hongo M, Hidaka H, Sakaguchi S, et al. Association between serum uric acid levels and cardiometabolic risk factors among Japanese junior high school students. Circ J 2010;74:1570–7.
37. Feig DI, Soletsky B, Johnson RJ. Effect of allopurinol on blood pressure of adolescents with newly diagnosed essential hypertension: a randomized trial. JAMA 2008;300:924–32.
38. Soletsky B, Feig DI. Uric acid reduction rectifies prehypertension in obese adolescents. Hypertension 2012;60:1148–56.
39. Kanbay M, Huddam B, Azak A, et al. A randomized study of allopurinol on endothelial function and estimated glomerular filtration rate in asymptomatic hyperuricemic subjects with normal renal function. Clin J Am Soc Nephrol 2011;6: 1887–94.
40. Gois PH, Souza ER. Pharmacotherapy for hyperuricemia in hypertensive patients. Cochrane Database Syst Rev 2013;(1):CD008652.
41. Patetsios P, Rodino W, Wisselink W, et al. Identification of uric acid in aortic aneurysms and atherosclerotic artery. Ann N Y Acad Sci 1996;800:243–5.

42. Montalcini T, Gorgone G, Gazzaruso C, et al. Relation between serum uric acid and carotid intima-media thickness in healthy postmenopausal women. Intern Emerg Med 2007;2:19–23.
43. Tavil Y, Kaya MG, Oktar SO, et al. Uric acid level and its association with carotid intima-media thickness in patients with hypertension. Atherosclerosis 2008;197: 159–63.
44. Neogi T, Ellison RC, Hunt S, et al. Serum uric acid is associated with carotid plaques: the National Heart, Lung, and Blood Institute Family Heart Study. J Rheumatol 2009;36:378–84.
45. Neogi T, Terkeltaub R, Ellison RC, et al. Serum urate is not associated with coronary artery calcification: the NHLBI Family Heart Study. J Rheumatol 2011;38: 111–7.
46. Wang H, Jacobs DR Jr, Gaffo AL, et al. Longitudinal association between serum urate and subclinical atherosclerosis: the Coronary Artery Risk Development in Young Adults (CARDIA) study. J Intern Med 2013;274(6):594–609.
47. Rabelink TJ, Luscher TF. Endothelial nitric oxide synthase: host defense enzyme of the endothelium? Arterioscler Thromb Vasc Biol 2006;26:267–71.
48. Higgins P, Dawson J, Lees KR, et al. Xanthine oxidase inhibition for the treatment of cardiovascular disease: a systematic review and meta-analysis. Cardiovasc Ther 2012;30:217–26.
49. Culleton BF, Larson MG, Kannel WB, et al. Serum uric acid and risk for cardiovascular disease and death: the Framingham Heart Study. Ann Intern Med 1999;131:7–13.
50. De Vera MA, Rahman MM, Bhole V, et al. Independent impact of gout on the risk of acute myocardial infarction among elderly women: a population-based study. Ann Rheum Dis 2010;69:1162–4.
51. Kuo CF, Yu KH, See LC, et al. Risk of myocardial infarction among patients with gout: a nationwide population-based study. Rheumatology (Oxford) 2013;52:111–7.
52. Wheeler JG, Juzwishin KD, Eiriksdottir G, et al. Serum uric acid and coronary heart disease in 9,458 incident cases and 155,084 controls: prospective study and meta-analysis. PLoS Med 2005;2:e76.
53. Kim SY, Guevara JP, Kim KM, et al. Hyperuricemia and coronary heart disease: a systematic review and meta-analysis. Arthritis Care Res 2010;62:170–80.
54. Shankar A, Klein BE, Nieto FJ, et al. Association between serum uric acid level and peripheral arterial disease. Atherosclerosis 2008;196:749–55.
55. Baker JF, Schumacher HR, Krishnan E. Serum uric acid level and risk for peripheral arterial disease: analysis of data from the multiple risk factor intervention trial. Angiology 2007;58:450–7.
56. Langlois M, De Bacquer D, Duprez D, et al. Serum uric acid in hypertensive patients with and without peripheral arterial disease. Atherosclerosis 2003;168: 163–8.
57. Tseng CH. Independent association of uric acid levels with peripheral arterial disease in Taiwanese patients with type 2 diabetes. Diabet Med 2004;21:724–9.
58. Ekundayo OJ, Dell'Italia LJ, Sanders PW, et al. Association between hyperuricemia and incident heart failure among older adults: a propensity-matched study. Int J Cardiol 2010;142:279–87.
59. Krishnan E. Hyperuricemia and incident heart failure. Circ Heart Fail 2009;2: 556–62.
60. Strasak AM, Kelleher CC, Brant LJ, et al. Serum uric acid is an independent predictor for all major forms of cardiovascular death in 28,613 elderly women: a prospective 21-year follow-up study. Int J Cardiol 2008;125:232–9.

61. Strasak A, Ruttmann E, Brant L, et al. Serum uric acid and risk of cardiovascular mortality: a prospective long-term study of 83,683 Austrian men. Clin Chem 2008;54:273–84.
62. Chen JH, Chuang SY, Chen HJ, et al. Serum uric acid level as an independent risk factor for all-cause, cardiovascular, and ischemic stroke mortality: a Chinese cohort study. Arthritis Rheum 2009;61:225–32.
63. Filippatos GS, Ahmed MI, Gladden JD, et al. Hyperuricaemia, chronic kidney disease, and outcomes in heart failure: potential mechanistic insights from epidemiological data. Eur Heart J 2011;32:712–20.
64. Tamariz L, Harzand A, Palacio A, et al. Uric acid as a predictor of all-cause mortality in heart failure: a meta-analysis. Congest Heart Fail 2011;17:25–30.
65. Krishnan E. Gout and the risk for incident heart failure and systolic dysfunction. BMJ Open 2012;2:e000282.
66. Bergamini C, Cicoira M, Rossi A, et al. Oxidative stress and hyperuricaemia: pathophysiology, clinical relevance, and therapeutic implications in chronic heart failure. Eur J Heart Fail 2009;11:444–52.
67. Hare JM, Mangal B, Brown J, et al. Impact of oxypurinol in patients with symptomatic heart failure. Results of the OPT-CHF study. J Am Coll Cardiol 2008;51: 2301–9.
68. Cingolani HE, Plastino JA, Escudero EM, et al. The effect of xanthine oxidase inhibition upon ejection fraction in heart failure patients: La Plata Study. J Card Fail 2006;12:491–8.
69. George J, Carr E, Davies J, et al. High-dose allopurinol improves endothelial function by profoundly reducing vascular oxidative stress and not by lowering uric acid. Circulation 2006;114:2508–16.
70. Noman A, Ang DS, Ogston S, et al. Effect of high-dose allopurinol on exercise in patients with chronic stable angina: a randomised, placebo controlled crossover trial. Lancet 2010;375:2161–7.
71. Ogino K, Kato M, Furuse Y, et al. Uric acid-lowering treatment with benzbromarone in patients with heart failure: a double-blind placebo-controlled crossover preliminary study. Circ Heart Fail 2010;3:73–81.
72. Schretlen DJ, Inscore AB, Vannorsdall TD, et al. Serum uric acid and brain ischemia in normal elderly adults. Neurology 2007;69:1418–23.
73. Wong KY, MacWalter RS, Fraser HW, et al. Urate predicts subsequent cardiac death in stroke survivors. Eur Heart J 2002;23:788–93.
74. Weir CJ, Muir SW, Walters MR, et al. Serum urate as an independent predictor of poor outcome and future vascular events after acute stroke. Stroke 2003;34:1951–6.
75. Kim SY, Guevara JP, Kim KM, et al. Hyperuricemia and risk of stroke: a systematic review and meta-analysis. Arthritis Rheum 2009;61:885–92.
76. Muir SW, Harrow C, Dawson J, et al. Allopurinol use yields potentially beneficial effects on inflammatory indices in those with recent ischemic stroke: a randomized, double-blind, placebo-controlled trial. Stroke 2008;39:3303–7.
77. Khan F, George J, Wong K, et al. Allopurinol treatment reduces arterial wave reflection in stroke survivors. Cardiovasc Ther 2008;26:247–52.
78. Dawson J, Quinn TJ, Harrow C, et al. The effect of allopurinol on the cerebral vasculature of patients with subcortical stroke; a randomized trial. Br J Clin Pharmacol 2009;68:662–8.
79. Cameron JS. Uric acid and renal disease. Nucleosides Nucleotides Nucleic Acids 2006;25:1055–64.
80. Cameron MA, Sakhaee K. Uric acid nephrolithiasis. Urol Clin North Am 2007;34: 335–46.

81. Cameron JS, Moro F, Simmonds HA. Gout, uric acid and purine metabolism in paediatric nephrology. Pediatr Nephrol 1993;7:105–18.
82. Sanchez-Lozada LG, Soto V, Tapia E, et al. Role of oxidative stress in the renal abnormalities induced by experimental hyperuricemia. Am J Physiol Renal Physiol 2008;295:F1134–41.
83. Sanchez-Lozada LG, Tapia E, Lopez-Molina R, et al. Effects of acute and chronic L-arginine treatment in experimental hyperuricemia. Am J Physiol Renal Physiol 2007;292:F1238–44.
84. Nakagawa T, Mazzali M, Kang DH, et al. Hyperuricemia causes glomerular hypertrophy in the rat. Am J Nephrol 2003;23:2–7.
85. Sanchez-Lozada LG, Lanaspa MA, Cristobal-Garcia M, et al. Uric acid-induced endothelial dysfunction is associated with mitochondrial alterations and decreased intracellular ATP concentrations. Nephron Exp Nephrol 2012;121:e71–8.
86. Sautin YY, Nakagawa T, Zharikov S, et al. Adverse effects of the classic antioxidant uric acid in adipocytes: NADPH oxidase-mediated oxidative/nitrosative stress. Am J Physiol Cell Physiol 2007;293:C584–96.
87. Kanellis J, Watanabe S, Li JH, et al. Uric acid stimulates monocyte chemoattractant protein-1 production in vascular smooth muscle cells via mitogen-activated protein kinase and cyclooxygenase-2. Hypertension 2003;41:1287–93.
88. Ryu ES, Kim MJ, Shin HS, et al. Uric acid-induced phenotypic transition of renal tubular cells as a novel mechanism of chronic kidney disease. Am J Physiol Renal Physiol 2013;304:F471–80.
89. Zeisberg M, Kalluri R. The role of epithelial-to-mesenchymal transition in renal fibrosis. J Mol Med (Berl) 2004;82:175–81.
90. Kang DH, Nakagawa T, Feng L, et al. A role for uric acid in the progression of renal disease. J Am Soc Nephrol 2002;13:2888–97.
91. Mazali FC, Johnson RJ, Mazzali M. Use of uric acid-lowering agents limits experimental cyclosporine nephropathy. Nephron Exp Nephrol 2012;120:e12–9.
92. Mazzali M, Kim YG, Suga S, et al. Hyperuricemia exacerbates chronic cyclosporine nephropathy. Transplantation 2001;71:900–5.
93. Kosugi T, Nakayama T, Heinig M, et al. Effect of lowering uric acid on renal disease in the type 2 diabetic db/db mice. Am J Physiol Renal Physiol 2009;297:F481–8.
94. Hsu CY, Iribarren C, McCulloch CE, et al. Risk factors for end-stage renal disease: 25-year follow-up. Arch Intern Med 2009;169:342–50.
95. Obermayr RP, Temml C, Gutjahr G, et al. Elevated uric acid increases the risk for kidney disease. J Am Soc Nephrol 2008;19:2407–13.
96. Weiner DE, Tighiouart H, Elsayed EF, et al. Uric acid and incident kidney disease in the community. J Am Soc Nephrol 2008;19:1204–11.
97. Iseki K, Ikemiya Y, Inoue T, et al. Significance of hyperuricemia as a risk factor for developing ESRD in a screened cohort. Am J Kidney Dis 2004;44:642–50.
98. Iseki K, Oshiro S, Tozawa M, et al. Significance of hyperuricemia on the early detection of renal failure in a cohort of screened subjects. Hypertens Res 2001;24:691–7.
99. Ohno I, Hosoya T, Gomi H, et al. Serum uric acid and renal prognosis in patients with IgA nephropathy. Nephron 2001;87:333–9.
100. Syrjanen J, Mustonen J, Pasternack A. Hypertriglyceridaemia and hyperuricaemia are risk factors for progression of IgA nephropathy. Nephrol Dial Transplant 2000;15:34–42.

101. Shi Y, Chen W, Jalal D, et al. Clinical outcome of hyperuricemia in IgA nephropathy: a retrospective cohort study and randomized controlled trial. Kidney Blood Press Res 2012;35:153–60.
102. Hovind P, Rossing P, Tarnow L, et al. Serum uric acid as a predictor for development of diabetic nephropathy in type 1 diabetes: an inception cohort study. Diabetes 2009;58:1668–71.
103. Jalal DI, Rivard CJ, Johnson RJ, et al. Serum uric acid levels predict the development of albuminuria over 6 years in patients with type 1 diabetes: findings from the Coronary Artery Calcification in Type 1 Diabetes study. Nephrol Dial Transplant 2010;25:1865–9.
104. Ficociello LH, Rosolowsky ET, Niewczas MA, et al. High-normal serum uric acid increases risk of early progressive renal function loss in type 1 diabetes: results of a 6-year follow-up. Diabetes Care 2010;33:1337–43.
105. Zoppini G, Targher G, Chonchol M, et al. Serum uric acid levels and incident chronic kidney disease in patients with type 2 diabetes and preserved kidney function. Diabetes care 2012;35:99–104.
106. Chang HY, Tung CW, Lee PH, et al. Hyperuricemia as an independent risk factor of chronic kidney disease in middle-aged and elderly population. Am J Med Sci 2010;339:509–15.
107. Chonchol M, Shlipak MG, Katz R, et al. Relationship of uric acid with progression of kidney disease. Am J Kidney Dis 2007;50:239–47.
108. Madero M, Sarnak MJ, Wang X, et al. Uric acid and long-term outcomes in CKD. Am J Kidney Dis 2009;53:796–803.
109. Hunsicker LG, Adler S, Caggiula A, et al. Predictors of the progression of renal disease in the Modification of Diet in Renal Disease Study. Kidney Int 1997;51:1908–19.
110. Sturm G, Kollerits B, Neyer U, et al. Uric acid as a risk factor for progression of non-diabetic chronic kidney disease? The Mild to Moderate Kidney Disease (MMKD) Study. Exp Gerontol 2008;43:347–52.
111. Gustafsson D, Unwin R. The pathophysiology of hyperuricaemia and its possible relationship to cardiovascular disease, morbidity and mortality. BMC Nephrol 2013;14:164.
112. Kanbay M, Ozkara A, Selcoki Y, et al. Effect of treatment of hyperuricemia with allopurinol on blood pressure, creatinine clearance, and proteinuria in patients with normal renal functions. Int Urol Nephrol 2007;39:1227–33.
113. Siu YP, Leung KT, Tong MK, et al. Use of allopurinol in slowing the progression of renal disease through its ability to lower serum uric acid level. Am J Kidney Dis 2006;47:51–9.
114. Goicoechea M, de Vinuesa SG, Verdalles U, et al. Effect of allopurinol in chronic kidney disease progression and cardiovascular risk. Clin J Am Soc Nephrol 2010;5:1388–93.
115. Talaat KM, el-Sheikh AR. The effect of mild hyperuricemia on urinary transforming growth factor beta and the progression of chronic kidney disease. Am J Nephrol 2007;27:435–40.
116. Miao Y, Ottenbros SA, Laverman GD, et al. Effect of a reduction in uric acid on renal outcomes during losartan treatment: a post hoc analysis of the reduction of endpoints in non-insulin-dependent diabetes mellitus with the Angiotensin II Antagonist Losartan Trial. Hypertension 2011;58:2–7.
117. Momeni A, Shahidi S, Seirafian S, et al. Effect of allopurinol in decreasing proteinuria in type 2 diabetic patients. Iran J Kidney Dis 2010;4:128–32.

118. Ejaz AA, Beaver TM, Shimada M, et al. Uric acid: a novel risk factor for acute kidney injury in high-risk cardiac surgery patients? Am J Nephrol 2009;30: 425–9.
119. Hillis GS, Cuthbertson BH, Gibson PH, et al. Uric acid levels and outcome from coronary artery bypass grafting. J Thorac Cardiovasc Surg 2009;138:200–5.
120. Lapsia V, Johnson RJ, Dass B, et al. Elevated uric acid increases the risk for acute kidney injury. Am J Med 2012;125:302.e9–17.
121. Ejaz AA, Dass B, Lingegowda V, et al. Effect of uric acid lowering therapy on the prevention of acute kidney injury in cardiovascular surgery. Int Urol Nephrol 2013;45:449–58.
122. Mehta TH, Goldfarb DS. Uric acid stones and hyperuricosuria. Adv Chronic Kidney Dis 2012;19:413–8.
123. Kamel KS, Cheema-Dhadli S, Halperin ML. Studies on the pathophysiology of the low urine pH in patients with uric acid stones. Kidney Int 2002;61:988–94.
124. Sakhaee K, Adams-Huet B, Moe OW, et al. Pathophysiologic basis for normouricosuric uric acid nephrolithiasis. Kidney Int 2002;62:971–9.
125. Kramer HJ, Choi HK, Atkinson K, et al. The association between gout and nephrolithiasis in men: the Health Professionals' Follow-Up Study. Kidney Int 2003;64: 1022–6.
126. Alvarez-Nemegyei J, Medina-Escobedo M, Villanueva-Jorge S, et al. Prevalence and risk factors for urolithiasis in primary gout: is a reappraisal needed? J Rheumatol 2005;32:2189–91.
127. Facchini F, Chen YD, Hollenbeck CB, et al. Relationship between resistance to insulin-mediated glucose uptake, urinary uric acid clearance, and plasma uric acid concentration. JAMA 1991;266:3008–11.
128. Reaven GM. The kidney: an unwilling accomplice in syndrome X. Am J Kidney Dis 1997;30:928–31.
129. Bray GA, Nielsen SJ, Popkin BM. Consumption of high-fructose corn syrup in beverages may play a role in the epidemic of obesity. Am J Clin Nutr 2004; 79:537–43.
130. Dhingra R, Sullivan L, Jacques PF, et al. Soft drink consumption and risk of developing cardiometabolic risk factors and the metabolic syndrome in middle-aged adults in the community. Circulation 2007;116:480–8.
131. Ludwig DS, Peterson KE, Gortmaker SL. Relation between consumption of sugar-sweetened drinks and childhood obesity: a prospective, observational analysis. Lancet 2001;357:505–8.
132. Nguyen S, Choi HK, Lustig RH, et al. Sugar-sweetened beverages, serum uric acid, and blood pressure in adolescents. J Pediatr 2009;154:807–13.
133. Malik VS, Popkin BM, Bray GA, et al. Sugar-sweetened beverages and risk of metabolic syndrome and type 2 diabetes: a meta-analysis. Diabetes Care 2010;33:2477–83.
134. Fox IH, Kelley WN. Studies on the mechanism of fructose-induced hyperuricemia in man. Metabolism 1972;21:713–21.
135. van den Berghe G, Bronfman M, Vanneste R, et al. The mechanism of adenosine triphosphate depletion in the liver after a load of fructose. A kinetic study of liver adenylate deaminase. Biochem J 1977;162:601–9.
136. Rho YH, Zhu Y, Choi HK. The epidemiology of uric acid and fructose. Semin Nephrol 2011;31:410–9.
137. Nakayama T, Kosugi T, Gersch M, et al. Dietary fructose causes tubulointerstitial injury in the normal rat kidney. Am J Physiol Renal Physiol 2010;298: F712–20.

138. Sanchez-Lozada LG, Tapia E, Jimenez A, et al. Fructose-induced metabolic syndrome is associated with glomerular hypertension and renal microvascular damage in rats. Am J Physiol Renal Physiol 2007;292:F423–9.
139. Nakagawa T, Hu H, Zharikov S, et al. A causal role for uric acid in fructose-induced metabolic syndrome. Am J Physiol Renal Physiol 2006;290:F625–31.
140. Sanchez-Lozada LG, Tapia E, Bautista-Garcia P, et al. Effects of febuxostat on metabolic and renal alterations in rats with fructose-induced metabolic syndrome. Am J Physiol Renal Physiol 2008;294:F710–8.
141. Lanaspa MA, Tapia E, Soto V, et al. Uric acid and fructose: potential biological mechanisms. Semin Nephrol 2011;31:426–32.
142. Ferrannini E. Is insulin resistance the cause of the metabolic syndrome? Annu Mediaev 2006;38:42–51.
143. Gallagher EJ, Leroith D, Karnieli E. Insulin resistance in obesity as the underlying cause for the metabolic syndrome. Mt Sinai J Med 2010;77:511–23.
144. Lann D, LeRoith D. Insulin resistance as the underlying cause for the metabolic syndrome. Med Clin North Am 2007;91:1063–77, viii.
145. Roy D, Perreault M, Marette A. Insulin stimulation of glucose uptake in skeletal muscles and adipose tissues in vivo is NO dependent. Am J Phys 1998;274:E692–9.
146. Simao AN, Lozovoy MA, Dichi I. The uric acid metabolism pathway as a therapeutic target in hyperuricemia related to metabolic syndrome. Expert Opin Ther Targets 2012;16:1175–87.
147. Baldwin W, McRae S, Marek G, et al. Hyperuricemia as a mediator of the proinflammatory endocrine imbalance in the adipose tissue in a murine model of the metabolic syndrome. Diabetes 2011;60:1258–69.
148. Furukawa S, Fujita T, Shimabukuro M, et al. Increased oxidative stress in obesity and its impact on metabolic syndrome. J Clin Invest 2004;114:1752–61.
149. Vuorinen-Markkola H, Yki-Jarvinen H. Hyperuricemia and insulin resistance. J Clin Endocrinol Metab 1994;78:25–9.
150. Meshkani R, Zargari M, Larijani B. The relationship between uric acid and metabolic syndrome in normal glucose tolerance and normal fasting glucose subjects. Acta Diabetol 2011;48:79–88.
151. Yoo TW, Sung KC, Shin HS, et al. Relationship between serum uric acid concentration and insulin resistance and metabolic syndrome. Circ J 2005;69:928–33.
152. Krishnan E, Pandya BJ, Chung L, et al. Hyperuricemia in young adults and risk of insulin resistance, prediabetes, and diabetes: a 15-year follow-up study. Am J Epidemiol 2012;176:108–16.
153. Carnethon MR, Fortmann SP, Palaniappan L, et al. Risk factors for progression to incident hyperinsulinemia: the Atherosclerosis Risk in Communities Study, 1987-1998. Am J Epidemiol 2003;158:1058–67.
154. Bhole V, Choi JW, Kim SW, et al. Serum uric acid levels and the risk of type 2 diabetes: a prospective study. Am J Med 2010;123:957–61.
155. Kramer CK, von Muhlen D, Jassal SK, et al. Serum uric acid levels improve prediction of incident type 2 diabetes in individuals with impaired fasting glucose: the Rancho Bernardo Study. Diabetes Care 2009;32:1272–3.
156. Niskanen L, Laaksonen DE, Lindstrom J, et al. Serum uric acid as a harbinger of metabolic outcome in subjects with impaired glucose tolerance: the Finnish Diabetes Prevention Study. Diabetes Care 2006;29:709–11.
157. Chien KL, Chen MF, Hsu HC, et al. Plasma uric acid and the risk of type 2 diabetes in a Chinese community. Clin Chem 2008;54:310–6.

158. Choi HK, De Vera MA, Krishnan E. Gout and the risk of type 2 diabetes among men with a high cardiovascular risk profile. Rheumatology (Oxford) 2008;47: 1567–70.
159. Taniguchi Y, Hayashi T, Tsumura K, et al. Serum uric acid and the risk for hypertension and type 2 diabetes in Japanese men: the Osaka Health Survey. J Hypertens 2001;19:1209–15.
160. Choi HK, Ford ES. Haemoglobin A1c, fasting glucose, serum C-peptide and insulin resistance in relation to serum uric acid levels–the Third National Health and Nutrition Examination Survey. Rheumatology (Oxford) 2008;47:713–7.
161. Rodriguez G, Soriano LC, Choi HK. Impact of diabetes against the future risk of developing gout. Ann Rheum Dis 2010;69:2090–4.
162. Bandaru P, Shankar A. Association between serum uric acid levels and diabetes mellitus. Int J Endocrinol 2011;2011:604715.
163. Ioachimescu AG, Brennan DM, Hoar BM, et al. Serum uric acid, mortality and glucose control in patients with type 2 diabetes mellitus: a PreCIS database study. Diabet Med 2007;24:1369–74.
164. Choi HK, Ford ES. Prevalence of the metabolic syndrome in individuals with hyperuricemia. Am J Med 2007;120:442–7.
165. Li Q, Yang Z, Lu B, et al. Serum uric acid level and its association with metabolic syndrome and carotid atherosclerosis in patients with type 2 diabetes. Cardiovasc Diabetol 2011;10:72.
166. Liu PW, Chang TY, Chen JD. Serum uric acid and metabolic syndrome in Taiwanese adults. Metabolism 2010;59:802–7.
167. Ford ES, Li C, Cook S, et al. Serum concentrations of uric acid and the metabolic syndrome among US children and adolescents. Circulation 2007;115:2526–32.
168. Hjortnaes J, Algra A, Olijhoek J, et al. Serum uric acid levels and risk for vascular diseases in patients with metabolic syndrome. J Rheumatol 2007;34: 1882–7.
169. Lee JM, Kim HC, Cho HM, et al. Association between serum uric acid level and metabolic syndrome. J Prev Med Public Health 2012;45:181–7.
170. Chiou WK, Huang DH, Wang MH, et al. Significance and association of serum uric acid (UA) levels with components of metabolic syndrome (MS) in the elderly. Arch Gerontol Geriatr 2012;55:724–8.
171. Ioachimescu AG, Brennan DM, Hoar BM, et al. Serum uric acid is an independent predictor of all-cause mortality in patients at high risk of cardiovascular disease: a preventive cardiology information system (PreCIS) database cohort study. Arthritis Rheum 2008;58:623–30.
172. Puig JG, Martinez MA, Mora M, et al. Serum urate, metabolic syndrome, and cardiovascular risk factors. A population-based study. Nucleosides Nucleotides Nucleic Acids 2008;27:620–3.
173. Juraschek SP, Miller ER 3rd, Gelber AC. Body mass index, obesity, and prevalent gout in the United States in 1988-1994 and 2007-2010. Arthritis Care Res 2013;65:127–32.
174. Simao AN, Lozovoy MA, Simao TN, et al. Adiponectinemia is associated with uricemia but not with proinflammatory status in women with metabolic syndrome. J Nutr Metab 2012;2012:418094.
175. Chen JH, Pan WH, Hsu CC, et al. Impact of obesity and hypertriglyceridemia on gout development with or without hyperuricemia: a prospective study. Arthritis Care Res 2013;65:133–40.
176. Cipriani S, Chen X, Schwarzschild MA. Urate: a novel biomarker of Parkinson's disease risk, diagnosis and prognosis. Biomark Med 2010;4:701–12.

177. Johnson RJ, Lanaspa MA, Gaucher EA. Uric acid: a danger signal from the RNA world that may have a role in the epidemic of obesity, metabolic syndrome, and cardiorenal disease: evolutionary considerations. Semin Nephrol 2011;31:394–9.

178. Orowan E. The origin of man. Nature 1955;175:683–4.

179. Ames BN, Cathcart R, Schwiers E, et al. Uric acid provides an antioxidant defense in humans against oxidant- and radical-caused aging and cancer: a hypothesis. Proc Natl Acad Sci U S A 1981;78:6858–62.

180. Whiteman M, Ketsawatsakul U, Halliwell B. A reassessment of the peroxynitrite scavenging activity of uric acid. Ann N Y Acad Sci 2002;962:242–59.

181. Regoli F, Winston GW. Quantification of total oxidant scavenging capacity of antioxidants for peroxynitrite, peroxyl radicals, and hydroxyl radicals. Toxicol Appl Pharmacol 1999;156:96–105.

182. Cohen AM, Aberdroth RE, Hochstein P. Inhibition of free radical-induced DNA damage by uric acid. FEBS Lett 1984;174:147–50.

183. Duan W, Ladenheim B, Cutler RG, et al. Dietary folate deficiency and elevated homocysteine levels endanger dopaminergic neurons in models of Parkinson's disease. J Neurochem 2002;80:101–10.

184. Guerreiro S, Ponceau A, Toulorge D, et al. Protection of midbrain dopaminergic neurons by the end-product of purine metabolism uric acid: potentiation by low-level depolarization. J Neurochem 2009;109:1118–28.

185. Church WH, Ward VL. Uric acid is reduced in the substantia nigra in Parkinson's disease: effect on dopamine oxidation. Brain Res Bull 1994;33:419–25.

186. Weisskopf MG, O'Reilly E, Chen H, et al. Plasma urate and risk of Parkinson's disease. Am J Epidemiol 2007;166:561–7.

187. Chen H, Mosley TH, Alonso A, et al. Plasma urate and Parkinson's disease in the Atherosclerosis Risk in Communities (ARIC) study. Am J Epidemiol 2009;169: 1064–9.

188. Alonso A, Rodriguez LA, Logroscino G, et al. Gout and risk of Parkinson disease: a prospective study. Neurology 2007;69:1696–700.

189. De Vera M, Rahman MM, Rankin J, et al. Gout and the risk of Parkinson's disease: a cohort study. Arthritis Rheum 2008;59:1549–54.

190. Toncev G, Milicic B, Toncev S, et al. Serum uric acid levels in multiple sclerosis patients correlate with activity of disease and blood-brain barrier dysfunction. Eur J Neurol 2002;9:221–6.

191. Auinger P, Kieburtz K, McDermott MP. The relationship between uric acid levels and Huntington's disease progression. Mov Disord 2010;25:224–8.

192. Spitsin S, Hooper DC, Leist T, et al. Inactivation of peroxynitrite in multiple sclerosis patients after oral administration of inosine may suggest possible approaches to therapy of the disease. Mult Scler 2001;7:313–9.

193. Macmullan P, McCarthy G. Treatment and management of pseudogout: insights for the clinician. Ther Adv Musculoskelet Dis 2012;4:121–31.

194. Salaffi F, Carotti M, Guglielmi G, et al. The crowned dens syndrome as a cause of neck pain: clinical and computed tomography study in patients with calcium pyrophosphate dihydrate deposition disease. Clin Exp Rheumatol 2008;26: 1040–6.

195. Felson DT, Anderson JJ, Naimark A, et al. The prevalence of chondrocalcinosis in the elderly and its association with knee osteoarthritis: the Framingham Study. J Rheumatol 1989;16:1241–5.

196. Sanmarti R, Panella D, Brancos MA, et al. Prevalence of articular chondrocalcinosis in elderly subjects in a rural area of Catalonia. Ann Rheum Dis 1993;52: 418–22.

197. Neame RL, Carr AJ, Muir K, et al. UK community prevalence of knee chondro-calcinosis: evidence that correlation with osteoarthritis is through a shared asso-ciation with osteophyte. Ann Rheum Dis 2003;62:513–8.
198. Ramonda R, Musacchio E, Perissinotto E, et al. Prevalence of chondrocalcinosis in Italian subjects from northeastern Italy. The Pro.V.A. (PROgetto Veneto Anziani) study. Clin Exp Rheumatol 2009;27:981–4.
199. Zhang W, Doherty M, Bardin T, et al. European League Against Rheumatism rec-ommendations for calcium pyrophosphate deposition. Part I: terminology and diagnosis. Ann Rheum Dis 2011;70:563–70.
200. Ciancio G, Bortoluzzi A, Govoni M. Epidemiology of gout and chondrocalcino-sis. Reumatismo 2011;63:207–20.
201. Nguyen C, Lieberherr M, Bordat C, et al. Intracellular calcium oscillations in articular chondrocytes induced by basic calcium phosphate crystals lead to cartilage degradation. Osteoarthr Cartil 2012;20:1399–408.
202. Rosenthal AK. Crystals, inflammation, and osteoarthritis. Curr Opin Rheumatol 2011;23:170–3.
203. Molloy ES, McCarthy GM. Basic calcium phosphate crystals: pathways to joint degeneration. Curr Opin Rheumatol 2006;18:187–92.
204. Netter P, Bardin T, Bianchi A, et al. The ANKH gene and familial calcium pyro-phosphate dihydrate deposition disease. Joint Bone Spine 2004;71:365–8.
205. Sun Y, Mauerhan DR, Honeycutt PR, et al. Calcium deposition in osteoarthritic meniscus and meniscal cell culture. Arthritis Res Ther 2010;12:R56.
206. Neogi T, Nevitt M, Niu J, et al. Lack of association between chondrocalcinosis and increased risk of cartilage loss in knees with osteoarthritis: results of two prospective longitudinal magnetic resonance imaging studies. Arthritis Rheum 2006;54:1822–8.
207. Pawlotsky Y, Le Dantec P, Moirand R, et al. Elevated parathyroid hormone 44-68 and osteoarticular changes in patients with genetic hemochromatosis. Arthritis Rheum 1999;42:799–806.
208. Dymock IW, Hamilton EB, Laws JW, et al. Arthropathy of haemochromatosis. Clinical and radiological analysis of 63 patients with iron overload. Ann Rheum Dis 1970;29:469–76.
209. Timms AE, Sathananthan R, Bradbury L, et al. Genetic testing for haemochro-matosis in patients with chondrocalcinosis. Ann Rheum Dis 2002;61:745–7.
210. Yashiro T, Okamoto T, Tanaka R, et al. Prevalence of chondrocalcinosis in pa-tients with primary hyperparathyroidism in Japan. Endocrinol Jpn 1991;38:457–64.
211. Rubin MR, Silverberg SJ. Rheumatic manifestations of primary hyperparathy-roidism and parathyroid hormone therapy. Curr Rheumatol Rep 2002;4:179–85.
212. Richette P, Ayoub G, Lahalle S, et al. Hypomagnesemia associated with chon-drocalcinosis: a cross-sectional study. Arthritis Rheum 2007;57:1496–501.
213. Cobeta-Garcia JC, Gascon A, Iglesias E, et al. Chondrocalcinosis and Gitel-man's syndrome. A new association? Ann Rheum Dis 1998;57:748–9.
214. Punzi L, Calo L, Schiavon F, et al. Chondrocalcinosis is a feature of Gitelman's variant of Bartter's syndrome. A new look at the hypomagnesemia associated with calcium pyrophosphate dihydrate crystal deposition disease. Rev Rhum Engl Ed 1998;65:571–4.
215. Favero M, Calo LA, Schiavon F, et al. Miscellaneous non-inflammatory musculo-skeletal conditions. Bartter's and Gitelman's diseases. Best Pract Res Clin Rheu-matol 2011;25:637–48.

216. Jones AC, Chuck AJ, Arie EA, et al. Diseases associated with calcium pyro-phosphate deposition disease. Semin Arthritis Rheum 1992;22:188–202.
217. Feig DI, Kang DH, Johnson RJ. Uric acid and cardiovascular risk. N Engl J Med 2008;359:1811–21.

The Genetic Basis of Gout

Tony R. Merriman, PhD[a],*, Hyon K. Choi, MD, DrPH[b],
Nicola Dalbeth, MBChB, MD, FRACP[c]

KEYWORDS

- Gout • Urate • Gene • Association • Genome-wide association studies • *SLC2A9*
- *ABCG2*

KEY POINTS

- Genome-wide association studies for serum urate have identified 28 loci influencing serum urate levels.
- The largest genetic effects on serum urate are within genes encoding transporters that excrete uric acid in the kidney and gut.
- Other genetic effects are within glycolysis genes.
- There are interactions between genes, and environmental influences on serum urate (diuretics, alcohol, sugar-sweetened beverages).
- Genome-wide association studies are required in gout using well-phenotyped cases to identify loci controlling progression from hyperuricemia to inflammatory gout.

INTRODUCTION

The central feature of gout is deposition of inflammatory monosodium urate (MSU) monohydrate microcrystals, which can lead to acute inflammatory arthritis, tendonitis, cartilage damage, and bone remodeling. Several checkpoints exist in the pathogenesis of gout (reviewed in Refs.[1,2]). Central to the development of gout is elevated tissue concentrations of urate, which in some individuals lead to formation of MSU crystals. Elevated serum urate levels (hyperuricemia) occur as a result of increased production of hepatic urate through the purine synthesis de novo and salvage pathways; however, renal underexcretion of uric acid is a dominant contributor, with reduced fractional excretion of uric acid in hyperuricemia and gout.[3–5] Once formed, MSU crystals may induce an acute inflammatory response leading to acute gouty arthritis and/or a chronic granulomatous response with formation of tophi. Although hyperuricemia is present in virtually all people with gout, this biochemical abnormality is not sufficient for the development of clinically apparent joint disease, as most people with hyperuricemia do not develop gout.[6]

[a] Department of Biochemistry, University of Otago, Dunedin 9012, New Zealand; [b] Section of Rheumatology and Clinical Epidemiology Unit, Boston University School of Medicine, Boston, MA 02118, USA; [c] Department of Medicine, University of Auckland, Auckland 1023, New Zealand
* Corresponding author.
E-mail address: tony.merriman@otago.ac.nz

Rheum Dis Clin N Am 40 (2014) 279–290
http://dx.doi.org/10.1016/j.rdc.2014.01.009
0889-857X/14/$ – see front matter © 2014 Elsevier Inc. All rights reserved.

Monogenic inborn errors of purine metabolism such as hypoxanthine-guanine phosphoribosyltransferase deficiency (Lesch-Nyhan syndrome) and 5-phosphoribo-syl-1-pyrophosphate synthetase superactivity lead to rare pediatric syndromes of hyperuricemia, associated with neurodevelopmental disorders, early-onset gout, and kidney stones. In addition, familial juvenile hyperuricemic nephropathy is an autosomal dominant disorder of renal uric acid underexcretion caused by mutations in the uromodulin gene that leads to severe underexcretion-type hyperuricemia, early-onset gout, and chronic kidney disease. These rare monogenic disorders provide important insights into physiologic purine metabolism and uric acid excretion mechanisms, but do not account for the vast majority of hyperuricemia or gout observed in the general population. Renal uric handling of acid and hyperuricemia have a large heritable component (87% for fractional excretion of uric acid,[7] 60% for serum urate).[8] Consistent with these observations, genome-wide association studies (GWAS) have revealed that a polygenic component of common inherited variants[9] contributes to the development of gout in the general population with, excepting the PRPSAP1 locus, little overlap with monogenic syndromes. This review focuses on recent insights into these common genetic variants that contribute to the development of gout, and their potential interaction with environmental risk factors.

GENOME-WIDE ASSOCIATION STUDY FINDINGS FOR SERUM URATE

Over the past 8 years, GWAS and subsequent meta-analyses have led to a considerable expansion in the knowledge of common genetic loci that are associated with hyperuricemia and gout in Europeans. Two meta-analyses, each involving more than 28,000 participants, found genome-wide genetic loci that are reproducibly associated with serum urate levels or gout (**Table 1**).[10,11] In 2009, a meta-analysis by Kolz and colleagues[10] reported associations between 9 common genetic variant loci and serum urate concentrations: SLC2A9, ABCG2, SLC22A12, SLC17A1, SLC22A11, SLC16A9, GCKR, LRRC16A, and near PDZK1. In 2010, a meta-analysis of the CHARGE consortium by Yang and colleagues[11] reconfirmed 6 of these loci (SLC2A9, ABCG2, SLC17A1, SLC22A11, GCKR, and PDZK1) and additionally identified the R3HDM2-INHBC region and RREB1 loci with genome-wide significance. The genetic urate risk score was strongly associated with the risk of gout. An Icelandic GWAS for serum urate, using whole genome sequence data in 15,506 individuals, identified 4 loci with a genome-wide level of significance[12] at SLC2A9, ABCG2, PDZK1, and ALDH16A1. The variant underlying the ALDH16A1 association appears to be a previously unreported Icelandic-specific genetic variation present at a frequency of 1.8%, which encodes a proline to arginine amino acid change in the ALDH16A1 protein. It was estimated that the variant explained 0.5% of variance in serum urate in the Icelandic population.[12]

In other ancestral groups, a meta-analysis[13] and a GWAS[14] have demonstrated that 10 of the 11 loci that have been shown to influence serum urate levels in individuals with European ancestry were also significantly associated with serum urate or gout in African American sample sets. The GWAS in African Americans also identified a novel locus influencing serum urate near the SLC2A12 gene on chromosome 6.[13] This gene is a good candidate, as it is a glucose transporter and a member of the same family as SLC2A9, which has a very strong influence on serum urate across populations.[9,13,15] Another GWAS among East Asians by Okada and colleagues[15] in 2012 showed genome-wide significance of serum urate levels with SLC2A9, ABCG2, SLC22A12, and MAF; all of these loci overlap with those identified in Europeans (see below). A previous study in Japanese had identified SLC2A9, ABCG2,

Table 1
GWAS meta-analyses of loci associated with serum urate and gout

	Kolz et al,[10] 2009	Yang et al,[11] 2010	Tin et al,[13] 2011	Okada et al,[15] 2012	Köttgen et al,[9] 2013
Sample size	28,141	28,283	14,706	71,149	>140,000 (primary data)
Population	European	European	African American	East Asian	European (primary data), African American, Indian, Japanese
Loci associated with serum urate with genome-wide significance	9 loci: *SLC2A9, ABCG2, SLC17A1, SLC22A11, SLC22A12, SLC16A9, GCKR, LRRC16A, PDZK1*	8 loci: *SLC2A9, ABCG2, SLC17A1, SLC22A11, GCKR, R3HDM2-INHBC region, RREB1, PDZK1*	3 loci: *SLC2A9, SLC22A12, SGK1-SLC2A12 region*	4 loci: *SLC2A9, ABCG2, SLC22A12, MAF*	28 loci: 10 previously described: *SLC2A9, ABCG2, SLC17A3, SLC16A9, SLC22A11, SLC22A12, GCKR, INHBC, RREB1, PDZK1* 18 new loci: *TRIM46, INHBB, SFMBT1, TMEM171, VEGFA, BAZ1B, PRKAG2, STC1, HNF4G, A1CF, ATXN2, UBE2Q2, IGF1R, NFAT5, MAF, HLF, ACVR1B-ACVRL1, B3GNT4*
Association with gout	Not reported	The genetic urate risk score was strongly and linearly associated with serum urate (multivariable adjusted $P<4.5 \times 10^{-308}$)	Directionally consistent effects on serum urate and gout were observed (P-binomial <.0001)	Not reported	Correlation between the effect on urate and the odds of gout for the replicated loci (Pearson correlation = 0.93); 17 of the replicated serum urate–associated SNPs reached statistical significance with gout ($P<.05$)

SLC22A12, and *LRP2* as being associated with serum urate at a genome-wide level of significance.[16] LRP2 (lipoprotein receptor-related protein 2) has not been associated with urate in Europeans.

Most recently, by combining data from more than 140,000 individuals of European ancestry within the Global Urate Genetics Consortium (GUGC), Köttgen and colleagues[9] have identified and replicated 28 genome-wide significant loci for serum urate. These loci included the 10 previously identified regions (as described above) and 18 new regions (in or near *TRIM46, INHBB, SFMBT1, TMEM171, VEGFA, BAZ1B, PRKAG2, STC1, HNF4G, A1CF, ATXN2, UBE2Q2, IGF1R, NFAT5, MAF, HLF, ACVR1B-ACVRL1,* and *B3GNT4*) (see **Table 1**). Furthermore, the meta-analysis also studied 8340 individuals of Indian ancestry, 5820 African Americans, and 15,286 Japanese, and found that the serum urate effects were direction-consistent with similar magnitude for most single-nucleotide polymorphisms (SNPs), although allele frequencies at the index SNPs varied considerably across the groups.

In all gout samples combined (3151 cases and 68,350 controls) in the study by Köttgen and colleagues,[9] 17 of 26 of the replicated urate concentration–associated SNPs showed nominal association with gout ($P<.05$; see **Table 1**). Of note, these gout cases included 1036 cases of incident gout (meeting the American College of Rheumatology classification criteria[17]) over a period of up to 22 years in prospective cohort studies.[18,19] The serum urate effects of these loci showed a positive linear correlation with the log odds of gout (Pearson correlation = 0.93), and genetic urate risk scores (created based on the number of risk alleles of serum urate–associated genes) were significantly associated with increased odds of prevalent gout (odds ratio [OR] = 1.11 per risk score unit increase) and incident gout over a period of up to 22 years (OR = 1.10, 95% confidence interval = 1.08–1.13). This study also evaluated the association with the fractional excretion of uric acid (FEUA, n = 6799) and found that SNPs at 10 replicated loci showed directionally consistent, significant association with FEUA (ie, *SLC2A9, GCKR, ABCG2, RREB1, SLC22A11, NRXN2/SLC22A12, UBE2Q2, IGFIR, NFAT5,* and *HLF*).

Notably in the same study, 2 novel regions of *B3GNT4* and *ACVR1B-ACVRL1* were discovered and replicated through a systematic functional association network analysis approach that incorporated previous knowledge on molecular interactions through which the gene products of implicated genes operate.[9] Furthermore, the functional association network analysis also highlighted a specific subnetwork from the analysis around the inhibins-activins pathway. Finally, pathway analyses showed functional network associations with gene expression, cellular organization, carbohydrate metabolism, molecular transport, and endocrine system disorders (lowest $P = 1 \times 10^{-28}$).

Most of the initially identified novel loci by GWAS studies and meta-analyses appear to encode proteins that are involved in the renal urate transport system (see **Table 1**).[2,20] These findings appear to be consistent with reduced renal excretion of urate being the dominant cause of hyperuricemia and gout in most individuals.[4] Nevertheless, new candidate genes for serum urate concentration, as reported by the meta-analysis by Köttgen and colleagues,[9] highlight the importance of metabolic control of urate production (in addition to urate excretion) in the pathogenesis of gout.

INSIGHTS INTO MECHANISM

Apart from uric acid transporters, little is understood about how the other genes identified in the various GWAS regulate urate, largely because the causal genes have not been identified. Extensive correlation between genetic markers (linkage disequilibrium) encompassing more than 1 gene at each locus means that the gene cannot be inferred from the position of the associated marker. However, at the major urate and gout risk loci (*SLC2A9* and *ABCG2*), progress has been made into the functional role of the genetically associated variants (see later discussion). Data from other loci (*PDZK1, SLC22A12*) are specifically discussed here, illustrating an apparent exception to the expectation that serum urate–increasing genetic variants also increase the risk of gout. The *GCKR* gene and other glycolytic genes are also discussed. Finally, a locus (*PRPSAP1*) in a pathway implicated in monogenic urate overproduction syndromes is mentioned.

SLC2A9

Genetic variation within introns 3 to 7 of *SLC2A9* explains about 3.5% of variation in serum urate concentration in European Caucasians,[9] an extremely large effect in the context of genetics of complex phenotypes. These variants are also strongly associated with gout, with effect sizes for the risk allele greater than OR 1.5 (eg, Refs.[9,21]). *SLC2A9* is a voltage-dependent transporter believed to be responsible for reabsorption of uric acid into the circulation via the proximal renal tubule.[22] The serum urate–associated intronic genetic variants are tightly correlated, which makes it very difficult to identify the causative variant. However, it is likely that the causative serum urate–raising variant increases the expression levels of an *SLC2A9* isoform (*SLC2A9b* [GLUT9S]) with a 28-residue portion missing from the N-terminus that is predominantly expressed on the apical (urine) membrane, presumably increasing reabsorption of uric acid from the filtered urine.[23,24] A portion of the group of intronic variants associated with urate and gout in Europeans is essentially monomorphic in Asian populations (risk allele >99%), and has not been shown to influence urate levels or gout in Asian samples. However, other SNPs (eg, *rs3775948*) are strongly associated with serum urate in Asians[15] and, importantly, these SNPs overlap with the associated intronic SNPs in Europeans. Thus the Asian data define a subset of associated SNPs and illustrate how transancestral mapping should allow fine-mapping of the etiologic variant at *SLC2A9*.

ABCG2

The nonsynonymous Gln141Lys (Q141K) variant of *ABCG2* explains about 0.5% of the variation in serum urate levels in Europeans,[9] and is almost certainly the etiological variant, with the lysine allele associated with increased serum urate levels.[25] Predictably the same allele increases the risk of gout in European, Chinese, Japanese, and New Zealand Pacific sample sets (OR ~2) but, for unclear reasons, not in New Zealand Māori, despite an allele frequency similar to that of Europeans (reviewed in Ref.[26]).

ABCG2, highly expressed in intestinal epithelial cells and also expressed in the apical membrane of the kidney proximal tubule, is an adenosine triphosphate (ATP)-dependent uric acid secretory molecule. The lysine allele encodes a molecule with approximately 50% reduced ability to transport uric acid,[25] which results from instability in the nucleotide-binding domain and decreased protein expression.[27] The defects in expression and function can be rescued by a histone deacetylase inhibitor approved by the Food and Drug Administration,[27] revealing a possible new urate-lowering therapy for evaluation.

ABCG2 functions predominantly as a gut secretory uric acid transporter. With high expression of *ABCG2* in extrarenal tissues (including the liver), this observation has led to the proposal that *ABCG2* dysfunction encoded by the 141K allele and subsequent gut underexcretion of uric acid is a significant contributor to the overproduction of urate in the serum. This process results in the urate-increasing lysine allele, paradoxically, being associated with increased urinary excretion of uric acid[4] as the renal uric acid excretion machinery physiologically adjusts to the lysine allele-mediated urate overproduction.

PDZK1 and SLC22A12

The *PDZK1* gene encodes a PDZ domain–containing scaffold protein known to bind uric acid transporters and, presumably, arrange their cell-surface localization for optimal uric acid transport.[28] *PDZK1* is strongly associated with serum urate levels; however, the same variants had no effect on the risk of gout in a large well-powered European meta-analysis of cases nested within population-based cohorts (OR = 1.03).[9] Why this is the case is unclear; however, it is notable that the same allele of the variant in *PDZK1* that associates with increased serum urate is also associated with decreased blood pressure.[29] The gout cases analyzed by Köttgen and colleagues[9] would have included a significant proportion of cases secondary to diuretic medication (for hypertension). Thus, it is possible that any increased risk of primary gout (ie, owing to increased urate with no obvious secondary cause) mediated by the allele of *PDZK1* via increased serum urate levels was negated by inclusion of cases with gout secondary to hypertension treatment, in which the other (serum urate–lowering) allele of *PDZK1* was overrepresented. Of possible relevance for understanding the relationship between hyperuricemia and other metabolic conditions,[30] PDZK1 also interacts with other molecules, including the high-density lipoprotein receptor known as scavenger receptor class B type 1, which is important in cholesterol metabolism.[31]

The *SLC22A12* gene encodes the canonical renal uric acid transporter URAT1. It is an example of a second locus with a strong genetic effect on serum urate, yet common variants are not associated with gout in Europeans,[9] with inconsistent associations in other populations.[32,33] For both *PDZK1* and *SLC22A12* the statistical power of the gout-association studies is unlikely to be an issue, as loci with a similar effect on serum urate are strongly associated with gout in the same samples (eg, *GCKR*, *SLC22A11*, *INHBC*).[9]

Glycolytic Genes

The glucokinase regulatory protein gene (*GCKR*) highlights a serum urate–controlling pathway probably distinct from renal (and gut) excretion of uric acid, providing some clues to the etiologic links between gout and other associated metabolic conditions such as diabetes and dyslipidemia. It is strongly associated with serum urate in Europeans,[9] and has been consistently associated with gout in Europeans and Chinese.[29,34] Genetic variation in *GCKR* has also been associated with concentrations of triglyceride and fasting glucose, and the risk of type 2 diabetes.[35] The association of *GCKR* with serum urate is weakened when triglyceride levels are accounted for[29] and the same *GCKR* allele is also associated with triglyceride levels. The most plausible explanation for this observation is that *GCKR* affects both serum urate and triglyceride levels by a common unconfirmed mediator that could be glucose-6-phosphate.[29] GCKR controls the hepatic production of glucose-6-phosphate, which is catabolized for triglyceride synthesis via glycolysis, pyruvate, and acetyl coenzyme A, while glucose-6-phosphate is also a precursor of de novo purine (uric acid) synthesis. Other loci encoding glycolysis genes are *PKLR* (encodes pyruvate kinase that catalyzes the final step of glycolysis, producing ATP and pyruvate), *MLXIPL* (encodes a glucose-responsive transcriptional factor that regulates *PKLR* expression), *PRKAG2* (encodes the regulatory subunit γ2 of the adenosine monophosphate [AMP]-activated protein kinase, which senses cellular AMP:ATP ratio and activates glucose uptake and catabolism), *NFAT5* (encodes a transcription factor that can influence glucose flux and the pentose phosphate pathway), and *HNF4G* (encodes a transcription factor responding to nutrient signals).

How the glucokinase regulatory protein and other glycolysis genes influence serum urate levels is unclear. It has been proposed[9] that this could occur by altering the flux of glucose-6-phosphate through the pentose phosphate pathway that generates ribose-5-phosphate (a precursor of de novo purine synthesis and subsequent urate production) and/or altering the amount of lactate available physiologically, given that lactate influences excretion of renal uric acid, likely through a role as a cotransporter molecule for uric acid transporters.[36] The observation that the *GCKR* and *NFAT5* loci also associate with FEUA[9] supports the latter possibility.

PRPSAP1

Of the 28 loci that influence serum urate levels, the phosphoribosylpyrophosphate synthetase–associated protein 1 gene (*PRPSAP1*) has the most obvious role in modifying urate levels, as it is part of the pentose phosphate pathway and de novo synthesis of purines. Other genes in the pathway (phosphoribosylpyrophosphate synthetases and *PRPS1*) cause urate overproduction in purine-related Mendelian syndromes that include gout and neurodevelopmental abnormalities in their symptoms.[37]

RELATIONSHIP BETWEEN GENETIC EFFECT ON SERUM URATE AND RISK OF GOUT

The *PDZK1* and *SLC22A12* genes illustrate the concept that there is not a straightforward relationship between an influence on serum urate and a subsequent risk of gout. Therefore, genetic variants associated with serum urate levels require testing for association with gout, preferably in sample sets where gout is ascertained by the American Rheumatology Association clinical classification criteria[17] or the gold-standard method of microscopic demonstration of MSU crystals. Identifying the loci that deviate from the expectation of an increased risk of gout from an effect on serum urate and then understanding the reason for such deviation will provide novel insights into the etiology of gout.

One apparent discrepancy is the comparative effect size on gout between *SLC2A9* and *ABCG2* which, if understood, could lead to novel knowledge on the etiology of gout. The risk allele at each of these genes increases serum urate by an average of 0.373 mg/dL and 0.217 mg/dL, respectively, in Europeans.[9] However, despite *SLC2A9* having a 1.7-fold stronger effect on serum urate levels, the effect size on gout is consistently stronger at *ABCG2* than at *SLC2A9* (ln(OR) is 0.536 ± 0.045 and 0.451 ± 0.045, respectively, in Europeans[9]). The reason for this is unclear; however, it is logical to speculate that either or both loci may also play a role in the progression from hyperuricemia to acute gout. This hypothesis would be readily verifiable by testing both loci for association with gout, using people with asymptomatic hyperuricemia as controls.

INTERACTIONS BETWEEN ENVIRONMENTAL AND GENETIC RISK FACTORS

In addition to the genetic factors outlined herein, several environmental risk factors contribute to the development of gout, including high intake of purine-rich beverages such as beer, purine-rich foods such as red meat and seafood, and sugar-sweetened beverages, including those sweetened with high-fructose corn syrup.[18,38–40] These dietary factors lead to increased purine synthesis through the hepatic salvage pathways, which in turn leads to increased urate production. The presence of high circulating insulin levels in individuals with metabolic syndrome also promotes renal underexcretion of uric acid.[41] Diuretic agents are a further important environmental cause of hyperuricemia and gout, through potent effects on renal handling of uric acid.[42] GWAS technology is a powerful tool with which to examine the relationship between allele and outcome but, owing to power considerations and availability of appropriate environmental exposure data, it is less amenable to analysis of interactions between genetic and environmental risk factors. Such interactions may be of particular importance when considering hyperuricemia and gout, in which environmental risk factors play an important role in the development of disease. Recent studies have explored these interactions in hyperuricemia and gout.

Alcohol

In a GWAS of the Japanese population, variation in *LRP2*, encoding low-density lipoprotein receptor-related protein 2 (megalin), was associated with higher serum urate concentrations.[16] A subsequent validation study confirmed this association in men, and also demonstrated an interaction between alcohol intake and the *LRP2* risk allele in men, particularly in those with homozygosity for the risk allele who were drinking 5 times or more per week.[43] The underlying mechanisms of this interaction are currently unclear; megalin is expressed in many tissues including the liver and renal tubule, and it is possible that variation in *LRP2* may influence serum urate in the context of alcohol intake because of activation of purine degradation pathways in the liver or underexcretion of uric acid in the renal tubule. The ALDH16A1 protein, identified as being associated with serum urate in the Icelandic GWAS,[12] is known to be involved in the metabolism of alcohol. Alcohol intake is known to increase serum urate levels and to trigger gout attacks.[39,44] This finding is interesting given a previous report of association of *ALDH2* with gout.[45] The *ALDH2* allele that increased the risk of gout also correlated with increased production of xanthine (a purine precursor of urate) on consumption of alcohol.[45]

Diuretics

The association between diuretics and the development of hyperuricemia/gout is thought to be due to interactions between diuretics and urate transporters in the proximal renal tubule. Analysis of the Atherosclerosis Risk in Communities (ARIC) study database has demonstrated that genetic variation in renal urate transporters, particularly *SLC2A9* (encoding GLUT9) and *SLC22A11* (encoding organic anion transporter 4, OAT4), interacts with diuretics to increase the risk of developing incident gout.[46] This study, however, did not report gene-diuretic relationships using serum urate or FEUA as end points.

Fructose

The interactions between fructose intake and variation in *SLC2A9*, encoding the urate transporter that is also reported to transport fructose and glucose,[47] have been explored in a short-term fructose-feeding study of healthy volunteers without gout.[48] The presence of the *SLC2A9* urate-lowering allele was associated with an attenuated hyperuricemic response and increased FEUA following the fructose load. Participants without the protective allele were more likely to have a sustained serum urate concentration above saturation levels at baseline and following fructose intake. This effect was strongly observed in the European Caucasian ancestral subgroup, but not the New Zealand Māori and Pacific ancestral subgroup, which is of particular interest given the high rates of hyperuricemia and gout that is well documented in Polynesian populations.[49] These data suggest a complex interaction between known risk factors for gout, including specific genetic variants in urate transporters, ancestry, and environmental factors.

In a separate case-control study from New Zealand examining genetic and environmental risk factors for gout, interactions between *SLC2A9* genotype and consumption of sugar-sweetened beverages was examined.[38] In this study, intake of sugar-sweetened beverages increased the risk of gout. With each extra daily sugar-sweetened beverage serving, carriage of the *SLC2A9* gout protective allele associated with a higher increase in gout risk in comparison with noncarriers. A similar trend for serum urate concentrations was noted in the United States Atherosclerosis Risk in Communities dataset. These interaction data indicate that *SLC2A9*-mediated renal uric acid excretion is physiologically influenced by intake of simple sugars derived from a sugar-sweetened beverage, with chronic sugar-sweetened beverage exposure negating the gout-risk discrimination of *SLC2A9*.

ASCERTAINMENT OF GOUT CASES AND IMPLICATIONS FOR DESIGN OF GENOME-WIDE ASSOCIATION STUDIES IN GOUT

In contrast to the knowledge about genetic control of serum urate levels (and subsequent risk of gout) that has come from GWAS, there are no robust and replicated associations of inflammatory loci with gout. The best strategy to identify such loci is GWAS with gout as the phenotype, using well-ascertained cases, which is an important methodological issue in large genetics studies. In many GWAS analyses, gout has been ascertained by a combination of self-report or use of allopurinol (which may be used for other indications including prevention of tumor lysis syndrome, nephrolithiasis and, in some countries, asymptomatic hyperuricemia). Inevitably this will result in inclusion of nongout cases in the case samples[50] and a negative impact on power to detect association in GWAS. An example that illustrates the weakness of this approach is the *SLC17A1* locus, which has the third strongest effect on serum urate,[9] and has been consistently and strongly associated with gout in candidate gene studies using Japanese and New Zealand European and Polynesian sample sets ascertained by clinical examination according to the American College of Rheumatology classification criteria,[17] with an OR of approximately 1.5.[51,52] However, the effect size for *SLC17A1* in the GWAS by Köttgen and colleagues[9] was considerably weaker (OR = 1.16). Although there was significant association (P = .01) with *SLC17A1* when the locus was specifically examined, the weaker effect meant that the association signal was completely hidden in the statistical noise. Thus there is a pressing need for gout GWAS in properly phenotyped (clinically ascertained) sample sets to identify immune genetic risk factors for gout. Such loci are likely to have a weak effect (OR <1.3) and will be undetectable using cases ascertained by self-report and allopurinol, resulting in case sample sets with a significant proportion of noncases.[50] Internationally there is a dearth of such sample sets. Large international collaborative efforts are currently under way to address this deficit.

A well-powered study design (in a defined ancestral group) would be a GWAS of 2000 cases and at least 2000 controls, with replication of genome-wide significant associations in an ancestrally matched sample set of equivalent size. If detection of inflammatory loci was the primary aim, a consideration would be to use asymptomatic hyperuricemic individuals as controls. However, this may result in a loss of power if there were latent cases within such controls, and if the biological mechanisms leading to hyperuricemia and the inflammatory pathways in gout are not independent.

REFERENCES

1. Choi HK, Mount DB, Reginato AM. Pathogenesis of gout. Ann Intern Med 2005; 143:499–516.

2. Merriman TR, Dalbeth N. The genetic basis of hyperuricaemia and gout. Joint Bone Spine 2011;78:35–40.
3. Gibson T, Waterworth R, Hatfield P, et al. Hyperuricaemia, gout and kidney function in New Zealand Maori men. Br J Rheumatol 1984;23:276–82.
4. Ichida K, Matsuo H, Takada T, et al. Decreased extra-renal urate excretion is a common cause of hyperuricemia. Nat Commun 2012;3:764.
5. Simmonds HA, McBride MB, Hatfield PJ, et al. Polynesian women are also at risk for hyperuricaemia and gout because of a genetic defect in renal urate handling. Br J Rheumatol 1994;33:932–7.
6. Campion EW, Glynn RJ, DeLabry LO. Asymptomatic hyperuricemia. Risks and consequences in the Normative Aging Study. Am J Med 1987;82:421–6.
7. Emmerson BT, Nagel SL, Duffy DL, et al. Genetic control of the renal clearance of urate: a study of twins. Ann Rheum Dis 1992;51:375–7.
8. Krishnan E, Lessov-Schlaggar CN, Krasnow RE, et al. Nature versus nurture in gout: a twin study. Am J Med 2012;125:499–504.
9. Köttgen A, Albrecht E, Teumer A, et al. Genome-wide association analyses identify 18 new loci associated with serum urate concentrations. Nat Genet 2013;45: 145–54.
10. Kolz M, Johnson T, Sanna S, et al. Meta-analysis of 28,141 individuals identifies common variants within five new loci that influence uric acid concentrations. PLoS Genet 2009;5:e1000504.
11. Yang Q, Köttgen A, Dehghan A, et al. Multiple genetic loci influence serum urate levels and their relationship with gout and cardiovascular disease risk factors. Circ Cardiovasc Genet 2010;3:523–30.
12. Sulem P, Gudbjartsson DF, Walters GB, et al. Identification of low-frequency variants associated with gout and serum uric acid levels. Nat Genet 2011;43: 1127–30.
13. Tin A, Woodward OM, Kao WHL, et al. Genome-wide association study for serum urate concentrations and gout among African Americans identifies genomic risk loci and a novel URAT1 loss-of-function allele. Hum Mol Genet 2011;20:4056–68.
14. Charles BA, Shriner D, Doumatey A, et al. A genome-wide association study of serum uric acid in African Americans. BMC Med Genomics 2011;4:17.
15. Okada Y, Sim X, Go MJ, et al. Meta-analysis identifies multiple loci associated with kidney function-related traits in east Asian populations. Nat Genet 2012;44:904–9.
16. Kamatani Y, Matsuda K, Okada Y, et al. Genome-wide association study of hematological and biochemical traits in a Japanese population. Nat Genet 2010; 42:210–5.
17. Wallace SL, Robinson H, Masi AT, et al. Preliminary criteria for the classification of the acute arthritis of primary gout. Arthritis Rheum 1977;20:895–900.
18. Choi HK, Atkinson K, Karlson EW, et al. Purine-rich foods, dairy and protein intake, and the risk of gout in men. N Engl J Med 2004;350:1093–103.
19. Choi HK, Willett W, Curhan G. Fructose-rich beverages and risk of gout in women. JAMA 2010;304:2270–8.
20. Reginato AM, Mount DB, Yang I, et al. The genetics of hyperuricaemia and gout. Nat Rev Rheumatol 2012;8:610–21.
21. Hollis-Moffatt JE, Xu X, Dalbeth N, et al. Role of the urate transporter SLC2A9 gene in susceptibility to gout in New Zealand Maori, Pacific Island, and Caucasian case-control sample sets. Arthritis Rheum 2009;60:3485–92.
22. Caulfield MJ, Munroe PB, O'Neill D, et al. SLC2A9 is a high-capacity urate transporter in humans. PLoS Med 2008;7:e197.

23. Doring A, Gieger C, Mehta D, et al. SLC2A9 influences uric acid concentrations with pronounced sex-specific effects. Nat Genet 2008;40:430–6.
24. Vitart V, Rudan I, Hayward C, et al. SLC2A9 is a newly identified urate transporter influencing serum urate concentration, urate excretion and gout. Nat Genet 2008;40:437–42.
25. Woodward OM, Köttgen A, Coresh J, et al. Identification of a urate transporter, ABCG2, with a common functional polymorphism causing gout. Proc Natl Acad Sci U S A 2009;106:10338–42.
26. Merriman TR. Population heterogeneity in the genetic control of serum urate. Semin Nephrol 2011;31:420–5.
27. Woodward OM, Tukaye DN, Cui J, et al. Gout-causing Q141K mutation in ABCG2 leads to instability of the nucleotide-binding domain and can be corrected with small molecules. Proc Natl Acad Sci U S A 2013;110:5223–8.
28. Anzai N, Endou H. Urate transporters: an evolving field. Semin Nephrol 2011;31: 400–9.
29. van der Harst P, Bakker SJ, de Boer RA, et al. Replication of the five novel loci for uric acid concentrations and potential mediating mechanisms. Hum Mol Genet 2010;19:387–95.
30. Choi HK, Ford ES, Li C, et al. Prevalence of the metabolic syndrome in patients with gout: the Third National Health and Nutrition Examination Survey. Arthritis Rheum 2007;57:109–15.
31. Tsukamoto K, Wales TE, Daniels K, et al. Noncanonical role of the PDZ4 domain of the adaptor protein PDZK1 in the regulation of the hepatic high density lipoprotein receptor scavenger receptor class B, type I (SR-BI). J Biol Chem 2013; 288:19845–60.
32. Guan M, Zhang J, Chen Y, et al. High-resolution melting analysis for the rapid detection of an intronic single nucleotide polymorphism in SLC22A12 in male patients with primary gout in China. Scand J Rheumatol 2009;38: 276–81.
33. Tu HP, Chen CJ, Lee CH, et al. The SLC22A12 gene is associated with gout in Han Chinese and Solomon Islanders. Ann Rheum Dis 2010;69:1252–4.
34. Wang J, Liu S, Wang B, et al. Association between gout and polymorphisms in GCKR in male Han Chinese. Hum Genet 2012;131:1261–5.
35. Vaxillaire M, Cavalcanti-Proenca C, Dechaume A, et al. The common P446L polymorphism in GCKR inversely modulates fasting glucose and triglyceride levels and reduces type 2 diabetes risk in the DESIR prospective general French population. Diabetes 2008;57:2253–7.
36. Taniguchi A, Kamatani N. Control of renal uric acid excretion and gout. Curr Opin Rheumatol 2008;20:192–7.
37. Roessler BJ, Nosal JM, Smith PR, et al. Human X-linked phosphoribosylpyrophosphate synthetase superactivity is associated with distinct point mutations in the PRPS1 gene. J Biol Chem 1993;268:26476–81.
38. Batt C, Phipps-Green A, Black MA, et al. Sugar-sweetened beverage consumption: a risk factor for prevalent gout with SLC2A9 genotype-specific effects on serum urate and risk of gout. Ann Rheum Dis 2013. [Epub ahead of print].
39. Choi HK, Curhan G. Beer, liquor, and wine consumption and serum uric acid level: the Third National Health and Nutrition Examination Survey. Arthritis Rheum 2004;51:1023–9.
40. Choi HK, Curhan G. Soft drinks, fructose consumption, and the risk of gout in men: prospective cohort study. BMJ 2008;336:309–12.

41. Facchini F, Chen YD, Hollenbeck CB, et al. Relationship between resistance to insulin-mediated glucose uptake, urinary uric acid clearance, and plasma uric acid concentration. JAMA 1991;266:3008–11.

42. Choi HK, Soriano LC, Zhang Y, et al. Antihypertensive drugs and risk of incident gout among patients with hypertension: population based case-control study. BMJ 2012;344:d8190.

43. Hamajima N, Naito M, Okada R, et al. Significant interaction between LRP2 rs2544390 in intron 1 and alcohol drinking for serum uric acid levels among a Japanese population. Gene 2012;503:131–6.

44. Zhang Y, Woods R, Chaisson CE, et al. Alcohol consumption as a trigger of recurrent gout attacks. Am J Med 2006;119:800.e11.

45. Yamanaka H, Kamatani N, Hakoda M, et al. Analysis of the genotypes for aldehyde dehydrogenase 2 in Japanese patients with primary gout. Adv Exp Med Biol 1994;370:53–6.

46. McAdams-Demarco MA, Maynard JW, Baer AN, et al. A urate gene-by-diuretic interaction and gout risk in participants with hypertension: results from the ARIC study. Ann Rheum Dis 2013;72:701–6.

47. Witkowska K, Smith KM, Yao SY, et al. Human SLC2A9a and SLC2A9b isoforms mediate electrogenic transport of urate with different characteristics in the presence of hexoses. Am J Physiol Renal Physiol 2012;15:F527–39.

48. Dalbeth N, House ME, Gamble GD, et al. Population-specific influence of SLC2A9 genotype on the acute hyperuricaemic response to a fructose load. Ann Rheum Dis 2013;72(11):1868–73.

49. Winnard D, Wright C, Taylor WJ, et al. National prevalence of gout derived from administrative health data in Aotearoa New Zealand. Rheumatology (Oxford) 2012;51:901–9.

50. Taylor W. Diagnosis of gout: considering clinical and research settings. Curr Rheumatol Rev 2011;7:97–105.

51. Hollis-Moffatt JE, Phipps-Green AJ, Chapman B, et al. The renal urate transporter SLC17A1 locus: confirmation of association with gout. Arthritis Res Ther 2012;14(2):R92.

52. Urano W, Taniguchi A, Anzai N, et al. Sodium-dependent phosphate cotransporter type 1 sequence polymorphisms in male patients with gout. Ann Rheum Dis 2010;69:1232–4.

Structural Joint Damage in Gout

Ashika Chhana, PhD, Nicola Dalbeth, MBChB, MD, FRACP*

KEYWORDS

• Gout • Urate crystal • Bone • Cartilage • Tendon

KEY POINTS

- Patients with chronic tophaceous gout often have structural damage in affected joints.
- Characteristic features of joint damage in gout include bone erosion, new bone formation, deposition of tophi within tendons, focal cartilage loss, and eventually complete destruction of the joint. There is a strong relationship between these structural changes and the presence of tophi at sites of joint damage.
- Increased osteoclast formation and activity and reduced osteoblast viability, function, and differentiation contribute to bone erosion in gout.
- Cartilage damage in gout is a result of reduced chondrocyte viability and matrix production and increased catabolic enzyme activity and inflammation.
- Research is needed to determine the effectiveness of urate-lowering therapy, anti–interleukin-1 treatment and antiosteoclast agents in preventing and/or repairing joint damage in gout.

INTRODUCTION

Advanced gout is associated with structural damage that can lead to joint deformity and disability.[1] Characteristic features of joint damage in chronic gout include bone erosion; new bone formation, such as spur formation and sclerosis; deposition of tophi within tendons; focal cartilage loss; and eventually complete destruction of the joint. The deposition of monosodium urate monohydrate (MSU) crystals is the central feature of gout and is likely to play a central role in the progression of bone, cartilage, and tendon damage in people with gout (**Fig. 1**).

This review summarizes the mechanisms of bone erosion, cartilage damage, and tendon involvement in gout, with a particular focus on the role of joint cells within this process. Understanding the mechanisms of damage in advanced gout is necessary to help identify potential therapeutic strategies for the prevention and treatment of joint damage in gout.

The authors have nothing to disclose.
Bone & Joint Research Group, Department of Medicine, Faculty of Medical & Health Sciences, University of Auckland, 85 Park Road, Grafton, Auckland 1023, New Zealand
* Corresponding author.
E-mail address: n.dalbeth@auckland.ac.nz

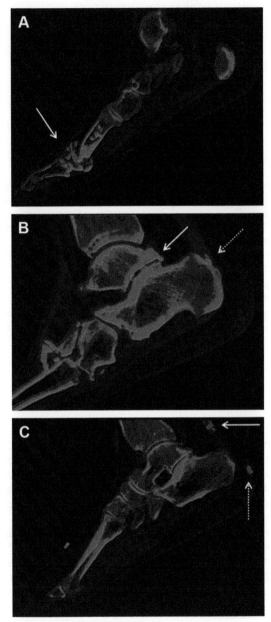

Fig. 1. Dual-energy computed tomography images of the feet from patients with tophaceous gout showing MSU crystals (*red*) (*A*) present within a bone erosion (*arrow*), (*B*) deposited on articular cartilage of the subtalar joint (*solid arrow*) and at the Achilles tendon enthesis (*dashed arrow*), and (*C*) within the Achilles tendon (*solid arrow*) and subcutaneous tissue (*dashed arrow*).

BONE EROSION IN GOUT

On plain radiography, bone changes in tophaceous gout typically consist of well-defined punched out focal erosions with sclerotic margins (**Fig. 2**).[2,3] Joint space widening and subchondral bone collapse may also develop in very advanced disease.[4,5] Radiographic bone erosion in gout is usually detected at later stages of disease.[6] Advanced imaging modalities allow further understanding about the patterns and mechanisms of bone erosion in gout. Magnetic resonance imaging (MRI) has shown that tophi, but not bone marrow edema or synovitis, is independently associated with the presence of bone erosion.[7] Tophi have been identified at sites of erosion in patients with gout using ultrasonography (US).[8–10] Conventional computed tomography (CT) enables excellent visualization of intraarticular tophi and bone erosions in patients with gout.[11–14] CT has also demonstrated the close relationship between intraosseous tophi and bone erosion in patients with gout.[14] A strong relationship between erosion score and the number of joints with intraosseous tophi was shown; and tophus size and erosion size were also found to be closely associated. Collectively, these findings implicate tophus infiltration into subchondral bone as a dominant mechanism for the development of bone erosion in gout.[14] Dual-energy CT (DECT) is a relatively new technology and is able to color code different materials within the joint according to their chemical composition, allowing differentiation between uric acid and calcium (bone) in joints.[15–17] In the future, DECT may prove to be a useful tool for examining the relationship between MSU crystal deposition and bone damage in gout (see **Fig. 1**A).

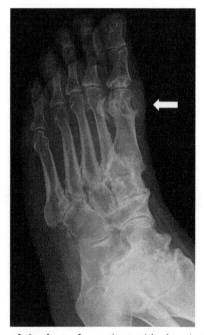

Fig. 2. Plain radiography of the foot of a patient with chronic tophaceous gout. Arrow shows an erosion at the first metatarsophalangeal joint with overlying soft tissue density (probable tophus). Features of new bone formation are also present with spur formation and bone sclerosis.

Cellular Mechanisms of Bone Erosion

Bone damage in chronic gout is closely associated with sites of MSU crystal deposition, with histologic and advanced imaging studies showing that crystals are often located adjacent to or within erosive lesions (see **Fig. 1A**).[14,18,19] MSU crystal deposits have been observed in histologic samples of subchondral bone in patients with gout,[19,20] indicating that bone cells, such as osteoclasts and osteoblasts, are in direct contact with MSU crystals following tophus infiltration into the bone.

The role of osteoclasts

As with other erosive arthropathies, such as rheumatoid arthritis and psoriatic arthritis,[21,22] the osteoclast has been identified as a key cellular mediator of localized bone loss in gout. Osteoclasts are multinucleated cells derived from hematopoietic stem cells; their main function is to resorb mineralized bone, helping to preserve a normal bone mass during physiological bone remodeling.[23] The differentiation of osteoclasts, or osteoclastogenesis, is a highly regulated process involving the interaction of receptor activator of nuclear factor-κB (RANK), expressed on osteoclast precursor cells, with receptor activator of nuclear factor-κB ligand (RANKL), which is expressed or secreted by mature osteoblasts (bone-forming cells) and activated T lymphocytes.[24] Osteoprotegerin (OPG) is a soluble decoy receptor for RANK secreted by osteoblasts and is a negative regulator of osteoclastogenesis.[24] Therefore, during bone remodeling, stromal cells have an important role in controlling osteoclastogenesis and subsequent bone resorption by determining the number of osteoclasts formed.

Histological analyses have demonstrated the presence of numerous osteoclast-like cells at sites of bone erosion in joint samples from patients with gout (**Fig. 3**).[25,26] These cells are positive for markers of active resorbing osteoclasts, such as tartrate-resistant acid phosphatase, the vitronectin receptor, and cathepsin K.[25,26] The increased numbers of osteoclasts in patients with tophaceous gout are most likely a result of enhanced osteoclastogenesis as these patients also have higher circulating levels of RANKL, monocyte colony-stimulating factor (M-CSF), and interleukin (IL)-6 receptor, factors critical for the development of mature osteoclasts.[25,27] Furthermore, peripheral blood mononuclear cells and synovial fluid mononuclear cells taken from patients with erosive gout preferentially formed osteoclast-like cells in the presence of RANKL and M-CSF.[25] The number of osteoclasts formed significantly correlated

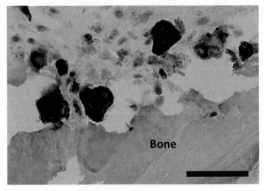

Bone

Fig. 3. Immunohistological analysis of bone from a gouty joint stained with cathepsin K demonstrating the presence of multinucleated osteoclasts (*stained brown*) at the bone-tophus interface. The bone surface is irregular and eroded with no osteoblasts or lining cells present (cathepsin K, original magnification × 200). Scale bar represents 50 μm.

with the number of tophi in the same patient. The direct culture of MSU crystals with osteoclast precursors did not increase osteoclast numbers,[25] although conditioned media from osteoblast-like cells cultured with MSU crystals did promote osteoclast formation from monocyte/macrophage precursors.[25] This finding indicates that MSU crystals may drive osteoclast formation by altering the balance of RANKL and OPG in stromal cells to favor osteoclastogenesis and bone resorption. Taken together, these reports suggest that enhanced osteoclast formation is an important mechanism for the development of bone erosion in gout.

The role of osteoblasts

Osteoblasts are responsible for new bone formation and are derived from mesen-chymal stem cells.[28] Osteoblasts may contribute to bone erosion in gout by promoting osteoclast formation. Human osteoblasts stimulated with MSU crystals and IL-1 showed upregulated expression of osteoclastogenesis promoters, such as prosta-glandin E_2 (PGE_2) and IL-6.[29] MSU crystals have also been shown to inhibit OPG gene and protein expression in an osteoblastic cell line, without significantly altering RANKL gene expression.[25] In addition, a recent study reported increased protein expression of RANKL in tophus samples from patients with gout, whereas OPG expression was largely absent.[26]

MSU crystals have also been shown to have direct effects on osteoblasts that may contribute to localized bone loss in gout that is not related to osteoclast activity. MSU crystals have a profound negative effect on osteoblast viability, function, and differen-tiation.[30] In vitro studies have demonstrated that MSU crystals reduced primary hu-man osteoblast viability in a dose-dependent manner; this finding was supported by the histological analysis of bone samples taken from the joints of patients with gout that had a relative paucity of bone lining cells and mature osteoblasts at sites of MSU crystal deposition and tophaceous material (see **Fig. 3**). The function and differ-entiation of osteoblasts is also impaired in the presence of MSU crystals. There was suppression of osteoblast activity markers osteocalcin and alkaline phosphatase following culture of human osteoblasts with MSU crystals and IL-1.[29] Long-term cul-ture of MSU crystals with osteoblast-like cells in vitro resulted in reduced mineraliza-tion and decreased expression of genes important for osteoblastogenesis, such as *Cbfa1* (Runx2), *Sp7* (osterix), *Ibsp* (bone sialoprotein), and *Bglap* (osteocalcin).[30]

To summarize, the available data suggest that osteoblasts contribute to bone loss in gout in 2 ways. Firstly, by modulating the RANKL/OPG axis to promote osteoclasto-genesis and bone resorption and, secondly, through the reduction of viability, differen-tiation, and function of osteoblasts following exposure to MSU crystals, leading to impaired mineralization and bone formation in joints affected by MSU crystal deposition.

Other mediators of bone erosion in gout

Other cell types are also likely to contribute to the joint damage observed in gout as the tophus contains numerous immune and stromal cells that produce a variety of soluble factors.[31] Cell-cell interactions between these various immune and stromal cells may contribute to joint damage in gout. An in vitro study investigating the interactions be-tween neutrophils and osteoblasts cultured on calcified matrix demonstrated that neu-trophils were able to induce osteoblast retraction in the presence of MSU crystals, which allowed osteoclast-like cells to resorb the newly exposed matrix surface below.[32] MSU crystals in the presence of IL-1β stimulated *Ptgs2* (cyclooxygenase-2 [COX-2]) gene expression and the release of PGE_2 protein from chondrocytes and synovial fibroblasts, which could enhance osteoclastogenesis.[24,33,34]

Other innate and adaptive immune cells present within the tophus, such as mono-nucleated and multinucleated macrophages and T and B lymphocytes[26,31] that come into contact with MSU crystals, are also likely to promote osteoclastogenesis through increased expression of RANKL, IL-1β, IL-6, tumor necrosis factor-α (TNF-α), and PGE$_2$.[26,35,36] T lymphocytes have been shown to be especially important, as osteo-clast formation from synovial fluid mononuclear cells derived from patients with chronic gout was inhibited in T-cell depleted cultures.[26]

Proinflammatory cytokines produced in the tophus, such as IL-1β, IL-6, and TNF-α,[26,31,37] as well as increasing osteoclastogenesis, are also likely to amplify bone resorption and joint damage by inducing degradative enzyme expression in stro-mal cells.[37–39] IL-1β is particularly important, as this cytokine is crucial for initiating inflammation during gouty flares[40,41] and it is also expressed within the tophus.[31] In addition to increasing osteoclastogenesis,[42] IL-1 has direct effects on bone cells, which may contribute to the bony changes seen in gout. IL-1 has been shown to in-crease osteoclast-like cell viability[43] and induce cytokine production in human osteo-blasts.[44] Human and mouse osteoblast-like cells cultured with IL-1 also demonstrated increased proliferation, reduced osteocalcin production, and inhibition of alkaline phosphatase activity.[45,46] IL-1 may also have similar effects on osteoblasts within the gouty joint.

Altered Bone Remodeling in Gout

From the data that are currently available on the role of bone cells in mediating bone erosion in gouty joints, the authors suggest that physiological bone remodeling is altered at the tophus-bone interface. In vitro and histological analyses have confirmed that there is excessive osteoclast formation and activity as well as reduced osteoblast viability and function at sites of MSU crystal deposition, overall resulting in localized bone loss (**Fig. 4**). The balance of bone resorption and bone formation at these sites is further disrupted because the inhibition of osteoblast differentiation from

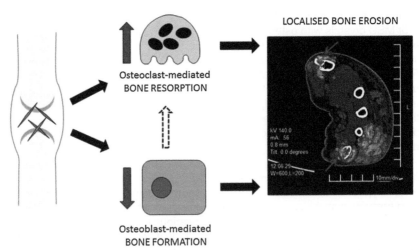

Osteoclast-mediated
BONE RESORPTION

LOCALISED BONE EROSION

Osteoblast-mediated
BONE FORMATION

Fig. 4. The presence of MSU crystals within gouty joints leads to increased osteoclast-mediated bone resorption and reduced osteoblast viability, differentiation, and function. This process results in localized bone erosion (*arrows*) at the site of tophus deposition. (*Adapted from* Dalbeth N, Clark B, Gregory K, et al. Mechanisms of bone erosion in gout: a quantitative analysis using plain radiography and computed tomography. Ann Rheum Dis 2009;68:1292; with permission.)

mesenchymal stem cells in the presence of MSU crystals leads to a decreased population of cells needed to replace and repair these erosive lesions with new bone. This model focuses entirely on the mechanism of bone loss (erosion) in response to MSU crystals. As discussed later, the mechanisms of new bone formation in joints affected by chronic gout require further study.

CARTILAGE DAMAGE IN GOUT

Normal adult articular cartilage is made up of an abundant extracellular matrix (ECM) composed mainly of type II collagen fibrils interspersed with types IX and XI collagens. Chondrocytes are derived from mesenchymal stem cells and comprise 2% to 5% of cartilage tissue volume. Chondrocytes have very low metabolic activity, partly because of low vascularization and innervation of cartilage tissues. Their principal function is to maintain the ECM by low turnover replacement of matrix components in response to mechanical stimuli, growth factors, and cytokines.[47,48] Cartilage loss tends to be a late feature of gouty arthropathy and, similar to bone erosion, is localized rather than diffuse. Cartilage damage is often associated with erosion and has been described as occurring in regions of biomechanical stress.[49,50]

Histopathological observations indicate that MSU crystals are deposited radially in the superficial layers of articular cartilage.[18,19] US studies have further demonstrated the close relationship between MSU crystals and articular cartilage as the double contour sign, which can be visualized over the superficial margin of the articular cartilage in gouty joints, and is thought to represent MSU crystal deposition.[8,51] DECT imaging may also be useful in identifying urate crystal deposits overlying cartilage in gouty joints (see **Fig. 1**B).

Mechanisms of Cartilage Damage

As with bone erosion in gout, MSU crystal deposition and tophus formation may also contribute to the loss of cartilage matrix in gout through the production of enzymes and other degradative products within and around the tophus region.

The role of chondrocytes

MSU crystals have negative effects on chondrocyte and cartilage viability and function.[52] The authors recently demonstrated that MSU crystals increase chondrocyte death in a dose-dependent manner in both isolated human chondrocytes and in human cartilage explants. This inhibitory effect was independent of crystal size, and soluble urate did not alter viability at similar concentrations. The ability of chondrocytes to produce matrix was also impaired following culture with MSU crystals, as both gene and protein expression of collagens was reduced. The gene expression of the matrix proteins aggrecan and versican was also reduced, suggesting that chondrocytes have limited repair capabilities in the presence of MSU crystals leading to compromised cartilage matrix. The potential clinical relevance of this in vitro work was further investigated through examination of cartilage in joints affected by tophaceous gout. Cartilage in these joints had abnormal morphology, with fewer live chondrocytes within lacunae. Notably, joints with extensive tophi had no intact hyaline articular cartilage; only small residual pieces of degenerate cartilage were remaining, almost entirely surrounded by tophaceous material (**Fig. 5**).[52] Chondrocytes have also been shown to actively contribute to cartilage degradation in gout. The authors reported that the gene expression of A disintegrin and metalloproteinase with thrombospondin motifs (ADAMTS)4 and ADAMTS5 aggrecanases was upregulated in human chondrocytes following culture with MSU crystals.[52]

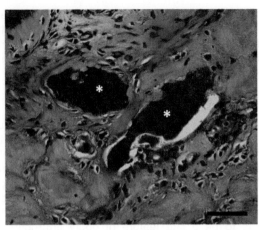

Fig. 5. Sample from the index finger distal interphalangeal joint of a cadaveric donor with microscopically proven gout showing 2 fragments of residual cartilage (*asterisks*) surrounded by tophaceous material (toluidine blue, original magnification × 400). Scale bar represents 50 µm.

Inflammation is also amplified by chondrocytes following culture with MSU crystals in vitro. MSU crystal binding to toll-like receptor 2 in bovine chondrocytes resulted in downstream NF-κβ activation through parallel intracellular signaling pathways involving MyD88, IL-1R–associated kinase 1, TNF receptor–associated factor 6, IκB kinase 2, and protein kinase Akt, eventually resulting in the release of nitric oxide.[53] This signaling may be upregulated in the context of elevated IL-1 within the tophus,[31] as knockdown of these signaling components in human chondrocytes inhibits IL-1 induced matrix metalloprotease (MMP)-13 gene expression.[54] IL-1β also inhibits proteoglycan synthesis and upregulates MMP-3 and MMP-13 expression in human chondrocytes and cartilage.[55] In another study, IL-1 treatment in rabbit articular chondrocytes also resulted in the release of large amounts of nitric oxide, which led to a decrease in DNA replication and proteoglycan synthesis.[56] High levels of nitric oxide can impair chondrocyte viability and may also enhance MMP activity,[57–59] leading to degradation of cartilage.

The role of degradative enzymes
MMPs are important for the maintenance of normal healthy cartilage. However, aberrant MMP activity is observed in other arthropathies and may be responsible for increased degradation of the ECM and compromised cartilage.[60,61] Furthermore, it is well known that the MMP activity is induced by and can be upregulated in the presence of IL-1.[62–66] As described earlier, IL-1β is essential for the initiation of acute gouty arthritis[40,41] and is expressed in the corona and fibrovascular zones within the tophus.[31] MMPs are also upregulated in gout by chondrocytes,[67] synovial fibroblasts,[33,68,69] and in macrophages isolated from gouty synovial tissue and within the tophus.[37,70]

TENDON INVOLVEMENT IN GOUT

Tendons connect muscle to bone and their main purpose is to transmit the force of muscle contraction to the skeleton and thus generate movement. Tendons also function to stabilize joints and are able to absorb large shocks, thereby protecting the muscle. The basic cellular units of tendons are tenocytes: fibroblastlike cells arranged in elongate rows within the collagen fibrils. Tenocytes produce collagens and other key matrix components of tendons.[71–73]

Several imaging modalities have been used to document the involvement of tendons in gout. An ultrasonographic analysis of 138 tophus-affected areas in 31 patients with gout reported tophus envelopment of the tendon as the most common finding, followed by presence of tophi at the enthesis, and lastly tophi adjacent to the tendon causing extrinsic compression.[74] MRI has demonstrated that tenosynovitis and tendinosis are seen in patients with gout.[75] US can also be used to identify hyperechoic aggregates within tendons, which can then be aspirated to confirm the presence of MSU crystals.[76] MSU crystal deposits have also been observed within the tendon and at the enthesis using CT in patients with gout.[13] Finally, a recent study using DECT in patients with tophaceous gout showed that 10.8% of tendon sites in the feet had MSU crystal deposition, with the Achilles tendon being the most commonly affected tendon of those assessed (see **Fig. 1**B, C).[77] Although tendon damage is not as clinically apparent as cartilage and bone damage in patients with advanced gout, cases of tendon rupture that may have been associated with the presence of MSU crystals or tophi have been reported.[78,79] Tophus infiltration into tendons has also been observed during surgery.[80–82]

The consequences of MSU crystal deposition and subsequent tophus formation on tendon function in patients with chronic gout are not fully known, but it is possible that larger crystal deposits may produce widening of the tendon and derangement of the normal linear tendon structure, which may have adverse effects on tendon function.[83] Examining the direct effects of MSU crystals on tenocytes will be of interest in the future to understand if these cells have a role in causing tendon damage in chronic gout. An initial study has shown that MSU crystals reduce the viability of both rat and human tenocytes in a dose-dependent manner.[84] IL-1β induces the expression of COX-2 and the degradative enzymes MMP-1, -3, and -13, and ADAMTS4 in human tenocytes.[85] Given that IL-1β is highly expressed in the tophus,[31] it is possible that these factors are also upregulated in tendons affected by gout, which would contribute to joint damage.

FUTURE RESEARCH DIRECTIONS
Mechanisms of New Bone Formation

Although bone erosion is the most pronounced feature observed in joints from patients with chronic gout, pathological new bone formation is also frequently observed.[5] The mechanisms behind new bone formation in gout are unknown. The features of new bone formation in gout have recently been described using plain radiography and CT.[86] The most common specific features of new bone formation in gout were bone sclerosis and bony spurs. Periosteal new bone formation was less common and ankylosis was rare. Osteophytes were also frequently observed. Joints with bone erosion and/or intraosseous tophi were more likely to have features of new bone formation, suggesting that there is a connection between bone erosion, the presence of tophi, and new bone formation during bone remodeling in gout.[86]

Bone morphogenic proteins (BMPs) and several Wnt signaling molecules have been implicated in pathological bone formation in other inflammatory arthropathies. Inhibition of the Wnt antagonist Dickkopf (DKK)-1 in a mouse model of rheumatoid arthritis demonstrated osteophyte formation, reduced bone erosion, and increased β-catenin expression in bone cells.[87,88] β-catenin is essential for osteoblast differentiation.[89] The anabolic Wnt factor DKK-2 has been shown to be upregulated in osteoarthritic osteoblasts[90] and was also shown to be involved in repair bone formation following resolution of inflammation in a mouse model of rheumatoid arthritis.[91] BMPs have been shown to promote osteogenesis and bone formation[92,93] and have a role in abnormal bone formation in ankylosing spondylitis.[94] Wnt signaling and BMPs may also play an important role in pathological new bone formation in chronic gout. The Wnt signaling pathway may also be involved in gouty cartilage degradation, as it is important for the cartilage changes that are observed in osteoarthritis (OA). β-catenin activation in chondrocytes results in increased MMP and ADAMTS expression as well as proteoglycan release. These effects were enhanced in the presence of IL-1β.[95] In an animal model of OA, β-catenin expression in chondrocytes was associated with age and degradation of cartilage. Other studies have shown that inhibition of Wnt signaling may contribute to cartilage destruction. The loss of DKK-1 function in a rodent model of OA inhibited chondrocyte apoptosis and impeded cartilage degradation and subchondral bone remodeling.[96] Conversely, upregulation of DKK-1 expression in a different model of OA was associated with increased expression of MMPs and proteinases and the loss of cartilage.[97] Studies investigating the changes in Wnt signaling in the context of gout will be useful in determining if this pathway contributes to the changes in bone, cartilage, and tendon observed in gouty joints.

The Link Between OA and Gout

A key unanswered question in gout pathogenesis is why MSU crystals preferentially form and deposit in certain joints. The first metatarsophalangeal joint is often the first and most common joint to suffer from a gouty attack.[98,99] Other than the known factors that contribute to the formation of MSU crystals, such as local temperature and pH, there is growing evidence to suggest that the presence of OA is related to MSU crystal formation and deposition. It is now well recognized that there is an association between gout and OA and that this relationship is likely to influence which joints are affected by gout.[100,101]

A histological study of 7855 cadaveric adult human tali demonstrated deposits of crystals on talar cartilage surfaces and the attached surrounding synovial tissue.[49] Further examination revealed that 67% of the sampled tali with surface crystals were actually deposits of MSU crystals and that these MSU crystal deposits were nearly always associated with cartilage lesions. MSU crystals were usually located on the surface of the superficial zone of cartilage but were also present within fissures that extended down into regions of degenerated cartilage.[49] Another recent study showed that synovial fluid urate levels were strongly and positively associated with OA severity in the knee, as measured by radiography and bone scintigraphy.[102] A smaller pilot study also found MSU crystal deposits on cartilage surfaces in patients with advanced OA undergoing knee replacement; these patients had no history of gout.[103]

Several reasons have been postulated as to why MSU crystals preferentially deposit in osteoarthritic cartilage,[101] such as the presence of nucleating factors, such as chondroitin sulfate from degraded cartilage, which lowers urate solubility and promotes MSU crystal formation.[104–106] Increased chondrocyte cell death in late-stage osteoarthritic cartilage,[107] which leads to locally elevated concentrations of urate in the joint from the degradation of nucleic acids,[108] may also promote MSU crystal precipitation. Biomechanical differences arising from differences in gait patterns in patients with OA and/or gout may also contribute to where MSU crystals form and deposit.[50,109] The relative preferential deposition of MSU crystals within the Achilles tendon and its enthesis compared with other sites of tendon involvement in gout[77,83] also supports the hypothesis that biomechanical strain contributes to the development of OA and subsequent MSU crystal formation.

Development of a Suitable In Vivo Model to Study Structural Changes in Gout

At present, a major limitation in understanding the mechanisms of joint damage in gout is the lack of a suitable in vivo model to study long-term chronic gout. Current rodent models of gout facilitate short-term studies that enable researchers to study acute gout. In these models, MSU crystals are most often injected into the peritoneal cavity[110] or membrane pouches in the dorsal subcutaneous tissue[111] as a substitute for the joint. Intraarticular models of gout whereby MSU crystals are injected into the ankle joints of rats or mice have been used to study acute gout. In these models, histological analyses have demonstrated that tissue edema and inflammation, including cytokine and chemokine production, occur rapidly following MSU crystal injection.[112,113] However, the presence of functional uricase in rodents is a limiting factor in the use of these models for studying chronic gout and although a uricase knockout animal model seems to be the likely answer to this problem, attempts to disrupt the urate oxidase gene in mice have led to high mortality rates and the development of urate nephropathy.[114] The development of an appropriate model in which chronic tophaceous gout can be induced, and in which articular spaces are used to represent human disease, is needed to allow further investigation into the mechanisms of joint damage in this disease. Importantly, this model would enable the study of joint structural changes over time and could help determine the sequence of events that leads to total destruction of the joint in gout, including whether cartilage degradation precedes bone erosion or whether both lesions occur simultaneously.

Therapeutic Strategies for Prevention and Treatment of Structural Joint Damage in Gout

Urate lowering therapy (ULT) is important in the long-term management of gout, and a serum urate concentration less than 360 μmol/L is the recommended target for most patients with gout.[115,116] Lower serum urate targets are recommended for people with severe tophaceous disease.[115] Given the strong relationship between bone erosion and intraosseous tophi, it seems likely that effective ULT, which can lead to resolution of tophi,[117,118] may prevent development or progression of bone erosion in people with gout. In a recent exploratory study whereby patients with tophaceous gout were treated with pegloticase, there was a significant reduction in radiographic joint damage after 1 year, with improvement in bone erosion scores.[119] Site-by-site analysis revealed regression of soft tissue masses, sclerosis, and filling in of erosive lesions with new bone, demonstrating that reducing serum urate to very low concentrations can alter the progression of radiographic damage.[119] As MSU crystals inhibit the function of osteoblasts within the gouty joint,[29,30] it seems reasonable to assume that while MSU crystals are still present within the joint, repair processes are limited, as the crystals continue to reduce the viability, differentiation, and function of the cells needed to form new replacement bone. The apparent healing of bone erosion following pegloticase treatment suggests that this may be possible.[119] It is currently unknown whether effective ULT can prevent joint damage in people with gout or what serum urate targets are required to achieve healing once bone erosion has developed.

Since the discovery that IL-1β is critical for initiation of MSU crystal-induced acute inflammation,[40,41] several clinical trials have demonstrated reduced inflammation and fewer gouty flares in patients with gout following treatment with inhibitors of IL-1 signaling, such as canakinumab, rilonacept, and anakinra.[120–123] As described earlier, IL-1 is also expressed within the tophus, and this cytokine has potent catabolic effects on bone and cartilage.[38,124,125] Longer-term studies are needed to determine whether

IL-1 inhibitors are effective in preventing development or progression of joint damage in people with gout.

Finally, given that osteoclast-mediated bone resorption is responsible for the focal bone erosions observed in gouty joints, therapies that aim to inhibit osteoclast activity may also be useful for preventing bone erosion in gouty joints. Bisphosphonates are widely available agents that have potent anti-osteoclast activity. Studies that assess the effects of bisphosphonates in the prevention of bone erosion in gout will be of interest.

A key issue in the assessment of therapies for prevention and treatment of structural damage is outcome measurement. With the exception of the small exploratory study of the potent urate-lowering drug pegloticase,[119] no clinical studies have shown improvement in structural damage in people with gout. The rate of structural damage in gout and the optimal time points for such studies are currently unknown. Several instruments have been developed for the assessment of structural damage in gout; these include a modified Sharp-van der Heijde scoring method for radiographic damage, which has been validated for gout,[6] and a scoring method for bone erosion in the feet using conventional CT.[126] The development and validation of US and MRI outcome measures for the assessment of structural joint damage in gout are also in progress.[7,76] The application of these tools in clinical trials specifically addressing structural damage in gout is needed to determine the optimal therapeutic strategy to prevent and treat these complications of the disease.

REFERENCES

1. Dalbeth N, Collis J, Gregory K, et al. Tophaceous joint disease strongly predicts hand function in patients with gout. Rheumatology (Oxford) 2007;46:1804–7.
2. Schlesinger N. Diagnosis of gout: clinical, laboratory, and radiologic findings. Am J Manag Care 2005;11:S443–50 [quiz: S65–8].
3. Buckley TJ. Radiologic features of gout. Am Fam Physician 1996;54:1232–8.
4. Resnick D, Broderick TW. Intraosseous calcifications in tophaceous gout. Am J Roentgenol 1981;137:1157–61.
5. Barthelemy CR, Nakayama DA, Carrera GF, et al. Gouty arthritis: a prospective radiographic evaluation of sixty patients. Skeletal Radiol 1984;11:1–8.
6. Dalbeth N, Clark B, McQueen F, et al. Validation of a radiographic damage index in chronic gout. Arthritis Rheum 2007;57:1067–73.
7. McQueen F, Doyle A, Reeves Q, et al. Bone erosions in patients with chronic gouty arthropathy are associated with tophi but not bone oedema or synovitis: new insights from a 3T MRI study. Rheumatology (Oxford) 2014;53(1):95–103.
8. Thiele RG, Schlesinger N. Diagnosis of gout by ultrasound. Rheumatology (Oxford) 2007;46:1116–21.
9. Wright SA, Filippucci E, McVeigh C, et al. High-resolution ultrasonography of the first metatarsal phalangeal joint in gout: a controlled study. Ann Rheum Dis 2007;66:859–64.
10. Schueller-Weidekamm C, Schueller G, Aringer M, et al. Impact of sonography in gouty arthritis: comparison with conventional radiography, clinical examination, and laboratory findings. Eur J Radiol 2007;62:437–43.
11. Gerster JC, Landry M, Dufresne L, et al. Imaging of tophaceous gout: computed tomography provides specific images compared with magnetic resonance imaging and ultrasonography. Ann Rheum Dis 2002;61:52–4.
12. Gerster JC, Landry M, Duvoisin B, et al. Computed tomography of the knee joint as an indicator of intraarticular tophi in gout. Arthritis Rheum 1996;39:1406–9.

13. Gerster JC, Landry M, Rappoport G, et al. Enthesopathy and tendinopathy in gout: computed tomographic assessment. Ann Rheum Dis 1996;55:921–3.
14. Dalbeth N, Clark B, Gregory K, et al. Mechanisms of bone erosion in gout: a quantitative analysis using plain radiography and computed tomography. Ann Rheum Dis 2009;68:1290–5.
15. Kim SK, Lee H, Kim JH, et al. Potential interest of dual-energy computed tomography in gout: focus on anatomical distribution and clinical association. Rheumatology (Oxford) 2013;52:402–3.
16. Johnson TR, Weckbach S, Kellner H, et al. Clinical image: dual-energy computed tomographic molecular imaging of gout. Arthritis Rheum 2007;56:2809.
17. Choi HK, Al-Arfaj AM, Eftekhari A, et al. Dual energy computed tomography in tophaceous gout. Ann Rheum Dis 2009;68:1609–12.
18. Sokoloff L. The pathology of gout. Metabolism 1957;6:230–43.
19. Levin MH, Lichtenstein L, Scott HW. Pathologic changes in gout; survey of eleven necropsied cases. Am J Pathol 1956;32:871–95.
20. Jaffe HL. Gout. In: Metabolic, degenerative, and inflammatory diseases of bones and joints. Philadelphia: Lea & Febiger; 1972. p. 482–4.
21. Redlich K, Hayer S, Ricci R, et al. Osteoclasts are essential for TNF-alpha-mediated joint destruction. J Clin Invest 2002;110:1419–27.
22. Ritchlin CT, Haas-Smith SA, Li P, et al. Mechanisms of TNF-alpha- and RANKL-mediated osteoclastogenesis and bone resorption in psoriatic arthritis. J Clin Invest 2003;111:821–31.
23. Dempster DW. Anatomy and functions of the adult skeleton. In: Favus MJ, Bikle DD, editors. Primer on the metabolic bone diseases and disorders of mineral metabolism. 6th edition. Washington, DC: The American Society for Bone and Mineral Research; 2006. p. 7–11.
24. Takahashi N, Udagawa N, Takami M, et al. Cells of bone. Osteoclast generation. In: Bilezikiam JP, Raisz LG, Rodan GA, editors. Principles of bone biology, vol. 1, 2nd edition. San Diego (CA): Academic Press; 2002. p. 109–26.
25. Dalbeth N, Smith T, Nicolson B, et al. Enhanced osteoclastogenesis in patients with tophaceous gout: urate crystals promote osteoclast development through interactions with stromal cells. Arthritis Rheum 2008;58:1854–65.
26. Lee SJ, Nam KI, Jin HM, et al. Bone destruction by receptor activator of nuclear factor kappaB ligand-expressing T cells in chronic gouty arthritis. Arthritis Res Ther 2011;13:R164.
27. Choe JY, Lee GH, Kim SK. Radiographic bone damage in chronic gout is negatively associated with the inflammatory cytokines soluble interleukin 6 receptor and osteoprotegerin. J Rheumatol 2011;38:485–91.
28. Aubin JE, Lian JB, Stein GS. Bone formation: maturation and functional activities of osteoblast lineage cells. In: Favus MJ, editor. Primer on the metabolic bone diseases and disorders of mineral metabolism. 6th edition. Washington, DC 20036-3309: The American Society for Bone and Mineral Research; 2006. p. 20–9.
29. Bouchard L, de Medicis R, Lussier A, et al. Inflammatory microcrystals alter the functional phenotype of human osteoblast-like cells in vitro: synergism with IL-1 to overexpress cyclooxygenase-2. J Immunol 2002;168:5310–7.
30. Chhana A, Callon KE, Pool B, et al. Monosodium urate monohydrate crystals inhibit osteoblast viability and function: implications for development of bone erosion in gout. Ann Rheum Dis 2011;70:1684–91.
31. Dalbeth N, Pool B, Gamble GD, et al. Cellular characterization of the gouty tophus: a quantitative analysis. Arthritis Rheum 2010;62:1549–56.

32. Allaeys I, Rusu D, Picard S, et al. Osteoblast retraction induced by adherent neutrophils promotes osteoclast bone resorption: implication for altered bone remodeling in chronic gout. Lab Invest 2011;91:905–20.

33. Hasselbacher P. Stimulation of synovial fibroblasts by calcium oxalate and monosodium urate monohydrate. A mechanism of connective tissue degradation in oxalosis and gout. J Lab Clin Med 1982;100:977–85.

34. Lee HS, Lee CH, Tsai HC, et al. Inhibition of cyclooxygenase 2 expression by diallyl sulfide on joint inflammation induced by urate crystal and IL-1beta. Osteoarthritis Cartilage 2009;17:91–9.

35. Alwan WH, Dieppe PA, Elson CJ, et al. Hydroxyapatite and urate crystal induced cytokine release by macrophages. Ann Rheum Dis 1989;48:476–82.

36. Pouliot M, James MJ, McColl SR, et al. Monosodium urate microcrystals induce cyclooxygenase-2 in human monocytes. Blood 1998;91:1769–76.

37. Schweyer S, Hemmerlein B, Radzun HJ, et al. Continuous recruitment, co-expression of tumour necrosis factor-alpha and matrix metalloproteinases, and apoptosis of macrophages in gout tophi. Virchows Arch 2000;437:534–9.

38. Zwerina J, Redlich K, Polzer K, et al. TNF-induced structural joint damage is mediated by IL-1. Proc Natl Acad Sci U S A 2007;104:11742–7.

39. Kim JH, Jin HM, Kim K, et al. The mechanism of osteoclast differentiation induced by IL-1. J Immunol 2009;183:1862–70.

40. Chen CJ, Shi Y, Hearn A, et al. MyD88-dependent IL-1 receptor signaling is essential for gouty inflammation stimulated by monosodium urate crystals. J Clin Invest 2006;116:2262–71.

41. Martinon F, Petrilli V, Mayor A, et al. Gout-associated uric acid crystals activate the NALP3 inflammasome. Nature 2006;440:237–41.

42. Ragab AA, Nalepka JL, Bi Y, et al. Cytokines synergistically induce osteoclast differentiation: support by immortalized or normal calvarial cells. Am J Physiol Cell Physiol 2002;283:C679–87.

43. Jimi E, Shuto T, Koga T. Macrophage colony-stimulating factor and interleukin-1 alpha maintain the survival of osteoclast-like cells. Endocrinology 1995;136: 808–11.

44. Chaudhary LR, Spelsberg TC, Riggs BL. Production of various cytokines by normal human osteoblast-like cells in response to interleukin-1 beta and tumor necrosis factor-alpha: lack of regulation by 17 beta-estradiol. Endocrinology 1992;130:2528–34.

45. Kim CH, Kang BS, Lee TK, et al. IL-1beta regulates cellular proliferation, prostaglandin E2 synthesis, plasminogen activator activity, osteocalcin production, and bone resorptive activity of the mouse calvarial bone cells. Immunopharmacol Immunotoxicol 2002;24:395–407.

46. Evans DB, Bunning RA, Russell RG. The effects of recombinant human interleukin-1 beta on cellular proliferation and the production of prostaglandin E2, plasminogen activator, osteocalcin and alkaline phosphatase by osteoblast-like cells derived from human bone. Biochem Biophys Res Commun 1990;166:208–16.

47. Goldring MB. Update on the biology of the chondrocyte and new approaches to treating cartilage diseases. Best Pract Res Clin Rheumatol 2006;20: 1003–25.

48. Goldring MB. Human chondrocyte cultures as models of cartilage-specific gene regulation. Methods Mol Med 1996;2:217–32.

49. Muehleman C, Li J, Aigner T, et al. Association between crystals and cartilage degeneration in the ankle. J Rheumatol 2008;35:1108–17.

50. Roddy E. Revisiting the pathogenesis of podagra: why does gout target the foot? J Foot Ankle Res 2011;4:13.
51. Grassi W, Meenagh G, Pascual E, et al. "Crystal clear"-sonographic assessment of gout and calcium pyrophosphate deposition disease. Semin Arthritis Rheum 2006;36:197–202.
52. Chhana A, Callon K, Pool B, et al. The effects of monosodium urate monohydrate crystals on chondrocyte viability and function: implications for development of cartilage damage in gout. J Rheumatol 2013;40(12):2067–74.
53. Liu-Bryan R, Pritzker K, Firestein GS, et al. TLR2 signaling in chondrocytes drives calcium pyrophosphate dihydrate and monosodium urate crystal-induced nitric oxide generation. J Immunol 2005;174:5016–23.
54. Ahmad R, Sylvester J, Zafarullah M. MyD88, IRAK1 and TRAF6 knockdown in human chondrocytes inhibits interleukin-1-induced matrix metalloproteinase-13 gene expression and promoter activity by impairing MAP kinase activation. Cell Signal 2007;19:2549–57.
55. Terkeltaub R, Yang B, Lotz M, et al. Chondrocyte AMP-activated protein kinase activity suppresses matrix degradation responses to proinflammatory cytokines interleukin-1beta and tumor necrosis factor alpha. Arthritis Rheum 2011;63: 1928–37.
56. Tamura T, Nakanishi T, Kimura Y, et al. Nitric oxide mediates interleukin-1-induced matrix degradation and basic fibroblast growth factor release in cultured rabbit articular chondrocytes: a possible mechanism of pathological neovascularization in arthritis. Endocrinology 1996;137:3729–37.
57. Blanco FJ, Ochs RL, Schwarz H, et al. Chondrocyte apoptosis induced by nitric oxide. Am J Pathol 1995;146:75–85.
58. Taskiran D, Stefanovic-Racic M, Georgescu H, et al. Nitric oxide mediates suppression of cartilage proteoglycan synthesis by interleukin-1. Biochem Biophys Res Commun 1994;200:142–8.
59. Murrell GA, Jang D, Williams RJ. Nitric oxide activates metalloprotease enzymes in articular cartilage. Biochem Biophys Res Commun 1995;206:15–21.
60. Giannelli G, Erriquez R, Iannone F, et al. MMP-2, MMP-9, TIMP-1 and TIMP-2 levels in patients with rheumatoid arthritis and psoriatic arthritis. Clin Exp Rheumatol 2004;22:335–8.
61. Yoshihara Y, Obata K, Fujimoto N, et al. Increased levels of stromelysin-1 and tissue inhibitor of metalloproteinases-1 in sera from patients with rheumatoid arthritis. Arthritis Rheum 1995;38:969–75.
62. Aida Y, Maeno M, Suzuki N, et al. The effect of IL-1beta on the expression of matrix metalloproteinases and tissue inhibitors of matrix metalloproteinases in human chondrocytes. Life Sci 2005;77:3210–21.
63. Koshy PJ, Lundy CJ, Rowan AD, et al. The modulation of matrix metalloproteinase and ADAM gene expression in human chondrocytes by interleukin-1 and oncostatin M: a time-course study using real-time quantitative reverse transcription-polymerase chain reaction. Arthritis Rheum 2002;46:961–7.
64. Shinmei M, Masuda K, Kikuchi T, et al. Production of cytokines by chondrocytes and its role in proteoglycan degradation. J Rheumatol Suppl 1991;27:89–91.
65. Tetlow LC, Adlam DJ, Woolley DE. Matrix metalloproteinase and proinflammatory cytokine production by chondrocytes of human osteoarthritic cartilage: associations with degenerative changes. Arthritis Rheum 2001;44:585–94.
66. Ainola MM, Mandelin JA, Liljestrom MP, et al. Pannus invasion and cartilage degradation in rheumatoid arthritis: involvement of MMP-3 and interleukin-1beta. Clin Exp Rheumatol 2005;23:644–50.

67. Liu R, Liote F, Rose DM, et al. Proline-rich tyrosine kinase 2 and Src kinase signaling transduce monosodium urate crystal-induced nitric oxide production and matrix metalloproteinase 3 expression in chondrocytes. Arthritis Rheum 2004;50:247–58.

68. McMillan RM, Vater CA, Hasselbacher P, et al. Induction of collagenase and prostaglandin synthesis in synovial fibroblasts treated with monosodium urate crystals. J Pharm Pharmacol 1981;33:382–3.

69. Hasselbacher P, McMillan RM, Vater CA, et al. Stimulation of secretion of collagenase and prostaglandin E2 by synovial fibroblasts in response to crystals of monosodium urate monohydrate: a model for joint destruction in gout. Trans Assoc Am Physicians 1981;94:243–52.

70. Hsieh MS, Ho HC, Chou DT, et al. Expression of matrix metalloproteinase-9 (gelatinase B) in gouty arthritis and stimulation of MMP-9 by urate crystals in macrophages. J Cell Biochem 2003;89:791–9.

71. Liu CF, Aschbacher-Smith L, Barthelery NJ, et al. What we should know before using tissue engineering techniques to repair injured tendons: a developmental biology perspective. Tissue Eng Part B Rev 2011;17:165–76.

72. Riley G. Tendinopathy–from basic science to treatment. Nat Clin Pract Rheumatol 2008;4:82–9.

73. Benjamin M, Ralphs JR. The cell and developmental biology of tendons and ligaments. Int Rev Cytol 2000;196:85–130.

74. de Avila Fernandes E, Sandim GB, Mitraud SA, et al. Sonographic description and classification of tendinous involvement in relation to tophi in chronic tophaceous gout. Insights Imaging 2010;1:143–8.

75. Poh YJ, Dalbeth N, Doyle A, et al. Magnetic resonance imaging bone edema is not a major feature of gout unless there is concomitant osteomyelitis: 10-year findings from a high-prevalence population. J Rheumatol 2011;38:2475–81.

76. Naredo E, Uson J, Jiménez-Palop M, et al. Ultrasound-detected musculoskeletal urate crystal deposition: which joints and what findings should be assessed for diagnosing gout? Ann Rheum Dis 2013. [Epub ahead of print].

77. Dalbeth N, Kalluru R, Aati O, et al. Tendon involvement in the feet of patients with gout: a dual-energy CT study. Ann Rheum Dis 2013;72(9):1545–8.

78. Hernandez-Cortes P, Caba M, Gomez-Sanchez R, et al. Digital flexion contracture and severe carpal tunnel syndrome due to tophaceous infiltration of wrist flexor tendon: first manifestation of gout. Orthopedics 2011;34:e797–9.

79. Radice F, Monckeberg JE, Carcuro G. Longitudinal tears of peroneus longus and brevis tendons: a gouty infiltration. J Foot Ankle Surg 2011;50:751–3.

80. Therimadasamy A, Peng YP, Putti TC, et al. Carpal tunnel syndrome caused by gouty tophus of the flexor tendons of the fingers: sonographic features. J Clin Ultrasound 2011;39:463–5.

81. Rand B, McBride TJ, Dias RG. Combined triggering at the wrist and severe carpal tunnel syndrome caused by gouty infiltration of a flexor tendon. J Hand Surg Eur Vol 2010;35:240–2.

82. Sano K, Kohakura Y, Kimura K, et al. Atypical triggering at the wrist due to intratendinous infiltration of tophaceous gout. Hand (N Y) 2009;4:78–80.

83. Pascual E, Martinez A, Ordonez S. Gout: the mechanism of urate crystal nucleation and growth. A hypothesis based in facts. Joint Bone Spine 2013;80:1–4.

84. Chhana A, Callon K, Pool B, et al. Monosodium urate crystals inhibit tenocyte viability and function: implications for periarticular involvement in chronic gout [abstract]. Arthritis Rheum 2012;64(Suppl 10):137.

85. Tsuzaki M, Guyton G, Garrett W, et al. IL-1 beta induces COX2, MMP-1, -3 and -13, ADAMTS-4, IL-1 beta and IL-6 in human tendon cells. J Orthop Res 2003; 21:256–64.
86. Dalbeth N, Milligan A, Doyle A, et al. Characterization of new bone formation in gout: a quantitative site-by-site analysis using plain radiography and computed tomography. Arthritis Res Ther 2012;14:R165.
87. Diarra D, Stolina M, Polzer K, et al. Dickkopf-1 is a master regulator of joint remodeling. Nat Med 2007;13:156–63.
88. Heiland GR, Zwerina K, Baum W, et al. Neutralisation of Dkk-1 protects from systemic bone loss during inflammation and reduces sclerostin expression. Ann Rheum Dis 2010;69:2152–9.
89. Hill TP, Später D, Taketo MM, et al. Canonical Wnt/β-Catenin signaling prevents osteoblasts from differentiating into chondrocytes. Dev Cell 2005;8: 727–38.
90. Chan TF, Couchourel D, Abed E, et al. Elevated Dickkopf-2 levels contribute to the abnormal phenotype of human osteoarthritic osteoblasts. J Bone Miner Res 2011;26:1399–410.
91. Matzelle MM, Gallant MA, Condon KW, et al. Resolution of inflammation induces osteoblast function and regulates the Wnt signaling pathway. Arthritis Rheum 2012;64:1540–50.
92. Cheng H, Jiang W, Phillips FM, et al. Osteogenic activity of the fourteen types of human bone morphogenetic proteins (BMPs). J Bone Joint Surg Am 2003;85: 1544–52.
93. Wozney JM, Rosen V, Celeste AJ, et al. Novel regulators of bone formation: molecular clones and activities. Science 1988;242:1528–34.
94. Lories RJ, Derese I, Luyten FP. Modulation of bone morphogenetic protein signaling inhibits the onset and progression of ankylosing enthesitis. J Clin Invest 2005;115:1571–9.
95. Yuasa T, Otani T, Koike T, et al. Wnt/beta-catenin signaling stimulates matrix catabolic genes and activity in articular chondrocytes: its possible role in joint degeneration. Lab Invest 2008;88:264–74.
96. Weng LH, Wang CJ, Ko JY, et al. Control of Dkk-1 ameliorates chondrocyte apoptosis, cartilage destruction, and subchondral bone deterioration in osteoarthritic knees. Arthritis Rheum 2010;62:1393–402.
97. Weng LH, Ko JY, Wang CJ, et al. Dickkopf-1 promotes angiogenic responses and cartilage matrix proteinase secretion in synovial fibroblasts of osteoarthritic joints. Arthritis Rheum 2012;64:3267–77.
98. Klemp P, Stansfield SA, Castle B, et al. Gout is on the increase in New Zealand. Ann Rheum Dis 1997;56:22–6.
99. Grahame R, Scott JT. Clinical survey of 354 patients with gout. Ann Rheum Dis 1970;29:461–8.
100. Roddy E, Zhang W, Doherty M. Are joints affected by gout also affected by osteoarthritis? Ann Rheum Dis 2007;66:1374–7.
101. Roddy E, Doherty M. Gout and osteoarthritis: a pathogenetic link? Joint Bone Spine 2012;79:425–7.
102. Denoble AE, Huffman KM, Stabler TV, et al. Uric acid is a danger signal of increasing risk for osteoarthritis through inflammasome activation. Proc Natl Acad Sci U S A 2011;108:2088–93.
103. Bongartz T, Andre OM, Sierra RJ, et al. Cartilaginous uric acid deposition in advanced osteoarthritis: innocent bystander or promoter of cartilage destruction? [abstract]. Ann Rheum Dis 2013;72(Suppl 3):701.

104. Katz WA, Schubert M. The interaction of monosodium urate with connective tissue components. J Clin Invest 1970;49:1783–9.

105. Laurent TC. Solubility of sodium urate in the presence of chondroitin-4-sulphate. Nature 1964;202:1334.

106. Burt HM, Dutt YC. Growth of monosodium urate monohydrate crystals: effect of cartilage and synovial fluid components on in vitro growth rates. Ann Rheum Dis 1986;45:858–64.

107. Aigner T, Hemmel M, Neureiter D, et al. Apoptotic cell death is not a widespread phenomenon in normal aging and osteoarthritis human articular knee cartilage: a study of proliferation, programmed cell death (apoptosis), and viability of chondrocytes in normal and osteoarthritic human knee cartilage. Arthritis Rheum 2001;44:1304–12.

108. Shi Y, Evans JE, Rock KL. Molecular identification of a danger signal that alerts the immune system to dying cells. Nature 2003;425:516–21.

109. Rome K, Survepalli D, Sanders A, et al. Functional and biomechanical characteristics of foot disease in chronic gout: a case-control study. Clin Biomech 2011;26:90–4.

110. Getting SJ, Flower RJ, Parente L, et al. Molecular determinants of monosodium urate crystal-induced murine peritonitis: a role for endogenous mast cells and a distinct requirement for endothelial-derived selectins. J Pharmacol Exp Ther 1997;283:123–30.

111. Pessler F, Mayer C, Jung S, et al. Identification of novel monosodium urate crystal regulated mRNAs by transcript profiling of dissected murine air pouch membranes. Arthritis Res Ther 2008;10:R64.

112. Coderre TJ, Wall PD. Ankle joint urate arthritis (AJUA) in rats: an alternative animal model of arthritis to that produced by Freund's adjuvant. Pain 1987;28: 379–93.

113. Torres R, Macdonald L, Croll SD, et al. Hyperalgesia, synovitis and multiple biomarkers of inflammation are suppressed by interleukin 1 inhibition in a novel animal model of gouty arthritis. Ann Rheum Dis 2009;68:1602–8.

114. Wu X, Wakamiya M, Vaishnav S, et al. Hyperuricemia and urate nephropathy in urate oxidase-deficient mice. Proc Natl Acad Sci U S A 1994;91:742–6.

115. Khanna D, Fitzgerald JD, Khanna PP, et al. 2012 American College of Rheumatology guidelines for management of gout. Part 1: systematic nonpharmacologic and pharmacologic therapeutic approaches to hyperuricemia. Arthritis Care Res 2012;64:1431–46.

116. Zhang W, Doherty M, Bardin T, et al. EULAR evidence based recommendations for gout. Part II: management. Report of a task force of the EULAR Standing Committee For International Clinical Studies Including Therapeutics (ESCISIT). Ann Rheum Dis 2006;65:1312–24.

117. Perez-Ruiz F, Calabozo M, Pijoan JI, et al. Effect of urate-lowering therapy on the velocity of size reduction of tophi in chronic gout. Arthritis Rheum 2002;47:356–60.

118. Perez-Ruiz F, Martin I, Canteli B. Ultrasonographic measurement of tophi as an outcome measure for chronic gout. J Rheumatol 2007;34:1888–93.

119. Dalbeth N, Doyle AJ, McQueen FM, et al. Exploratory study of radiographic change in patients with tophaceous gout treated with intensive urate-lowering therapy. Arthritis Care Res (Hoboken) 2014;66(1):82–5.

120. Schlesinger N, Alten RE, Bardin T, et al. Canakinumab for acute gouty arthritis in patients with limited treatment options: results from two randomised, multicentre, active-controlled, double-blind trials and their initial extensions. Ann Rheum Dis 2012;71:1839–48.

121. Terkeltaub R, Sundy JS, Schumacher HR, et al. The interleukin 1 inhibitor rilonacept in treatment of chronic gouty arthritis: results of a placebo-controlled, monosequence crossover, non-randomised, single-blind pilot study. Ann Rheum Dis 2009;68:1613–7.
122. Terkeltaub RA, Schumacher HR, Carter JD, et al. Rilonacept in the treatment of acute gouty arthritis: a randomized, controlled clinical trial using indomethacin as the active comparator. Arthritis Res Ther 2013;15:R25.
123. So A, De Smedt T, Revaz S, et al. A pilot study of IL-1 inhibition by anakinra in acute gout. Arthritis Res Ther 2007;9:R28.
124. Joosten LA, Helsen MM, Saxne T, et al. IL-1 alpha beta blockade prevents cartilage and bone destruction in murine type II collagen-induced arthritis, whereas TNF-alpha blockade only ameliorates joint inflammation. J Immunol 1999;163: 5049–55.
125. Stolina M, Schett G, Dwyer D, et al. RANKL inhibition by osteoprotegerin prevents bone loss without affecting local or systemic inflammation parameters in two rat arthritis models: comparison with anti-TNF-alpha or anti-IL-1 therapies. Arthritis Res Ther 2009;11:R187.
126. Dalbeth N, Doyle A, Boyer L, et al. Development of a computed tomography method of scoring bone erosion in patients with gout: validation and clinical implications. Rheumatology (Oxford) 2011;50:410–6.

The Structural Consequences of Calcium Crystal Deposition

Laura Durcan, MD[a], Ferdia Bolster, MD[b],
Eoin C. Kavanagh, MB BCh, FRCSI[b],
Geraldine M. McCarthy, MD, FRCPI[a],*

KEYWORDS

- Calcium crystals • Basic calcium phosphate • Calcium pyrophosphate dihydrate
- Arthritis • Vascular calcification • Atherosclerosis

KEY POINTS

- Calcium pyrophosphate dihydrate and basic calcium phosphate crystals are the most common calcium-containing crystals associated with articular and periarticular disorders.
- Common clinical manifestations of calcium crystal include acute or chronic inflammatory and degenerative arthritides and certain forms of periarthritis.
- Current evidence suggests that calcium deposition, in its various forms, contributes directly to joint degeneration and causes inflammation.

INTRODUCTION

Calcium pyrophosphate dihydrate (CPP) and basic calcium phosphate (BCP) crystals are the most common calcium-containing crystals associated with articular and periarticular disorders. Deposition of these crystals is frequently asymptomatic but it can be intermittently symptomatic. However, common clinical manifestations of calcium crystal deposition include acute or chronic inflammatory and degenerative arthritides and certain forms of periarthritis. Current evidence suggests that calcium deposition, in its various forms, contributes directly to joint degeneration and causes inflammation. Although ample in vitro and recent in vivo evidence show the potent biological effects of calcium-containing crystals, controversy still exists as to whether these crystals play a causal role or are a consequence of joint destruction.[1] Vascular calcification is a common finding in aging, diabetes, chronic renal failure, and atherosclerosis. Although arterial calcification is now accepted to be an active and highly

None of the authors have any conflict of interest.
[a] Division of Rheumatology, Mater Misericordiae University Hospital, Eccles Street, Dublin 7, Ireland; [b] Department of Radiology, Mater Misericordiae University Hospital, Eccles Street, Dublin 7, Ireland
* Corresponding author.
E-mail address: g.mccarthy@ucd.ie

Rheum Dis Clin N Am 40 (2014) 311–328
http://dx.doi.org/10.1016/j.rdc.2014.01.007
0889-857X/14/$ – see front matter © 2014 Elsevier Inc. All rights reserved.

regulated process similar to that of bone ossification, the level of calcification has tended to be seen as a surrogate marker for the burden of atherosclerotic disease rather than a contributor to disease progression.[2] In this regard, investigations into the size and distribution of calcified deposits in atherosclerotic plaques have suggested that small, diffuse, speckled or spotty deposits cause local plaque stress and plaque instability, whereas large platelike areas of calcification correlate with stable plaques. This article reviews the clinical, radiographic, vascular, and cellular consequences of calcium crystal deposition.

CALCIUM CRYSTAL STRUCTURE AND IDENTIFICATION

CPP crystals have rhomboid or parallelelepedic morphology. They are typically described as weakly birefringent, but it has been noted that some CPP crystals lack birefringence under polarized light microscopy (PLM).[3] Nonetheless, they are generally readily identifiable by PLM of synovial fluid.

BCP crystals are composed mostly of partly carbonate-substituted hydroxyapatite but also include octacalcium phosphate, tricalcium phosphate, and magnesium whitlockite.[4] Although BCP crystals are common, particularly in osteoarthritis (OA), their presence in synovial fluid is recognized infrequently because of the lack of a simple, reliable test for detection. BCP crystals have no features that allow identification using light microscopy. They do not show any birefringence and are therefore not visible using PLM.[5]

Individual crystals are typically less than 1 μm (20–100 nm) and aggregate in synovial fluid to form amorphous-looking clumps.[6] The most widely used stain for detecting BCP crystals is alizarin red S, which indiscriminately stains calcium-containing particulates. These particulates appear orange or red using compensated PLM. This method leads to a high rate of false-positives.[7] As a result of this, more specific methods have been used, including ^{14}C-ethane-1-hydroxy-1,1-diphosphonate binding assay and tetracycline staining.[8] BCP crystals can also be imaged using several different methods including, but not limited to, scanning electron and atomic force microscopy and Fourier transform infrared and Raman spectroscopy. These methods are limited by availability and cost.[8]

CLINICAL MANIFESTATIONS OF CALCIUM CRYSTAL DEPOSITION

Calcium crystal deposition is often asymptomatic but can be associated with a wide spectrum of clinical manifestations (Table 1). A more comprehensive review of diagnosis and epidemiology are presented elsewhere in this issue.

Intra-articular CPP crystals can cause pseudogout. This condition is an acute crystal-induced synovitis. It is possibly the most common cause of acute monoarthritis in the elderly.[9] Any joint may be involved, but the knees (Fig. 1) and wrists are the commonest sites. The attack is self-limiting.

Several provocative factors have been recognized, the most common being stress response to intercurrent illness or surgery, including lavage of the affected joint. The incidence of pseudogout following arthroscopic lavage in knee OA with preexisting chondrocalcinosis is estimated to be 26%.[10] It has also been suggested that bisphosphonates[11,12] and intra-articular hyaluronan[13] can trigger pseudogout attacks. The mechanism by which these might induce acute synovitis mediated by CPP crystals remains unclear. Other clinical presentations associated with calcium pyrophosphate dehydrate (CPPD) include OA with CPPD and chronic CPP inflammatory arthritis.[14]

Table 1
Common clinical syndromes associated with the deposition of calcium crystals

Periarticular deposits of BCP crystals	Asymptomatic, incidental finding
	Acute calcific periarthritis
	Chronic periarticular pain and/or joint dysfunction
Intra-articular deposits of BCP crystals	Asymptomatic, incidental finding
	Acute synovitis
	Severe OA
	Destructive arthropathy (eg, Milwaukee shoulder syndrome)
Intra-articular CPP crystals	Asymptomatic, incidental finding
	Acute CPP crystal arthritis (pseudogout)
	Chronic CPP inflammatory arthritis
	OA with CPP

Underscoring the association of CPP and adverse structural consequences in the joint is the presence of CPP in patients without neurologic abnormalities who present with a painful mononeuropathy similar to that seen in neuropathic joints. Dramatic destructive radiographic changes are typical.[15]

Extra-articular calcium-containing crystals can cause tenosynovitis and nerve and spinal cord compression. Pseudotumoral deposition has also been described.[4,16,17] Both CPPD and BCP crystal deposition around the odontoid process can cause the so-called crowned dens syndrome, which is characterized by acute cervical pain and stiffness associated with fever.[18]

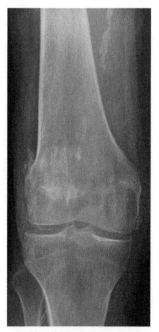

Fig. 1. Anteroposterior (AP) radiograph of the right knee showing calcification of the subarticular cartilage and of the menisci bilaterally. Also note calcified atherosclerosis of the superficial femoral artery.

Periarticular BCP crystal deposition can lead to calcific tendinitis, periarthritis, bursitis, and bone erosions.[19] Intra-articular BCP crystals are associated with a variety of degenerative manifestations, most notably the Milwaukee shoulder syndrome (MSS) (**Figs. 2–5**).[20,21] MSS is the prototypical example of the structural consequences of calcium crystal–associated joint destruction. It is associated with rotator cuff defects and numerous aggregates of BCP crystals in the synovial fluid. Fifty percent of these fluids also contain CPP crystals. MSS is characterized by large joint effusions. Rupture of the effusion can lead to a massive extravasation of blood and synovial fluid into the surrounding tissues (see **Fig. 2**). The synovial aspirate is frequently blood tinged and contains a low, predominantly mononuclear, cell count. In some fluids, collagenolytic enzyme activity is detected. There has been debate as to the role of BCP crystals in the pathogenesis of MSS. It has been proposed that the presence of intra-articular BCP crystals is the consequence of advanced degeneration and a product of denuded bone. However, the scarcity of BCP crystals in advanced secondary degenerative arthropathies, such as those resulting from rheumatoid arthritis, argues against the concept of BCP as simply an epiphenomenon in MSS.[22] Knee joints can also be affected.[23]

BCP crystals are frequently found in osteoarthritic cartilage, synovium, and synovial fluid. Apatite crystals have been found in between 30% and 67% of synovial fluid samples from patients with knee joint OA.[24–26] This detection rate depends on the sensitivity of the various techniques used. It has been suggested that many OA joint fluids contain clusters of BCP crystals that are too small or too few in number to be identified by conventional techniques.[22] Fuerst and colleagues[27] showed that human knee and hip cartilage harvested at the time of joint replacement contained BCP crystals in 100% of cases and CPPD in 20%. The exact prevalence of intra-articular BCP in normal joints or those with early OA remains difficult to ascertain, because BCP

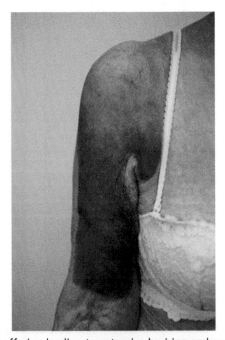

Fig. 2. MSS. Ruptured effusion leading to extensive bruising and swelling.

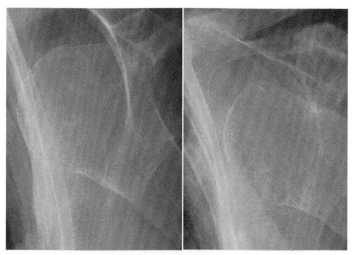

Fig. 3. Frontal radiographs taken 4 years apart of left shoulder in a patient with MSS. The left shoulder is dislocated anteriorly and there has been progressive resorption and deformity of the humeral head.

crystals are very small even when present in aggregates. Nalbant and colleagues[26] found the crystals in 52% of 330 synovial samples obtained from knees with OA, regardless of the OA grade. The menisci can also be involved. Sun and colleagues[28] reported calcium deposition in 100% of OA menisci harvested at the time of joint replacement surgery.

RADIOGRAPHIC AND DIAGNOSTIC IMAGING CHANGES ASSOCIATED WITH CALCIUM CRYSTAL DEPOSITION

The structural consequences of calcium crystal deposition are easily and often dramatically apparent on diagnostic imaging. Intra-articular BCP deposits are rarely detectable using plain radiography, whereas CPPD crystals are often visible.

Chondrocalcinosis predominantly results from CPP.[29] In CPPD, chondrocalcinosis can occur in both hyaline and fibrocartilage.[30] It is a common finding in plain film evaluation and occurs in 3.7% of persons aged 50 to 59 years and in 17.5% of those aged more than 80 years.[9] The Framingham study examined 1425 participants more than the age of 63 years and found an 8.1% prevalence of CPPD.[31] There is significant ethnic variation in the prevalence of chondrocalcinosis. A study by Zhang and colleagues[32] compared differences in the prevalence of chondrocalcinosis between Chinese subjects in Beijing and white subjects in the Framingham cohort. The Chinese subjects had a lower prevalence of knee chondrocalcinosis (1.8% in men, 2.7% in women) than white subjects (6.2% in men, 7.7% in women). Radiographic wrist chondrocalcinosis was rare in Chinese subjects.

Calcification of articular cartilage is a well-known and frequently observed phenomenon in late-stage OA.[33,34] Pathologic mineralization of articular cartilage is also described in association with various genetic and metabolic disorders.[35] There is ample evidence that hereditary hemochromatosis, hyperparathyroidism, and hypomagnesaemia predispose to chondrocalcinosis. CPP can also occur as a familial monogenic disorder with varying phenotype.[36] Familial CPPD has been recognized in many countries. Molecular genetics studies have identified 2 genetic locations: one (CCAL1) related to a mutation in the long arm of chromosome 8 (8q) and

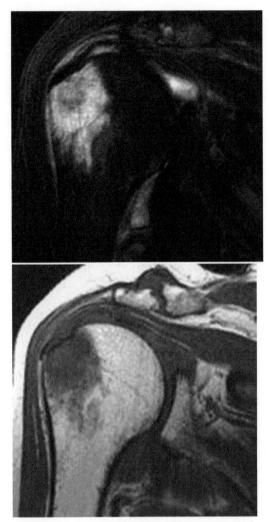

Fig. 4. Sagittal magnetic resonance imaging (MRI) (short tau inversion recovery [STIR] [*top panel*] and proton density [*bottom panel*]) of a right shoulder with early changes consistent with MSS. There is a complex joint effusion with subchondral edema and erosive change at the humeral head.

associated with severe OA, and the other (CCAL2) resulting from a mutation on the short arm of chromosome 5 (5p). The responsible gene at the CCAL2 locus has been identified as the ANKH (ankylosis human) gene, which codes for a transmembrane protein (ANKH). This protein regulates transport of inorganic pyrophosphate out of cells. However, these genetic mutations and metabolic derangements are rare and most chondrocalcinosis is sporadic. All epidemiologic studies evaluating chondrocalcinosis agree that aging is the most important risk factor and that, in those who present with chondrocalcinosis at a young age, screening for an underlying metabolic cause should be considered.[37]

In CPPD, fibrocartilaginous calcifications are most commonly seen in the menisci of the knee, triangular fibrocartilage of the wrist,[38] symphysis pubis, annulus fibrosis of

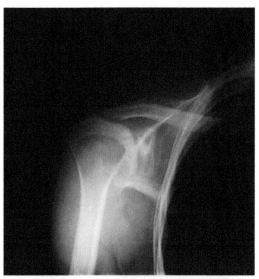

Fig. 5. Frontal radiograph of right shoulder in a patient with MSS. There is marked narrowing of the acromiohumeral interval with remodeling of the undersurface of the acromion consistent with chronic rotator cuff tear. The humeral head is flattened and sclerotic consistent with secondary avascular necrosis.

the intervertebral disc, and acetabular and glenoid labra.[39] Calcific deposits can also be visualized within the fibrocartilage of the sternoclavicular and acromioclavicular joints.[40,41] Hyaline cartilage deposits are seen most commonly in the knee, wrist, hip, elbow, and shoulder. These deposits are usually thin, punctate or linear, and are parallel to but separated from the subchondral bone plate. Capsular calcification is most frequently seen in the elbow, knee, and metacarpophalangeal and glenohumeral joints. Calcification of tendons, bursae, and ligaments has also been described as features of CPPD.[42] The most commonly involved tendons include the Achilles, triceps, quadriceps, gastrocnemius (**Fig. 6**), popliteus, and occasionally the tendons of the rotator cuff. Commonly involved ligaments include the intercarpal and cruciate ligaments. Soft tissue calcification can be seen in CPPD, in particular around the elbows, pelvis, and wrist. Plain radiography often fails to correlate with the symptoms and clinical features of CPP deposition. One study found a correlation of only 39.2% between radiographic and arthroscopic findings.[43]

Radiographically visible BCP deposition is predominantly periarticular with calcifications occurring near the insertion of supraspinatus (**Figs. 7** and **8**), in the flexor carpi ulnaris, near pisiform, and in the metacarpophalangeal joints. In the MSS, plain film of the affected joint commonly shows capsular calcification, subchondral sclerosis with cyst formation, destruction of subchondral bone, soft tissue swelling, and intra-articular loose bodies.[44] Using magnetic resonance imaging (MRI), the findings mirror those seen with plain film and include large joint effusion, rotator cuff tears, narrowing of the glenohumeral joint, thinning of cartilage, and destruction of subchondral bone (see **Fig. 4**).

An individual can be screened for CPPD using plain film by obtaining an anteroposterior (AP) view of each knee, an AP view of the pelvis, and posterior-anterior (PA) views of the hands, ensuring visualization of both wrists. It was previously accepted that screening for CPPD could be done by plain film AP view of the knees alone.

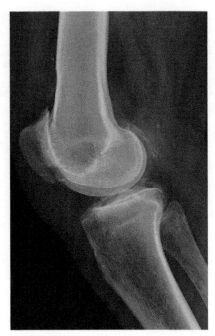

Fig. 6. Lateral radiograph of the left knee. There is severe narrowing of the patellofemoral joint, chondrocalcinosis and calcification of the gastrocnemius and quadriceps tendons consistent with CPPD arthropathy.

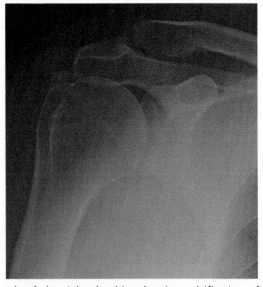

Fig. 7. AP radiograph of the right shoulder showing calcification of the supraspinatus tendon.

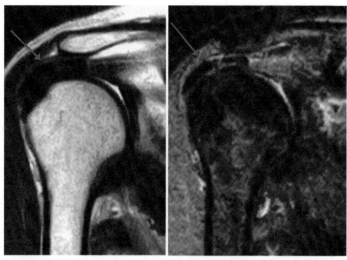

Fig. 8. Proton density (*left*) and STIR (*right*) MRI of right shoulder. Images show diffuse hypointense signal (*arrows*) in the supraspinatus tendon consistent with calcific tendinopathy.

However, the usefulness of this method was brought into question by the findings of the Genetics and Osteoarthritis and Lifestyle (GOAL) study. In the GOAL study, 42% of participants with chondrocalcinosis of hip, wrist, metacarpophalangeal joints, or pubic symphysis had no chondrocalcinosis on plain film evaluation of the knees. Another clinically useful lesson from the GOAL study was the finding that in the presence of metacarpophalangeal chondrocalcinosis more than 90% of participants had involvement elsewhere.[45,46]

Using ultrasonography (US), CPPD can be easily detected.[47] In contrast with gout, the crystals commonly lie within the substance of the hyaline cartilage. In fibrocartilage, calcific deposits in CPPD appear as hyperechoic rounded or amorphous areas.[48]

These aggregates can be easily identified in the menisci of the knee and in the triangular ligament of the wrist. A study by Foldes[49] determined the US features in 34 patients with CPPD disease diagnosed by joint aspiration. Articular chondrocalcinosis produces rounded hyperechoic foci that correlate with the radiographic images. Tendinous calcifications are also readily detectible using US. These are visible as hyperechoic lines of calcification running parallel to the tendon fibers. They are a common finding in patients with chondrocalcinosis and are frequently asymptomatic.

Frediani and colleagues[50] in 2005 evaluated the diagnostic criteria for chondrocalcinosis. Hyperechoic images were considered to reflect CPPD deposits if they had one of the following patterns: thin hyperechoic band parallel to the surface of the hyaline cartilage (often seen at the knee), punctate pattern of hyperechoic spots (seen chiefly in fibrocartilage and tendons), and/or homogeneous hyperechoic nodular or oval deposits in the bursae and articular recesses (frequently mobile).

These criteria were assessed by performing a US scan of the femoral head, menisci, and triangular fibrocartilage complex in 11 patients with known chondrocalcinosis and 13 controls. The findings were compared with those of the joint fluid examination. The 11 patients had US findings of chondrocalcinosis and CPPD crystals in joint fluid. None of the controls had any of the chondrocalcinosis US patterns, and none had CPPD crystals in synovial aspirate. A 2007 study compared patients with chondrocalcinosis diagnosed by US with controls to assess the diagnostic performance of US.[51]

The US findings were compared with the results of the joint fluid examination for CPPD crystals. US detected calcifications with 96.4% sensitivity and 86.7% specificity. In a 2009 study by Filippucci and colleagues,[52] 48 patients meeting McCarty criteria for chondrocalcinosis were compared with 32 patients with gout and 52 patients with rheumatoid arthritis, psoriatic arthritis, or OA. There was double contour sign in 14 patients with gout and 1 with chondrocalcinosis, with intra-cartilaginous hyperechoic spots in 68.7% with chondrocalcinosis and 2 control subjects.

In BCP deposition, US is also useful and has been studied most in calcific shoulder syndromes.[53] BCP deposits near the insertion of the supraspinatus tendon can be readily assessed sonographically. They frequently affect the critical zone, which is a poorly vascularized area of the supraspinatus tendon 0.5 to 1 cm proximal to its insertion. CPPD deposition over the humeral head is also easily identifiable using US.[39]

US also has role in guiding therapy in BCP crystal–associated arthropathies. A study by del Cura and colleagues[54] reported that US-guided percutaneous needle aspiration and lavage in calcific tendinitis of the shoulder provides significant improvement in shoulder motion, pain, and disability. For those patients with calcific tendinitis of the shoulder requiring surgery, preoperative marking of calcific deposits using US significantly improves the clinical results of arthroscopic surgery.[55]

The role of computed tomography in the calcium crystal arthropathies is limited, although this modality is useful in the diagnosis and assessment of disease at unusual sites, including the previously mentioned crowned dens syndrome and spinal CPPD.

Because MRI creates images by detecting H^+ ions rather than the Ca^{2+} ions that are detected by radiography, calcific deposits are typically associated with loss of signal intensity. For CPPD crystal deposition in the knee, plain film evaluation has been shown to have greater sensitivity that MRI.[48] MRI has also been shown to have poor sensitivity, specificity, and reproducibility compared with plain radiography for diagnosis of calcific tendinitis of the shoulder.[56]

A promising area in crystal arthropathies is dual-energy computed tomography (DECT). This modality has been studied for the most part in the setting of monosodium urate crystal deposition,[57,58] in which an image is acquired simultaneously using 2 X-ray tubes with different voltages and aligned at 90° to one another. Because materials act differently at different energies depending on their chemical composition, differences in composition can be shown and color coded. This method has been well studied in gouty arthritis and in the evaluation of tophus burden but has rarely been used in calcium crystal deposition. DECT has been used in the evaluation of renal calculi and can show calcium-predominant renal stones.[59] It is hoped that it will be a useful tool in CPPD-related and BCP-related arthritis, although it has yet to be studied in detail.

PATHOGENESIS OF JOINT DESTRUCTION IN CRYSTAL DEPOSITION

BCP crystals are frequently found in OA cartilage, synovium, and synovial fluid. Ample data exist to support the role of BCP crystals in the promotion of cartilage degeneration. Their presence correlates strongly with the severity of radiographic change.[60] The concept that the presence of BCP crystals associates with more severe disease is also supported by the findings of an increased prevalence of crystal-positive joint aspirates with advancing disease. In a study by Nalbant and colleagues,[26] BCP crystals were found in 23% of joints at the first aspiration, but in 58% at the final aspiration (at a mean interval of 3.6 years), suggesting that BCP crystals may be generated as part of the pathologic process in OA. Furthermore, joints with BCP crystals have larger effusions than those without.[61] In contrast, the suggestion that intra-articular CPP may represent a marker for a poor prognosis in patients with knee OA has not been validated in longitudinal studies.[62,63]

Calcium crystals are actively involved in the pathogenesis of a wide spectrum of joint disorders. However, they are still considered by some clinicians to be simply a byproduct of joint destruction rather than an active component of an inflammatory process. BCP crystals have been shown in numerous studies to have multiple biological effects on articular cells such as chondrocytes and synovial fibroblasts (**Fig. 9**). In vitro, they induce cellular proliferation, stimulate matrix metalloproteinases (MMP),[64] increase nitric oxide production, and upregulate inflammatory cytokines such as tumor necrosis factor alpha (TNF-α) and interleukin (IL) 1-beta (IL-1β). BCP crystals are unusual in that they upregulate both cyclooxygenase-1 and cyclooxygenase-2 followed by increased prostaglandin E_2 in human fibroblasts.[65] They induce apoptosis in synovial fibroblasts and articular chondrocytes.[4,66,67] These combined processes lead to an imbalance in anabolic versus catabolic mediators of cartilage turnover, and ultimately to extracellular matrix degradation.

IL-1β in particular has been identified as a key driver of destructive and inflammatory responses in OA as a result of its ability to upregulate aggrecanases and MMPs while also suppressing the biosynthesis of extracellular matrix.[68] In keeping with this, IL-1β has been shown to be increased in the cartilage and synovial fluid of patients with OA.[69,70] BCP crystals initiate IL-1β–mediated inflammatory processes through NLRP3 (NACHT, LRR, and PYD containing protein 3) inflammasome-dependent as well as inflammasome-independent pathways.[71,72] Cunningham and colleagues[73] showed that lipopolysaccharide (LPS)-primed murine macrophages incubated with BCP produce high levels of IL-1β as well as IL-18, also an important cytokine in propagating joint damage. More importantly, longer incubation of non–LPS-primed macrophages with BCP crystals resulted in production of S100A8, a well-described damage-associated molecule that may further activate the macrophages through

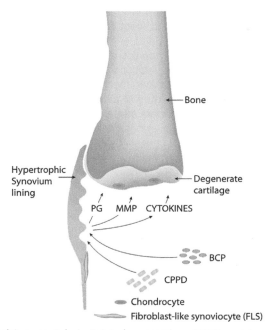

Fig. 9. Role of calcium crystals in joint degeneration. MMP, matrix metalloproteinases; PG, prostaglandins.

Toll-like receptors leading to production of IL-1β. Therefore BCP may cause the production of IL-1β both directly and indirectly through the autocrine effect of S100A8.

The signaling pathways that lead to the production of proinflammatory cytokines by BCP were further characterized. The spleen tyrosine kinase (Syk) and PI3 kinase are necessary for the induction of IL-1β following macrophage activation by BCP crystals. Pharmacologic inhibition of Syk and PI3K resulted in complete abrogation of BCP crystal–induced proinflammatory cytokine production by these cells. The exact mechanism whereby BCP-induced Syk activation occurs remains obscure. BCP crystals might be endocytosed and activate the kinase in the cytosol, or might interact with an unknown receptor on the surface of the cells.[73]

CPPD crystals are considered to be more proinflammatory than BCP crystals.[74] In lapine models, weekly injection of CPPD crystals into knees, which were rendered osteoarthritic by partial meniscectomy and section of the collateral ligament, worsened OA cartilage destruction.[75] Intra-articular BCP crystals in murine knees similarly induce synovial inflammation, cartilage degradation, and chondrocyte apoptosis.[76]

CHONDROCALCINOSIS AND ATHEROSCLEROSIS

Vascular calcification is a common finding associated with aging, diabetes, chronic renal failure, and atherosclerosis. Coronary artery calcification occurs as part of the atherosclerotic process, and is caused by the deposition of BCP crystals in the arterial intima.[77]

In a recent study by Abhishek and colleagues[78] the relationship between bone mineral density (BMD) and vascular calcification was examined in 431 cases of chondrocalcinosis, which were compared with 2708 controls as part of the GOAL study. Chondrocalcinosis was defined as linear calcification or spotty calcification arranged in a linear fashion in fibrocartilage or hyaline articular cartilage of the knees, wrists, hips, and symphysis pubis; or as synovial/capsular calcification or linear hyaline articular cartilage calcification at the metacarpophalangeal joints. Calcaneal BMD z scores were calculated and participants were characterized according to whether their BMD was high (z>1), medium (z between −1 and +1), or low (z<−1). Age, OA, periarticular knee calcification, low BMD, and pelvic vascular calcification were associated with chondrocalcinosis. There may be a relationship between chondrocalcinosis and vascular calcification because of a common mechanism mediating both.

Coronary artery calcification is a feature of atherosclerosis because of the intimal deposition of BCP crystals. BCP crystals can elicit the release of TNF-α and other proinflammatory cytokines from human monocyte-derived macrophages in vitro. Human macrophages interact with BCP crystals by internalizing them into vacuoles with the subsequent production of proinflammatory cytokines.[79] TNF-α in turn can promote calcification of smooth muscle calls. Thus there is a potential cycle of crystal-induced inflammation and calcification of vessel walls.

It has also been shown that small BCP crystals may be more biologically active than large crystals. Crystals with diameters 1 to 2 μm were shown to be the most biologically active by Nadra and colleagues.[80] This finding is in keeping with the clinical finding that larger calcific deposits in vessel walls tend to be stable and inert and are less prone to plaque rupture with subsequent thrombosis. Microscopic calcific deposits in the early stages of atherosclerosis may pose a greater inflammatory risk to the plaque than macroscopically or radiologically visible deposits in more advanced lesions.[2] BCP crystals also induce cell death in human vascular smooth muscle cells, potentially destabilizing atherosclerotic plaques.[81]

Deficiency of physiologic calcification inhibitors, as described by Luo and colleagues,[82] may be of particular interest in explaining the interplay between vascular calcification and calcific arthropathy. The matrix-GLA protein knockout mice have vascular calcification, cartilage calcification, and osteoporosis, a similar phenotype to that shown in the GOAL study.[78] Some of the findings may similarly be mediated by low osteoprotegerin. Osteoprotegerin is a decoy receptor for the receptor activator of nuclear factor kappa B ligand. It can reduce the production of osteoclasts by inhibiting the differentiation of osteoclast precursors into osteoclasts and also regulates the resorption of osteoclasts. Osteoprotegerin inhibits the differentiation of the osteoclast precursor into a mature osteoclast. Osteoprotegerin knockout mice show osteoporosis and vascular calcification.

There has been recent widespread concern that calcium supplementation could cause vascular calcification and in turn increase cardiovascular risk.[83,84] There is no consensus on this issue of vascular calcification and calcium supplementation. The Iowa Women's Health Study found a one-third reduction in deaths from cardiovascular events in women whose calcium intakes (dietary or supplementary) were in the highest fourth compared with those in the lowest fourth.[85] The Boston Nurse's Health Study found that women in the highest fifth for calcium intake had an adjusted relative risk of ischemic stroke of 0.69 compared with those in the lowest fifth.[86] A study in the United Kingdom reported a strong inverse relationship between calcium intake and standardized mortality ratios for ischemic heart disease,[87] which is contrary to the findings by Bolland and colleagues.[83,84] A recent Framingham study also found no association between coronary artery calcification and calcium intake.[88]

Calcium crystals are biologically active molecules playing a central role in both vascular and articular calcification. Whether dietary or supplementary calcium intake has any influence on this process is at present unknown. There is currently no consensus on calcium intake and the risk of vascular calcification.

SUMMARY

The structural consequences of calcium crystal deposition are manifold and not limited to the musculoskeletal system. These crystals are implicated in a broad spectrum of rheumatic conditions, in particular OA. Thus, calcium-containing crystal deposition diseases are associated with significant functional disability. There is at present no specific treatment of these conditions and so they remain a challenge both to the rheumatologist and to society. The role of these crystals as mediators of joint damage and inflammation in OA is of particular interest because they represent a potential therapeutic target. At present, options in the management of these patients are limited to interventions such as intra-articular corticosteroid injection or joint replacement.

In addition, although the presence of arterial calcification has historically been viewed solely as a marker of atherosclerotic disease progression, recent investigation suggests an active role for BCP crystals in the pathogenesis of atherosclerosis and plaque rupture.

REFERENCES

1. McCarthy GM, Cheung HS. Point: hydroxyapatite crystal deposition is intimately involved in the pathogenesis and progression of human osteoarthritis. Curr Rheumatol Rep 2009;11(2):141–7.
2. McCarthy GM. Inspirational calcification: how rheumatology research directs investigation in vascular biology. Curr Opin Rheumatol 2009;21(1):47–9.
3. Ivorra J, Rosas J, Pascual E. Most calcium pyrophosphate crystals appear as non-birefringent. Ann Rheum Dis 1999;58(9):582–4.

4. Molloy ES, McCarthy GM. Calcium crystal deposition diseases: update on pathogenesis and manifestations. Rheum Dis Clin North Am 2006;32(2): 383–400, vii.

5. Rosenthal AK, Fahey M, Gohr C, et al. Feasibility of a tetracycline-binding method for detecting synovial fluid basic calcium phosphate crystals. Arthritis Rheum 2008;58(10):3270–4.

6. Yavorskyy A, Hernandez-Santana A, McCarthy G, et al. Detection of calcium phosphate crystals in the joint fluid of patients with osteoarthritis – analytical approaches and challenges. Analyst 2008;133(3):302–18.

7. Lazcano O, Li CY, Pierre RV, et al. Clinical utility of the alizarin red S stain on permanent preparations to detect calcium-containing compounds in synovial fluid. Am J Clin Pathol 1993;99(1):90–6.

8. MacMullan P, McMahon G, McCarthy G. Detection of basic calcium phosphate crystals in osteoarthritis. Joint Bone Spine 2011;78(4):358–63.

9. Neame RL, Carr AJ, Muir K, et al. UK community prevalence of knee chondro-calcinosis: evidence that correlation with osteoarthritis is through a shared association with osteophyte. Ann Rheum Dis 2003;62(6):513–8.

10. Pasquetti P, Selvi E, Righeschi K, et al. Joint lavage and pseudogout. Ann Rheum Dis 2004;63(11):1529–30.

11. Watanabe H, Yamada S, Anayama S, et al. Pseudogout attack induced during etidronate disodium therapy. Mod Rheumatol 2006;16(2):117–9.

12. Young-Min SA, Herbert L, Dick M, et al. Weekly alendronate-induced acute pseudogout. Rheumatology (Oxford) 2005;44(1):131–2.

13. Halverson PB, Derfus BA. Calcium crystal-induced inflammation. Curr Opin Rheumatol 2001;13(3):221–4.

14. Zhang W, Doherty M, Bardin T, et al. European League Against Rheumatism recommendations for calcium pyrophosphate deposition. Part I: terminology and diagnosis. Ann Rheum Dis 2011;70(4):563–70.

15. Whelan BR, O'Shea F, McCarthy G. Pseudoneuropathic CPPD arthropathy: magnesium matters. Rheumatology (Oxford) 2008;47(4):551–2.

16. Rosenthal AK. Calcium crystal-associated arthritides. Curr Opin Rheumatol 1998;10(3):273–7.

17. Rosenthal AK. Crystal arthropathies and other unpopular rheumatic diseases. Curr Opin Rheumatol 2004;16(3):262.

18. Uh M, Dewar C, Spouge D, et al. Crowned dens syndrome: a rare cause of acute neck pain. Clin Rheumatol 2013;32(5):711–4.

19. Fritz P, Bardin T, Laredo JD, et al. Paradiaphyseal calcific tendinitis with cortical bone erosion. Arthritis Rheum 1994;37(5):718–23.

20. McCarty DJ, Halverson PB, Carrera GF, et al. "Milwaukee shoulder"–association of microspheroids containing hydroxyapatite crystals, active collagenase, and neutral protease with rotator cuff defects. I. Clinical aspects. Arthritis Rheum 1981;24(3):464–73.

21. Halverson PB, Cheung HS, McCarty DJ, et al. "Milwaukee shoulder"–association of microspheroids containing hydroxyapatite crystals, active collagenase, and neutral protease with rotator cuff defects. II. Synovial fluid studies. Arthritis Rheum 1981;24(3):474–83.

22. Swan A, Chapman B, Heap P, et al. Submicroscopic crystals in osteoarthritic synovial fluids. Ann Rheum Dis 1994;53(7):467–70.

23. Halverson PB, Carrera GF, McCarty DJ. Milwaukee shoulder syndrome. Fifteen additional cases and a description of contributing factors. Arch Intern Med 1990;150(3):677–82.

24. Dieppe PA, Crocker PR, Corke CF, et al. Synovial fluid crystals. Q J Med 1979; 48(192):533–53.
25. Gibilisco PA, Schumacher HR, Hollander JL, et al. Synovial fluid crystals in osteoarthritis. Arthritis Rheum 1985;28(5):511–5.
26. Nalbant S, Martinez JA, Kitumnuaypong T, et al. Synovial fluid features and their relations to osteoarthritis severity: new findings from sequential studies. Osteoarthritis Cartilage 2003;11(1):50–4.
27. Fuerst M, Bertrand J, Lammers L, et al. Calcification of articular cartilage in human osteoarthritis. Arthritis Rheum 2009;60(9):2694–703.
28. Sun Y, Mauerhan DR, Honeycutt PR, et al. Calcium deposition in osteoarthritic meniscus and meniscal cell culture. Arthritis Res Ther 2010;12(2):R56.
29. Resnick D, Niwayama G, Goergen TG, et al. Clinical, radiographic and pathologic abnormalities in calcium pyrophosphate dihydrate deposition disease (CPPD): pseudogout. Radiology 1977;122(1):1–15.
30. McCarty DJ, Haskin ME. The roentgenographic aspects of pseudogout (articular chondrocalcinosis). An analysis of 20 cases. Am J Roentgenol Radium Ther Nucl Med 1963;90:1248–57.
31. Felson DT, Anderson JJ, Naimark A, et al. The prevalence of chondrocalcinosis in the elderly and its association with knee osteoarthritis: the Framingham Study. J Rheumatol 1989;16(9):1241–5.
32. Zhang Y, Terkeltaub R, Nevitt M, et al. Lower prevalence of chondrocalcinosis in Chinese subjects in Beijing than in white subjects in the United States: the Beijing Osteoarthritis Study. Arthritis Rheum 2006;54(11):3508–12.
33. Mitsuyama H, Healey RM, Terkeltaub RA, et al. Calcification of human articular knee cartilage is primarily an effect of aging rather than osteoarthritis. Osteoarthritis Cartilage 2007;15(5):559–65.
34. Gordon GV, Villanueva T, Schumacher HR, et al. Autopsy study correlating degree of osteoarthritis, synovitis and evidence of articular calcification. J Rheumatol 1984;11(5):681–6.
35. Caswell A, Guilland-Cumming DF, Hearn PR, et al. Pathogenesis of chondrocalcinosis and pseudogout. Metabolism of inorganic pyrophosphate and production of calcium pyrophosphate dihydrate crystals. Ann Rheum Dis 1983; 42(Suppl 1):27–37.
36. Netter P, Bardin T, Bianchi A, et al. The ANKH gene and familial calcium pyrophosphate dihydrate deposition disease. Joint Bone Spine 2004;71(5): 365–8.
37. Richette P, Bardin T, Doherty M. An update on the epidemiology of calcium pyrophosphate dihydrate crystal deposition disease. Rheumatology (Oxford) 2009;48(7):711–5.
38. Donich AS, Lektrakul N, Liu CC, et al. Calcium pyrophosphate dihydrate crystal deposition disease of the wrist: trapezioscaphoid joint abnormality. J Rheumatol 2000;27(11):2628–34.
39. Terkeltaub R. Gout and other crystal arthropathies. Philadelphia: Elsevier; 2012. p. 240–81.
40. Huang GS, Bachmann D, Taylor JA, et al. Calcium pyrophosphate dihydrate crystal deposition disease and pseudogout of the acromioclavicular joint: radiographic and pathologic features. J Rheumatol 1993;20(12):2077–82.
41. Resnik CS, Resnick D. Crystal deposition disease. Semin Arthritis Rheum 1983; 12(4):390–403.
42. Steinbach LS, Resnick D. Calcium pyrophosphate dihydrate crystal deposition disease: imaging perspectives. Curr Probl Diagn Radiol 2000;29(6):209–29.

43. Fisseler-Eckhoff A, Müller KM. Arthroscopy and chondrocalcinosis. Arthroscopy 1992;8(1):98–104.
44. Hayes CW, Conway WF. Calcium hydroxyapatite deposition disease. Radiographics 1990;10(6):1031–48.
45. Abhishek A, Doherty S, Maciewicz R, et al. Chondrocalcinosis is common in the absence of knee involvement. Arthritis Res Ther 2012;14(5):R205.
46. Abhishek A, Doherty S, Maciewicz R, et al. Evidence of a systemic predisposition to chondrocalcinosis and association between chondrocalcinosis and osteoarthritis at distant joints: a cross-sectional study. Arthritis Care Res (Hoboken) 2013;65(7):1052–8.
47. Dufauret-Lombard C, Vergne-Salle P, Simon A, et al. Ultrasonography in chondrocalcinosis. Joint Bone Spine 2010;77(3):218–21.
48. Abreu M, Johnson K, Chung CB, et al. Calcification in calcium pyrophosphate dihydrate (CPPD) crystalline deposits in the knee: anatomic, radiographic, MR imaging, and histologic study in cadavers. Skeletal Radiol 2004;33(7):392–8.
49. Foldes K. Knee chondrocalcinosis: an ultrasonographic study of the hyalin cartilage. Clin Imaging 2002;26(3):194–6.
50. Frediani B, Filippou G, Falsetti P, et al. Diagnosis of calcium pyrophosphate dihydrate crystal deposition disease: ultrasonographic criteria proposed. Ann Rheum Dis 2005;64(4):638–40.
51. Filippou G, Frediani B, Gallo A, et al. A "new" technique for the diagnosis of chondrocalcinosis of the knee: sensitivity and specificity of high-frequency ultrasonography. Ann Rheum Dis 2007;66(8):1126–8.
52. Filippucci E, Riveros MG, Georgescu D, et al. Hyaline cartilage involvement in patients with gout and calcium pyrophosphate deposition disease. An ultrasound study. Osteoarthritis Cartilage 2009;17(2):178–81.
53. Le Goff B, Berthelot JM, Guillot P, et al. Assessment of calcific tendonitis of rotator cuff by ultrasonography: comparison between symptomatic and asymptomatic shoulders. Joint Bone Spine 2010;77(3):258–63.
54. del Cura JL, Torre I, Zabala R, et al. Sonographically guided percutaneous needle lavage in calcific tendinitis of the shoulder: short- and long-term results. AJR Am J Roentgenol 2007;189(3):W128–34.
55. Kayser R, Hampf S, Seeber E, et al. Value of preoperative ultrasound marking of calcium deposits in patients who require surgical treatment of calcific tendinitis of the shoulder. Arthroscopy 2007;23(1):43–50.
56. Zubler C, Mengiardi B, Schmid MR, et al. MR arthrography in calcific tendinitis of the shoulder: diagnostic performance and pitfalls. Eur Radiol 2007;17(6):1603–10.
57. Dalbeth N, Doyle A, McQueen FM. Imaging in gout: insights into the pathological features of disease. Curr Opin Rheumatol 2012;24(2):132–8.
58. Dalbeth N, Choi HK. Dual-energy computed tomography for gout diagnosis and management. Curr Rheumatol Rep 2013;15(1):301.
59. Hidas G, Eliahou R, Duvdevani M, et al. Determination of renal stone composition with dual-energy CT: in vivo analysis and comparison with x-ray diffraction. Radiology 2010;257(2):394–401.
60. Halverson PB, McCarty DJ. Patterns of radiographic abnormalities associated with basic calcium phosphate and calcium pyrophosphate dihydrate crystal deposition in the knee. Ann Rheum Dis 1986;45(7):603–5.
61. Carroll GJ, Stuart RA, Armstrong JA, et al. Hydroxyapatite crystals are a frequent finding in osteoarthritic synovial fluid, but are not related to increased concentrations of keratan sulfate or interleukin 1 beta. J Rheumatol 1991;18(6):861–6.

62. Neogi T, Nevitt M, Niu J, et al. Lack of association between chondrocalcinosis and increased risk of cartilage loss in knees with osteoarthritis: results of two prospective longitudinal magnetic resonance imaging studies. Arthritis Rheum 2006;54(6):1822–8.

63. Doherty M, Dieppe P, Watt I. Pyrophosphate arthropathy: a prospective study. Br J Rheumatol 1993;32(3):189–96.

64. McCarthy GM, Mitchell PG, Cheung HS. The mitogenic response to stimulation with basic calcium phosphate crystals is accompanied by induction and secretion of collagenase in human fibroblasts. Arthritis Rheum 1991;34(8): 1021–30.

65. Morgan MP, Whelan LC, Sallis JD, et al. Basic calcium phosphate crystal-induced prostaglandin E2 production in human fibroblasts: role of cyclooxygenase 1, cyclooxygenase 2, and interleukin-1beta. Arthritis Rheum 2004;50(5): 1642–9.

66. Ea HK, Uzan B, Rey C, et al. Octacalcium phosphate crystals directly stimulate expression of inducible nitric oxide synthase through p38 and JNK mitogen-activated protein kinases in articular chondrocytes. Arthritis Res Ther 2005; 7(5):R915–26.

67. Molloy ES, Morgan MP, Doherty GA, et al. Mechanism of basic calcium phosphate crystal-stimulated cyclo-oxygenase-1 up-regulation in osteoarthritic synovial fibroblasts. Rheumatology (Oxford) 2008;47(7):965–71.

68. Daheshia M, Yao JQ. The interleukin 1beta pathway in the pathogenesis of osteoarthritis. J Rheumatol 2008;35(12):2306–12.

69. Hussein MR, Fathi NA, El-Din AM, et al. Alterations of the CD4(+), CD8 (+) T cell subsets, interleukins-1beta, IL-10, IL-17, tumor necrosis factor-alpha and soluble intercellular adhesion molecule-1 in rheumatoid arthritis and osteoarthritis: preliminary observations. Pathol Oncol Res 2008;14(3):321–8.

70. Saha N, Moldovan F, Tardif G, et al. Interleukin-1beta-converting enzyme/ caspase-1 in human osteoarthritic tissues: localization and role in the maturation of interleukin-1beta and interleukin-18. Arthritis Rheum 1999;42(8): 1577–87.

71. Narayan S, Pazar B, Ea HK, et al. Octacalcium phosphate crystals induce inflammation in vivo through interleukin-1 but independent of the NLRP3 inflammasome in mice. Arthritis Rheum 2011;63(2):422–33.

72. Jin C, Frayssinet P, Pelker R, et al. NLRP3 inflammasome plays a critical role in the pathogenesis of hydroxyapatite-associated arthropathy. Proc Natl Acad Sci U S A 2011;108(36):14867–72.

73. Cunningham CC, Mills E, Mielke LA, et al. Osteoarthritis-associated basic calcium phosphate crystals induce pro-inflammatory cytokines and damage-associated molecules via activation of Syk and PI3 kinase. Clin Immunol 2012;144(3):228–36.

74. Ea HK, Lioté F. Advances in understanding calcium-containing crystal disease. Curr Opin Rheumatol 2009;21(2):150–7.

75. Fam AG, Morava-Protzner I, Purcell C, et al. Acceleration of experimental lapine osteoarthritis by calcium pyrophosphate microcrystalline synovitis. Arthritis Rheum 1995;38(2):201–10.

76. Ea HK, Chobaz V, Nguyen C, et al. Pathogenic role of basic calcium phosphate crystals in destructive arthropathies. PLoS One 2013;8(2):e57352.

77. Fitzpatrick LA, Severson A, Edwards WD, et al. Diffuse calcification in human coronary arteries. Association of osteopontin with atherosclerosis. J Clin Invest 1994;94(4):1597–604.

78. Abhishek A, Doherty S, Maciewicz R, et al. Association between low cortical bone mineral density, soft-tissue calcification, vascular calcification and chondrocalcinosis: a case-control study. Ann Rheum Dis 2013. [Epub ahead of print].

79. Nadra I, Mason JC, Philippidis P, et al. Proinflammatory activation of macrophages by basic calcium phosphate crystals via protein kinase C and MAP kinase pathways: a vicious cycle of inflammation and arterial calcification? Circ Res 2005;96(12):1248–56.

80. Nadra I, Boccaccini AR, Philippidis P, et al. Effect of particle size on hydroxyapatite crystal-induced tumor necrosis factor alpha secretion by macrophages. Atherosclerosis 2008;196(1):98–105.

81. Ewence AE, Bootman M, Roderick HL, et al. Calcium phosphate crystals induce cell death in human vascular smooth muscle cells: a potential mechanism in atherosclerotic plaque destabilization. Circ Res 2008;103(5):e28–34.

82. Luo G, Ducy P, McKee MD, et al. Spontaneous calcification of arteries and cartilage in mice lacking matrix GLA protein. Nature 1997;386(6620):78–81.

83. Bolland MJ, Barber PA, Doughty RN, et al. Vascular events in healthy older women receiving calcium supplementation: randomised controlled trial. BMJ 2008;336(7638):262–6.

84. Bolland MJ, Avenell A, Baron JA, et al. Effect of calcium supplements on risk of myocardial infarction and cardiovascular events: meta-analysis. BMJ 2010;341: c3691.

85. Bostick RM, Potter JD, Sellers TA, et al. Relation of calcium, vitamin D, and dairy food intake to incidence of colon cancer among older women. The Iowa Women's Health Study. Am J Epidemiol 1993;137(12):1302–17.

86. Iso H, Stampfer MJ, Manson JE, et al. Prospective study of calcium, potassium, and magnesium intake and risk of stroke in women. Stroke 1999;30(9):1772–9.

87. Knox EG. Ischaemic-heart-disease mortality and dietary intake of calcium. Lancet 1973;1(7818):1465–7.

88. Samelson EJ, Booth SL, Fox CS, et al. Calcium intake is not associated with increased coronary artery calcification: the Framingham Study. Am J Clin Nutr 2012;96(6):1274–80.

Treatment of Acute Gout

Naomi Schlesinger, MD

KEYWORDS

- Acute gout • Treatment • Monosodium urate

KEY POINTS

- Gout is due to excess uric acid pools in the body, leading to formation of monosodium urate crystals and their deposition in and around joints where they induce inflammation, leading to acute gout attacks.
- The goal of therapy in acute gout is prompt and safe termination of pain and inflammation.
- Recently published treatment guidelines and new drugs under development may provide needed alternatives for patients with gout who are intolerant of or refractory to available therapies.

INTRODUCTION

Gout, the most common inflammatory arthritis in adults, is caused by excess uric acid pools in the body, leading to formation of monosodium urate (MSU) crystals and their deposition in and around joints where they induce inflammation, leading to acute gout attacks. The extreme inflammatory burden and pain of an acute gout attack can be unbearable. A quote from Rev. Sydney Smith in a letter to Lady Gray in 1836 alludes to how painful acute gout is: "When I have gout, I feel as if I am walking on my eyeballs!"[1] The initial attacks are usually self-limiting, but recurrent acute attacks tend to become more frequent and prolonged.

The goal of therapy in acute gout is prompt and safe termination of pain and inflammation. In Bellamy's 7-day observational study that followed the natural course of an acute gout attack in patients presenting with acute podagra,[2] 2 of 11 patients withdrew because of severe pain 4 days after entering the study. By day 7, full resolution of pain was observed in only 3 of 9 (33%) patients. Thus, although without drug treatment the extreme pain of acute gout may resolve within a few days, it may last up to several weeks.

Anti-inflammatory drugs need to be initiated promptly and adequate doses be given for a long enough period of time to terminate an acute attack. The usual

Disclosures: Grants, Novartis; Advisory boards, Novartis, Takeda, Savient, Enzyme Rx, URL Pharma, Sobi; Speakers bureau, Novartis, Takeda, Savient; Consultant, Novartis, Sobi.
Division of Rheumatology, Department of Medicine, Rutgers – Robert Wood Johnson Medical School, One Robert Wood Johnson Place, PO Box 19, New Brunswick, NJ 08903-0019, USA
E-mail address: schlesna@rwjms.rutgers.edu

Rheum Dis Clin N Am 40 (2014) 329–341
http://dx.doi.org/10.1016/j.rdc.2014.01.008
0889-857X/14/$ – see front matter © 2014 Elsevier Inc. All rights reserved.

anti-inflammatory drugs used in acute gout are nonsteroidal anti-inflammatory drugs (NSAIDs), corticosteroids (CS), and/or colchicine.[3]

These are exciting times in the research field of acute gout. There is more awareness of the disease, its pathogenesis, and its diagnosis, including new imaging modalities helpful in aiding with the diagnosis. In addition, recently published treatment guidelines and new drugs under development may provide necessary alternatives for patients with gout who are intolerant of or refractory to available therapies.

NONPHARMACOLOGIC TREATMENT

Joint motion enhanced the severity of inflammation in experimentally induced gout in dogs, whereas rest may aid in its resolution.[4] In addition, it has been suggested that less medication is needed if the patient rests the inflamed joint(s) for 1 to 2 days.[5]

Topical ice applications may benefit patients with acute gout. In a small, prospective randomized study,[6] patients with acute gout treated with topical ice had a greater reduction in pain ($P = .021$), joint circumference, and synovial fluid volume compared with the control group. By contrast, in experimentally induced gout in dogs, heat application to the inflamed joints exacerbated MSU-induced synovitis.[7]

PHARMACOLOGIC TREATMENT

Several options are currently available for the treatment of acute gout, including NSAIDs, colchicine, CS, and corticotropin (adrenocorticotropic hormone [ACTH]). However, in many patients the available treatments are contraindicated (relative or absolute contraindication), largely owing to the presence of common comorbidities in patients with gout such as hypertension, cardiovascular disease, chronic kidney disease, and diabetes (see article elsewhere in this issue). It is important to consider these comorbidities when treating patients with acute gout.

Guidelines and recommendations by the European League Against Rheumatism (EULAR) and the American College of Rheumatology (ACR) Task Force Panels (TFP) have helped physicians in the treatment of acute gout (**Table 1**). The EULAR Standing Committee for International Clinical Studies Including Therapeutics (ESCISIT)[8] and the ACR TFP recommended oral colchicine and/or NSAIDs as first-line treatment for acute gout. The ACR TFP recommended combinations of these medications in severe or refractory attacks.

The ACR guidelines for the treatment of acute gout recommended initiating drug therapy within 24 hours of the onset of the acute attack (based on the consensus that early treatment leads to better outcomes). It is proposed that during the acute attack, urate-lowering therapy (ULT) be continued without interruption.[9]

It must be borne in mind that whereas several of the guidelines and recommendations of the EULAR and the ACR guidelines were based on randomized controlled trials (RCTs) or meta-analysis evaluating the efficacy of the various treatments for acute gout, many of these recommendations were based on the consensus opinion of experts, case studies, or standard of care.

Monotherapy

The ACR TFP[9] recommended that in mild to moderate acute gout (defined as pain ≤6 on a 0–10 visual analog scale [VAS]), monotherapy with NSAIDs, systemic CS, or oral colchicine be initiated. The ACR TFP did not rank one drug class over the other.

Colchicine and NSAIDs are the most commonly used drugs in the treatment of acute gout.[3] In an American survey study,[10] NSAIDs were reported to be the most commonly used monotherapy (77%). Of interest, in this study, intra-articular CS injections (47%)

Table 1
Pharmacologic treatment recommendations for acute gout

	2006 European League Against Rheumatism Recommendations[8]	2012 American College of Rheumatology Guidelines for Management of Gout[9]
First-line agents	Oral colchicine and/or NSAIDs	Oral colchicine, NSAIDs, or CS
Choice of drug	NSAIDs accepted option in absence of contraindications	Choice of drug depends on patient, physician preference, comorbidities, and contraindications Initiation within 12–24 h after attack onset Treatment may need to continue for 7–10 d
Low-dose oral colchicine	0.5 mg 3 times daily	1.2 mg administered as soon as possible, followed by 0.6 mg 1 h later; followed by 0.6 mg once or twice daily until attack resolves Initiation not recommended ≥36 h after attack onset Not recommended when attack in a patient taking colchicine prophylaxis
Intra-articular aspiration and long-acting CS injections	Effective and safe after septic arthritis ruled out	Effective and safe after sufficient precautions have been taken Intra-articular CS favored in attacks involving 1–2 joints
ULT started during an attack		ULT could be started during an attack, provided that inflammation is controlled Differs from common practice of starting ULT 2–4 wk from resolution of an attack before starting ULT
IL-1 inhibitors		Canakinumab, approved by the EMEA for treatment of adult patients with frequent gout attacks not included in recommendations
Combination treatment		Combination of colchicine and NSAIDs in severe attacks

Abbreviations: CS, corticosteroids; EMEA, European Medicines Agency; IL-1, interleukin-1; NSAIDs, nonsteroidal anti-inflammatory drugs; ULT, urate-lowering therapy.

and oral prednisone (42%) were reported to be more commonly than oral colchicine (37%) used to treat acute gout. Triamcinolone intramuscularly (11%) and ACTH intramuscularly (5%) were also reported to be used uncommonly. In the United States, oral CS were reported to be the most commonly used monotherapy by rheumatologists in a patient with chronic kidney disease, which is a common comorbidity seen in patients with gout.

In another American study,[11] monotherapy was used in 58% of hospitalized patients with acute gout. In the patients prescribed monotherapy, colchicine use (76%) exceeded NSAID (14%) and oral CS (10%) use. A recent Australian study[12] reported similar findings. Colchicine was the most common monotherapy (75%), followed by NSAIDs (32%), and oral CS (28%). Oral CS was used to treat acute gout in approximately 10% of patients. Of note, a recent Malaysian study[13] of primary care physicians found that oral CS were used to treat acute gout in approximately 10% of patients, as was suggested by the 2 other studies.

NSAIDs were the also the agents most commonly used for acute gout in other survey studies (**Table 2**). Among Canadian clinicians, only 11% of family physicians and 6% of rheumatologists said that they would use colchicine in the acute situation.[14] A similar preference for NSAIDs has been noted in Australia,[15] New Zealand,[16] and Malaysia.[13] By contrast, in a French survey study evaluating the treatment of gout,[17] colchicine as monotherapy was found to be the most commonly used drug. The most widely prescribed treatments for acute gout were colchicine alone (63%), colchicine with an NSAID (31.7%), and NSAID alone (5.2%). Survey studies in China,[18] Brazil,[19] Argentina,[20] and a recent American study[21] found colchicine to be the agent most commonly used for acute gout.

Colchicine

Colchicine is an alkaloid derived from extracts of meadow saffron (*Crocus autoimmale*). It is thought that colchicine relieves pain through its binding to tubulin dimers and by inhibiting β-tubulin polymerization into microtubules,[22] thus interfering with neutrophil functions including diapedesis (ameboid movement), mobilization, lysosomal degranulation, and, most importantly, leukocyte chemotaxis. In addition, colchicine suppresses MSU crystal–induced NALP3 inflammasome-driven caspase-1 activation and interleukin (IL)-1β processing.[23,24]

Colchicine is metabolized in the liver, and excreted in the urine and by the biliary tract. The half-life of oral colchicine in patients with normal renal and hepatic functions is approximately 9 hours, whereas in patients with renal failure it is approximately 24 hours, and in cirrhotic patients with renal failure it is up to 10 times normal (approximately 4 days) and is not removed via hemodialysis.[25]

Despite the widespread use of oral colchicine, it did not gain Food and Drug Administration (FDA) approval until August 2009 following the Acute Gout Flare Receiving Colchicine Evaluation (AGREE) trial.[26] The AGREE trial was a randomized, double-blind, placebo-controlled trial of 184 patients with acute gout treated within 12 hours of the onset of an attack. Low-dose colchicine (1.2 mg followed by 0.6 mg 1 hour later for a total of 1.8 mg) was found to be equally effective and better tolerated than high-dose colchicine (1.2 mg followed by 0.6 mg hourly × 6 hours for a total of 4.8 mg). There was a significantly higher incidence of gastrointestinal side effects such as diarrhea, nausea, and vomiting when high-dose colchicine was used, compared with low-dose colchicine and placebo.

Ahern and colleagues[27] studied 43 patients in an earlier placebo-controlled study of colchicine treatment in acute gout. Twenty-two patients were started on colchicine, 1 mg followed by 0.5 mg every 2 hours until complete response or toxicity, and 21 patients were enrolled in the placebo group. No NSAIDs were used during the study. Two-thirds of the colchicine-treated patients improved within 48 hours compared with only one-third of the patients receiving placebo. Colchicine was found to be more effective when used within 24 hours of an acute attack. The problem was the high incidence of adverse events, with more than 80% of patients in the colchicine group experiencing nausea, vomiting, diarrhea, and abdominal pain before full clinical improvement.[27]

The recommended doses of colchicine depend on renal and hepatic functions in addition to colchicine drug-drug interactions. Colchicine is a substrate for both the CYP3A4 enzyme and P-glycoprotein (P-gp) transporter. Therefore, coadministration with drugs known to inhibit CYP3A4 and/or P-gp increases the risk of colchicine-induced adverse events. These agents include cyclosporine, erythromycin, and calcium-channel antagonists such as verapamil and diltiazem. Other examples of P-gp and strong CYP3A4 inhibitors include telithromycin, ketoconazole, itraconazole,

Table 2
Treatment of acute gout: representative survey studies

Study,[Ref.] Year	Country	No. of Rheumatologists	Colchicine as Primary Agent (%)	Colchicine Plus NSAIDs (%)	NSAIDs Alone (%)	Corticosteroids (%)
Gnanentheran et al,[12] 2011	USA	518	37	32	27	42 (71 if CKD)
Yeap et al,[13] 2009	Malaysia	128 PCD	10.2		68	10
Bellamy et al,[14] 1988	Canada	71	6	?	?	
Stuart et al,[16] 1991	New Zealand	26	12	25	Indomethacin used in 73	
Rozenberg et al,[17] 1996	France	750	63	32	5	0
Fang et al,[18] 2006	China	82	77		17	1 (48 if CKD)
Ferraz et al,[19] 1994	Brazil		57			
Fara et al,[20] 2012	Argentina	33 52 IM 86 PCD	76	?	?	?
Harrold et al,[21] 2013	USA	444 FP 387 IM	59		51	45

Abbreviations: CKD, chronic kidney disease; FP, family practitioners; IM, internal medicine doctors; PCD, primary care physicians.

human immunodeficiency virus protease inhibitors, and nefazodone.[28] The FDA advises patients treated with P-gp or strong CYP3A4 inhibitor drugs within 14 days of colchicine use for acute gout to reduce the dose or stop colchicine treatment. For treatment of acute gout in patients with mild (glomerular filtration rate [GFR] 50–80 mL/min) to moderate (GFR 30–50 mL/min) kidney disease, adjustment of this recommended dose is not required. For patients with acute gout requiring repeated courses of colchicine, consideration should be given to alternative therapy. For patients undergoing dialysis, the total recommended dose for the treatment of acute gout should be reduced to a single dose of 0.6 mg (1 tablet), and the treatment should not be repeated more than once every 2 weeks. Treatment of gout attacks with colchicine is not recommended in patients with kidney disease receiving colchicine prophylaxis.[28]

A clinical response to colchicine is not pathognomonic for acute gout, and can be seen in other conditions such as acute pseudogout, psoriatic arthritis, and calcific tendonitis.

Oral nonsteroidal anti-inflammatory drugs

NSAIDs are among the most commonly prescribed drugs.[29] These agents differ in their structure and their pharmacokinetic and pharmacodynamic properties, but share the same mode of action. NSAIDs exert their anti-inflammatory action by inhibiting cyclooxygenase (COX), an enzyme that transforms phospholipid-derived arachidonic acid into prostaglandins. NSAIDs may be nonselective, inhibiting both COX-1 and COX-2 (eg, ibuprofen and naproxen), or may be more COX-1 (eg, aspirin) or COX-2 selective (eg, celecoxib).

NSAIDs are commonly used in patients with acute gout who do not have underlying comorbidities. The most important determinant of therapeutic success is not which NSAID is chosen, but rather how soon the NSAID is initiated, and that large enough dosages be given at the onset of symptoms and continued for a long enough period of time. Naproxen, indomethacin, and sulindac are FDA-approved for acute gout; however, several head-to-head studies, some of which were RCTs for acute gout, show equivalence between different NSAIDs. Most of these small trials[3] compared indomethacin with another NSAID including COX-2–selective drugs, which were also found to be effective.[30–32] In 2 studies comparing etoricoxib with indomethacin, etoricoxib 120 mg once daily was comparable with indomethacin 50 mg 3 times daily in treating acute gout. Studies comparing celecoxib (400 mg and 800 mg) and indomethacin 50 mg 3 times daily show equivalence between celecoxib and indomethacin.[32]

The use of NSAIDs is limited by their side effects.[29] NSAID-related gastrointestinal side effects may lead to bleeding, hospitalizations, and deaths. Coadministration of a proton-pump inhibitor may lessen gastrointestinal side effects. In addition, the use of NSAIDs in patients with heart disease or those thought to be at increased risk of heart disease should be cautioned. All patients taking NSAIDs should be carefully monitored for the development of high blood pressure, worsening heart disease, worsening renal function, fluid retention, gastrointestinal bleeding, and elevations in liver enzymes.

There are no RCTs comparing colchicine with NSAIDs, and such studies comparing their efficacy and adverse events are much needed.

Systemic corticosteroids

CS interfere with the proinflammatory signaling process,[33] suppress the immune response, and inhibit prostaglandins and leukotrienes. One of the most important anti-inflammatory effects of CS is directly inhibiting the activity of transcription factors by a transrepression mechanism, which results in protein-protein interaction. In addition, CS inhibit proinflammatory cytokines such as IL-1, IL-6, IL-8, and tumor necrosis factor α, and upregulate genes for lipocortin and vasocortin, which have anti-inflammatory effects by inhibiting phospholipase A2, thereby blocking eicosanoid production and inhibiting various leukocyte inflammatory functions (epithelial adhesion, diapedesis, chemotaxis, phagocytosis, and so forth).

CS can be given orally, intravenously, intramuscularly, and intra-articularly, and are commonly used in patients who cannot be treated with NSAIDs and/or colchicine. CS are commonly used, and often preferred, for polyarticular gout. The ACR TFP recommended oral prednisone or prednisolone at a dose of 0.5 mg/kg/d for 5 to 10 days, or for 2 to 5 days at this full dose followed by a 7- to 10-day taper.[9] It is unclear whether treatment with parenteral CS confers any advantage over other modes of treatment, unless the patient cannot take oral medications.

In a prospective case cohort using systemic CS for acute gout in 13 patients (15 attacks) who had contraindications to NSAIDs, Groff and colleagues[34] noted improvement within 12 to 48 hours. Complete resolution occurred in 11 of 15 attacks within 7 days. Patients with more than 5 involved joints required longer CS courses (mean 17 days).

Several studies compared oral prednisolone with NSAIDs, and found them equivalent for the treatment of acute gout. A study by Man and colleagues[35] compared oral indomethacin given as 50 mg 3 times daily for 2 days followed by 25 mg indomethacin 3 times daily for 3 days plus placebo prednisolone (n = 46), with prednisolone 30 mg daily for 5 days plus placebo indomethacin (n = 44); both arms also received a single dose of diclofenac, 75 mg intramuscularly, and acetaminophen, 1 g every 6 hours as needed over 5 days. In another RCT, Janssens and colleagues[36] compared prednisolone 35 mg daily (n = 60) with naproxen 500 mg twice daily (n = 60) for 5 days in acute gout among patients with MSU crystal–proven gout presenting within 24 hours of an attack. Although 216 subjects were potentially eligible for the trial, 96 were excluded mostly because of current use of NSAIDs or colchicine, or contraindications to NSAIDs. Oral prednisolone was found to be comparably effective with naproxen 500 mg twice daily in treating acute gout. At 90 hours, mean reductions in pain assessed on a VAS were similar in the naproxen and prednisolone groups. Adverse effects during treatment were minor and comparable between groups. At 3-week follow-up, all patients reported complete resolution of pain and disability.

Administration of a single intramuscular dose of triamcinolone acetonide (TA) was addressed in several studies. Alloway and colleagues[37] compared 60-mg intramuscular TA injections with oral indomethacin. Twenty-seven patients presenting within 5 days of the onset of an acute attack were included in the study. Fourteen patients received one 60-mg TA injection, 3 patients received a second injection 2 days after enrollment in the study, and 13 patients received oral indomethacin (50 mg 3 times daily). There was no statistical difference in responses, with resolution of all symptoms occurring at an average of 8 days for the indomethacin-treated patients and 7 days for patients treated with TA. Siegel and colleagues,[38] in a prospective, controlled, unblinded study, compared patients receiving a single 40-IU injection of ACTH intramuscularly (n = 16) with patients receiving a 60-mg intramuscular injection of TA (n = 15) in acute gout. The main efficacy outcome was the number of days to 100% symptom resolution. Both groups had similar mean times to resolution (7.9 and 7.6 days, respectively).

Intra-articular corticosteroids

Intra-articular CS are beneficial and useful in acute gout when 1 or 2 joints are inflamed. This approach is less favored when 2 or more joints are involved or when the involved joint is not easily amenable to aspiration. Ensuring that the joint is not infected before injecting intra-articular CS is of utmost importance. Intra-articular CS should be avoided if septic arthritis is suspected.

This modality has not been well studied, although in an uncontrolled trial[39] small intra-articular doses of TA (10 mg in knees and 8 mg in small joints) helped resolve 20 attacks of acute gout in 19 men. Joints involved were 11 knees, 4 metatarsophalangeal joints, 3 ankles, and 2 wrists. All had an MSU crystal–proven diagnosis. After one intra-articular injection of TA in 11 joints (55%) the attack of acute gout had resolved at 24 hours, and in 9 joints (45%) at 48 hours. All attacks in the 19 patients receiving intra-articular injections of CS improved within 48 hours.

Future studies are needed to compare different injectable CS suspensions and dosages to further the understanding of their efficacy and safety in treating acute gout.

Corticotropin (ACTH)

The exact mechanism of action of ACTH in gouty inflammation is not well understood. ACTH is secreted by the pituitary gland. It affects adrenal CS release, stimulating production of cortisol, corticosterone, and androgens by the pituitary. In addition, ACTH may inhibit gouty inflammation peripherally by activating the melanocortin type 3 receptor (MC3R).[40] Getting and colleagues[41] showed that small fragments of α–melanocyte-stimulating hormone (MSH) and β-MSH inhibit MSU crystal–induced neutrophil migration and release of proinflammatory cytokines and chemokines. These anti-inflammatory effects occurred in a corticosterone-independent manner, hence no reflex stimulation of the hypothalamic-pituitary-adrenal axis was observed.

A retrospective study of 33 patients who received ACTH for their acute gout or pseudogout attacks[42] found the most common regimen (90%) to be 40 IU administered intramuscularly every 8 hours. Duration of therapy was 1 to 14 days; a 97% resolution rate was reported. The mean time to complete resolution was 5.5 days, and a relapse rate of 11% (n = 4) was reported.

In a prospective controlled, unblinded study of 76 patients presenting within 24 hours of the onset of an attack of acute gout, Axelrod and Preston[43] compared intramuscular ACTH (40 IU) with oral indomethacin 50 mg 4 times daily, and found the mean pain interval from administration of the study drug to complete pain relief was 3 ± 1 hour for ACTH-treated patients versus 24 ± 10 hours for indomethacin-treated patients ($P<.0001$). The study concluded that patients treated with intramuscular ACTH experienced quicker pain relief than those treated with oral indomethacin for their acute attack.

No blinded RCTs have been conducted comparing ACTH with other modalities. It is not clear whether ACTH or CS are superior to one another or whether they have equivalent efficacy in acute gout. Future studies are needed to compare ACTH treatment with others for acute gout.

Interleukin-1β inhibitors (anakinra, canakinumab, rilonacept)

IL-1β is an important cytokine involved in gouty inflammation. MSU crystals stimulate IL-1 release by monocytes and synovial mononuclear cells,[44] and cause activation of the cryopyrin (NLRP3) inflammasome, an intracellular, multiprotein complex. Cryopyrin regulates the protease caspase-1 and controls IL-1β activation. Once caspase-1 becomes active it cleaves pro–IL-1β to release the mature p17 form of IL-1β, resulting in the active form of IL-1β.[23,45] IL-1 inhibition has now been shown to have a beneficial effect in gouty inflammation. Current IL-1 inhibitors in trials include anakinra, canakinumab, and rilonacept. Canakinumab is approved for use in acute gout by the European Medicines Agency (EMEA).

Anakinra is a no glycosylated recombinant human IL-1 receptor antagonist (IL-1Ra). IL-1Ra is an endogenous receptor antagonist for the IL-1 receptor (IL-1RI). It binds to IL-1RI and prevents it from associating with its accessory protein, IL-1RAcP, thus preventing signal transduction. Because of its short plasma half-life of approximately 4 to 6 hours following subcutaneous administration, anakinra is administered daily. Anakinra significantly relieved pain associated with acute gout in patients who could not tolerate or had failed standard anti-inflammatory therapies.[46] In an open-label pilot study, So and colleagues[47] studied 10 patients with gout, acute gout, and subacute gout, and their response to treatment with anakinra, 100 mg daily subcutaneously for 3 days. All patients responded and had relief of symptoms within 48 hours of the first anakinra injection. A complete resolution of symptoms was reported in 9 of the 10 patients on day 3 of the study. In a retrospective study of anakinra in the treatment of acute gout,[48] 15 hospitalized patients (22 attacks) who had failed CS treatment or had comorbid limitations to the use of CS were given anakinra, 100 mg daily subcutaneously for 3 days. In 19 of 22 attacks, pain reduction was reported within a day. Anakinra treatment was effective in recurrent acute attacks in the same patients, with no decrement in response to multiple anakinra courses observed.

Canakinumab, a fully selective human anti–IL-1β monoclonal antibody, does not bind IL-1α or IL-1Ra. Canakinumab has a long plasma half-life of 28 days. Two recently published phase III studies (n = 454 patients with gout) compared canakinumab, 150 mg subcutaneously with intramuscular TA. Both studies were 12 weeks long and had a 12-week extension.[49] Canakinumab, 150 mg was found to provide rapid pain relief in comparison with TA, 40 mg intramuscularly. A statistically significant dose response was observed at 72 hours for canakinumab, 150 mg subcutaneously. It was superior to 40 mg of TA intramuscularly in providing pain relief, starting at 24 hours. The median time to 50% reduction in pain was reached at 1 day with canakinumab 150 mg, compared with 2 days for the TA group ($P = .0006$).[49] Canakinumab is approved by the EMEA for the treatment of adult patients with frequent gout attacks (at least 3 attacks in the previous 12 months) in whom NSAIDs and colchicine are contraindicated, are not tolerated, or do not provide an adequate response, and in whom repeated courses of corticosteroids are not appropriate.[46]

Rilonacept (Arcalyst) is an IL-1 trap. It binds to IL-1α and IL-1β with high affinity, as well as IL-1Ra, thus preventing IL-1 from binding to the endogenous IL-1 receptor. Results of an acute gout study comparing indomethacin alone versus rilonacept with indomethacin versus rilonacept alone[50] reported that rilonacept, when combined with indomethacin and when used alone, failed to improve pain and inflammation more than indomethacin alone.

Combination Drug Treatment

In 1965, Gutman[51] suggested that there is an advantage to combining daily oxyphenbutazone (a metabolite of phenylbutazone), 800 mg with daily colchicine, 2 mg, in divided doses for the first 2 days of the gout attack followed by tapering of treatment. However, there are only a few other studies evaluating combination treatment in acute gout.

The ACR TFP[9] recommended that in severe disease, characterized by intense pain and often a polyarticular presentation, combination treatment should be used. Suggested combinations include colchicine with NSAIDs, oral corticosteroids with colchicine, or intra-articular CS with each of the other options. The use of combination anti-inflammatory drugs to treat acute gout is not described in most textbooks and reviews[3]; however, it may reflect what occurs in practice. In an American survey study evaluating gout treatment,[10] 64% of rheumatologists claimed to use combination treatment for acute gout, whereas American internists tended to use monotherapy ($P = .0005$). In this survey the most frequently used combination therapies for acute gout in an otherwise healthy patient were NSAIDs with intra-articular CS (43%), NSAIDs with oral CS (33%), and NSAIDs with oral colchicine (32%). In a study evaluating treatment of acute gout in hospitalized patients, combination treatment was used in more than 50% of patients.[11] In an Australian study,[12] combination treatment was used in 43% of patients. The most frequently used combination treatments in the Australian study were: colchicine with oral CS (35%); colchicine with an NSAID (39%); colchicine, an NSAID, and oral CS (16%); and NSAIDs with oral CS (10%).

There is little in the literature to support the use of combination anti-inflammatory drugs in acute gout. Most studies have evaluated monotherapy, despite the suspected common use of combination therapy in clinical practice. This common practice merits further study.

SUMMARY

The EULAR and ACR TFPs recently published recommendations and guidelines for the treatment of acute and chronic gout. Although these recommendations and guidelines are based on only few RCTs evaluating the efficacy of the various treatments of acute gout, they will assist individual clinicians in the management of acute gout and improvement of treatment.

The current treatment options for acute gout are NSAIDs, colchicine, systemic and intra-articular CS, and ACTH. Many use combination therapy to treat acute gout, a practice which merits study. In a patient without comorbidities, NSAIDs and colchicine are used. CS are often used in patients who have failed NSAID or colchicine treatment, or have contraindications to the use of NSAIDs and/or colchicine. IL-1 inhibition has been shown to have a beneficial effect on gouty inflammation. IL-1 inhibitors provide a treatment option for patients with acute gout who could not tolerate, have contraindications to, or were not responsive to current treatments. The most important determinant of therapeutic success is not only which drug is used but, more importantly, how soon the treatment is initiated and that the patient receives an adequate dose and for a long enough period.

These are exciting times in the research field of gout. The growing incidence and interest in gout combined with better understanding of gout pathogenesis has led to new drugs being developed for the treatment of this condition. Recent recommendations and guidelines combined with new drugs on the horizon will lead to improvement in the treatment of acute gout.

REFERENCES

1. Weede RP. Poison in the pot: the legacy of lead. Carbondale and Edwardsville (IL): Southern Illinois University Press; 1984. p. 83. In: Porter R, Rousseau GS, editors. Gout the patrician malady. Yale University Press; 1998.
2. Bellamy N, Downie WW, Buchanan WW. Observations on spontaneous improvement in patients with podagra: implications for therapeutic trials of nonsteroidal anti-inflammatory drugs. Br J Clin Pharmacol 1987;24:33–6.
3. Schlesinger N. Management of acute and chronic gouty arthritis: present state-of-the-art. Drugs 2004;64(21):2399–416.
4. Agudelo CA, Schumacher HR Jr, Phelps P. Effect of exercise on urate crystal-induced inflammation in canine joints. Arthritis Rheum 1972;15:609–16.
5. Schumacher HR Jr. Crystal induced arthritis: an overview. Am J Med 1996; 100(Suppl 2A):46–52.

6. Schlesinger N, Baker DG, Beutler AM, et al. Local ice therapy during bouts of acute gouty arthritis. J Rheumatol 2002;29:331–4.
7. Dorwart BB, Hansell JR, Schumacher HR Jr. Effects of cold and heat on urate-induced synovitis in dog. Arthritis Rheum 1974;17:563–71.
8. Zhang W, Doherty M, Bardin T, et al, EULAR Standing Committee for International Clinical Studies Including Therapeutics. EULAR evidence based recommendations for gout. Part II: management. Report of a task force of the EULAR Standing Committee For International Clinical Studies Including Therapeutics (ESCISIT). Ann Rheum Dis 2006;65:1312–24.
9. Khanna D, Khanna PP, Fitzgerald JD, et al. 2012 American College of Rheumatology guidelines for management of gout. Part 2: therapy and anti-inflammatory prophylaxis of acute gouty arthritis. Arthritis Care Res 2012;64(10):1447–61.
10. Schlesinger N, Moore DF, Sun JD, et al. A survey of current evaluation and treatment of gout. J Rheumatol 2006;33:2050–2.
11. Petersel D, Schlesinger N. Treatment of acute gout in hospitalized patients. J Rheumatol 2007;34:1566–8.
12. Gnanenthiran SR, Hassett GM, Gibson KA, et al. Acute gout management during hospitalisation: a need for a protocol. Intern Med J 2011;41(8):610–7.
13. Yeap SS, Goh EM, Gun SC. A survey on the management of gout in Malaysia. Int J Rheum Dis 2009;12:329–35.
14. Bellamy N, Gilbert JR, Brooks PM, et al. A survey of current prescribing practices of anti-inflammatory and urate lowering drugs in gouty arthritis in the Province of Ontario. J Rheumatol 1988;15:1841–71.
15. Bellamy N, Brooks PM, Gilbert RJ, et al. Survey of current prescribing practices of anti-inflammatory and urate lowering drugs in gouty arthritis in New South Wales and Queensland. Med J Aust 1989;151:537–51.
16. Stuart RA, Gow PJ, Bellamy N, et al. A survey of current prescribing practices of anti-inflammatory and urate-lowering drugs in gouty arthritis. N Z Med J 1991;104(908):115–7.
17. Rozenberg S, Lang T, Laatar A, et al. Diversity of opinions on the management of gout in France. A survey of 750 rheumatologists. Rev Rhum Engl Ed 1996;63:255–61.
18. Fang W, Zeng X, Li M, et al. The management of gout at an academic healthcare center in Beijing: a physician survey. J Rheumatol 2006;33:2041–9.
19. Ferraz MB, Sato EI, Nishie IA, et al. A survey of current prescribing practices in gouty arthritis and symptomatic hyperuricemia in San Paulo, Brazil. J Rheumatol 1994;21(2):374–5.
20. Fara N, Vázquez Mellado J, Sequeira G, et al. A survey on the current evaluation and treatment of gout in Buenos Aires, Argentina. Reumatol Clin 2012;8(6):306–9.
21. Harrold LR, Mazor KM, Negron A, et al. Primary care providers' knowledge, beliefs and treatment practices for gout: results of a physician questionnaire. Rheumatology (Oxford) 2013;52(9):1623–9.
22. Katzung BG, Furst DE. Nonsteroidal antiinflammatory drugs; disease-modifying antirheumatic drugs; nonopioid analgesics; drugs used in gout. In: Katzung BG, editor. Basic and Clinical Pharmacology. 7th edition. Stamford (CT): Appleton and Lange; 1998. p. 578–602.
23. Martinon F, Petrilli V, Mayor A, et al. Gout-associated uric acid crystals activate the NALP3 inflammasome. Nature 2006;440:237–41.
24. Levy M, Spino M, Read SE. Colchicine: a state-of-the-art review. Pharmacotherapy 1991;11:196–211.

25. Yang LP. Oral colchicine (Colcrys®) in the treatment and prophylaxis of gout. Drugs 2010;70(12):1603–13.
26. Terkeltaub RA, Furst DE, Bennett K, et al. High versus low dosing of oral colchicine for early acute gout flare: twenty-four-hour outcome of the first multicenter, randomized, double-blind, placebo-controlled, parallel-group, dose-comparison colchicine study. Arthritis Rheum 2010;63:1060–8.
27. Ahern MJ, Reid C, Gordon TP. Does colchicine work? Results of the first controlled study in gout. Aust N Z J Med 1987;17:301–4.
28. Available at: http://www.accessdata.fda.gov/scripts/cder/drugsatfda/index.cfm?fuseaction=Search.DrugDetails#.UvP36k3PMA8.email. Accessed February 6, 2014.
29. Vonkeman HE, van de Laar MA. Nonsteroidal anti-inflammatory drugs: adverse effects and their prevention. Semin Arthritis Rheum 2010;39(4):294–312.
30. Macagno A, Di Giorgio E, Romanowicz A. Effectiveness of etodolac (Lodine) compared with naproxen in patients with acute gout. Curr Med Res Opin 1991;12:423–9.
31. Rubin BR, Burton R, Navarra S, et al. Efficacy and safety profile of treatment with etoricoxib 120 mg once daily compared with indomethacin 50 mg three times daily in acute gout: a randomized controlled trial. Arthritis Rheum 2004;50:598–606.
32. Schumacher HR, Berger MF, Li-Yu J, et al. Efficacy and tolerability of celecoxib in the treatment of acute gouty arthritis: a randomized controlled trial. J Rheumatol 2012;39(9):1859–66.
33. Riccardi C, Bruscoli S, Migliorati G. Molecular mechanisms of immunomodulatory activity of glucocorticoids. Pharmacol Res 2002;45:361–8.
34. Groff GD, Franck WA, Raddatz DA. Systemic steroid therapy for acute gout: a clinical trial and review of the literature. Semin Arthritis Rheum 1990;19:329–36.
35. Man CY, Cheung IT, Cameron PA, et al. Comparison of oral prednisolone/paracetamol and oral indomethacin/paracetamol combination therapy in the treatment of acute goutlike arthritis: a double-blind, randomized, controlled trial. Ann Emerg Med 2007;49:670–7.
36. Janssens HJ, Janssen M, van de Lisdonk EH, et al. Use of oral prednisolone or naproxen for the treatment of gout arthritis: a double-blind, randomized equivalence trial. Lancet 2008;371:1854–60.
37. Alloway JA, Moriarty MJ, Hoogland YT, et al. Comparison of triamcinolone acetonide with indomethacin in the treatment of acute gouty arthritis. J Rheumatol 1993;20:111–3.
38. Seigel LB, Alloway JA, Nashel DJ. Comparison of adrenocorticotropic hormone and triamcinolone acetonide in the treatment of gouty arthritis. J Rheumatol 1994;21:1325–7.
39. Fernandez C, Noguera R, Gonzalez JA, et al. Treatment of acute attacks of gout with small doses of intraarticular triamcinolone acetonide. J Rheumatol 1999;26:2285–6.
40. Getting SJ, Christian HC, Flower RJ, et al. Activation of melanocortin type 3 receptor as a molecular mechanism for adrenocorticotropic hormone efficacy in gouty arthritis. Arthritis Rheum 2002;46(10):2765–75.
41. Getting SJ, Gibbs L, Clark AJ, et al. POMC gene derived peptides activate MC3R on murine macrophages, suppress cytokine release and inhibit neutrophil migration in acute experimental inflammation. J Immunol 1999;162:7446–53.

42. Ritter J, Kerr LD, Valeriano-Marcet J, et al. ACTH revisited: effective treatment for acute crystal induced synovitis in patients with multiple medical problems. J Rheumatol 1994;21:696–9.
43. Axelrod D, Preston S. Comparison of parenteral adrenocorticotropic hormone with oral indomethacin in the treatment of acute gout. Arthritis Rheum 1988; 31:803–5.
44. Di Giovine FS, Malawista SE, Nuki G, et al. Interleukin 1 (IL 1) as a mediator of crystal arthritis. Stimulation of T cell and synovial fibroblast mitogenesis by urate crystal-induced IL 1. J Immunol 1987;138:3213–8.
45. Cronstein RN, Terkeltaub R. The inflammatory process of gout and its treatment. Arthritis Res Ther 2006;8(Suppl 1):S3.
46. Available at: http://webcache.googleusercontent.com/search?q=cache: 2mNlWDW2pVMJ:www.ema.europa.eu/docs/en_GB/document_library/EPAR_-_ Assessment_Report_-_Variation/human/001109/WC500140963.pdf+Canakinu mab+is+approved+for+use+in+acute+gout+by+the+EMEA&cd=2&hl=en& ct=clnk&gl=us. Accessed February 6, 2014.
47. So A, De Smedt T, Revaz S, et al. A pilot study of IL-1 inhibition by anakinra in acute gout. Arthritis Res Ther 2007;9(2):R28.
48. Cho M, Ghosh P, Hans G, et al. The safety and efficacy of anakinra in the treatment of acute gout in hospitalized patients. Arthritis Rheum 2010;60(Suppl 9): S163.
49. Schlesinger N, Alten RE, Bardin T, et al. Canakinumab for acute gouty arthritis in patients with limited treatment options: results from two randomised, multi-centre, active-controlled, double-blind trials and their initial extensions. Ann Rheum Dis 2012;71:1839–48.
50. Terkeltaub RA, Schumacher HR, Carter JD, et al. Rilonacept in the treatment of acute gouty arthritis: a randomized, controlled clinical trial using indomethacin as the active comparator. Arthritis Res Ther 2013;15(1):R25.
51. Gutman AB. Treatment of primary gout: the present status. Arthritis Rheum 1965;8:911–20.

Nonpharmacologic and Pharmacologic Management of CPP Crystal Arthritis and BCP Arthropathy and Periarticular Syndromes

Ann K. Rosenthal, MD*, Lawrence M. Ryan, MD

KEYWORDS

- Calcium pyrophosphate • Pseudogout • Chondrocalcinosis
- Basic calcium phosphate • Hydroxyapatite • Therapy • Acute calcific tendinitis

KEY POINTS

- Calcium-containing crystals are commonly associated with painful musculoskeletal syndromes.
- Calcific tendonitis is treated with a variety of interventions designed to dissolve basic calcium phosphate crystals.
- A better understanding of why and how crystal deposits occur, more accurate diagnostic modalities and randomized controlled trials of available therapies will lead to the development of more specific and effective management strategies for patients with these conditions.

INTRODUCTION

Calcium crystal arthritis, including calcium pyrophosphate deposition (CPPD) and basic calcium phosphate (BCP) arthropathies and tendinitis, are common, underrecognized causes of arthritis and musculoskeletal pain for which there are few effective therapies. This article defines these syndromes, briefly describes existing diagnostic challenges, and discusses available and emerging management strategies for CPPD and BCP-associated musculoskeletal syndromes. These entities are considered separately although there is considerable overlap in the populations they affect and, in arthritis, both types of crystals may be simultaneously present in a single joint.[1]

Disclosures: Neither Dr A.K. Rosenthal nor Dr L.M. Ryan have any financial conflicts of interest to report in regard to this work.
Division of Rheumatology, Department of Medicine, Zablocki VA Medical Center and The Medical College of Wisconsin, FEOB 4th Floor, 9200 West Wisconsin Avenue, Milwaukee, WI 53226, USA
* Corresponding author.
E-mail address: arosenthal@mcw.edu

CPPD
Clinical Presentation and Epidemiology

CPPD comprises a clinically heterogeneous group of arthritides caused by the presence of calcium pyrophosphate (CPP) crystals in articular tissues (**Fig. 1**). CPP crystals produce a vigorous inflammatory response under certain conditions but are also present in noninflammatory settings. For example, CPP crystals were seen in 20% of unselected samples of cartilage and synovium examined at the time of knee replacement for osteoarthritis (OA).[2] The presence of CPP crystals is often suggested by the finding of chondrocalcinosis on radiographs of affected joints. Chondrocalcinosis typically appears as finely stippled lines of calcification in fibrocartilages such as menisci (**Fig. 2**), or outlines the bony contours in hyaline articular cartilage (**Fig. 3**).

The most commonly recognized clinical manifestation of CPPD is an acute inflammatory monoarthritis or oligoarthritis resembling gout. In acute CPPD (formerly known as pseudogout), the affected joint is erythematous and swollen, and synovial fluids can be inflammatory. The knee is the most commonly affected joint in acute CPPD.[3] CPPD also presents as a chronic noninflammatory arthritis similar to OA, although it often affects joints rarely affected in typical OA, such as shoulders, wrists, metacarpophalangeal joints, and ankles. Patients with CPPD may or may not have intermittent episodes of inflammation in these areas. Polyarticular chronic inflammatory involvement in CPPD may resemble rheumatoid arthritis. Unusual presentations of CPPD similar to those of neuropathic arthropathy have also been described.[4] Although tophaceous deposits of CPPD are unusual, they can be particularly symptomatic in the axial skeleton.[5]

Advanced age is the major risk factor for CPPD, and idiopathic CPPD is unusual in patients younger than 60 years of age. Familial forms of CPPD are well-described.[6] CPPD also occurs in association with a small number of metabolic diseases, including hyperparathyroidism, hemochromatosis, hypomagnesemia, and hypophosphatasia.[7] The association between CPPD and other common comorbidities such as diabetes, renal disease, and hypothyroidism, require further study for confirmation.[7]

Diagnostic Modalities

Because the clinical picture of CPPD may resemble other forms of arthritis, much of the challenge in management of CPPD lies in making an accurate diagnosis. The radiographic finding of chondrocalcinosis is suggestive but not diagnostic of the disease. Isolated chondrocalcinosis developing after meniscal tears in the knee is well-described[8] and is of uncertain clinical significance. In addition, CPP crystals are often

Fig. 1. CPPD crystals seen under polarizing light microscopy. These crystals appear as weakly positive birefringent rhomboidal crystals.

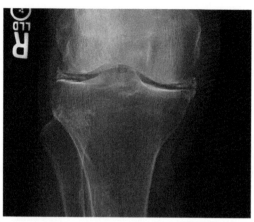

Fig. 2. Radiographic chondrocalcinosis. Dense deposits of CPPD are seen in this knee radiograph in the fibrocartilage of the meniscus.

seen in synovial fluids of joints without radiographically apparent chondrocalcinosis. Indeed, in histopathologic studies, chondrocalcinosis was present in only about 37% of subjects with articular CPP crystals.[2]

Diagnostic criteria for CPPD were proposed by Ryan and McCarty.[9] Although the presence of rhomboidal, positively-birefringent crystals in synovial fluid (see **Fig. 1**) is relied on to confirm this diagnosis, the presence of severe OA with an unusual distribution in addition to key radiographic findings may strongly suggest CPPD.[9] CPP crystals in synovial fluids can be difficult to identify because they are often quite small and only weakly birefringent.[10] Accurate and reproducible identification of CPP crystals in synovial fluid samples requires some expertise and careful thorough examinations of the samples.[11]

Studies including plain radiography, ultrasonography, and advanced imaging techniques such as CT and MRI scans can be suggestive of CPPD. In addition to chondrocalcinosis (see **Figs. 2** and **3**), CPPD is suggested by radiocarpal or patellofemoral predominant joint space narrowing, large or numerous subchondral cysts, severe progressive joint degeneration with bony collapse and fragmentation, variable osteophyte formation, tendon calcification, and unusual axial skeleton involvement.[9] The increasing use of musculoskeletal ultrasound as a readily available bedside technique provides an additional diagnostic tool for crystal arthritis. The double contour sign may correlate with radiographic chondrocalcinosis and small bright objects in synovial fluid

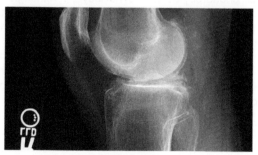

Fig. 3. Radiographic chondrocalcinosis. Dense deposits of CPPD are seen outlining the contours of the articular cartilage in this knee radiograph.

may reflect clusters of CPP crystals.[12] Ultrasound may be a useful screening tool to prompt studies that are more specific and may assist in more accurate and successful arthrocentesis. MRI is relatively insensitive to CPP deposits and presents particular difficulties in distinguishing tears and calcium deposits in menisci.[13] CT scanning more effectively identifies calcified deposits but is not commonly used to image painful joints.

TREATMENT STRATEGIES

CPPD lacks a clear cause and thus has no mechanistically targeted therapies. In addition, this field suffers from a paucity of randomized control trials of any commonly used therapies. Consequently, many of the treatment paradigms for CPPD lack a sound evidence base.

Causal Influences in Therapy

Although there is still much to learn about the pathogenesis of CPPD, it can be conceptualized in three stages. In the first stage, CPP crystals develop in the pericellular matrix of articular cartilage. It is known that overproduction of the anionic component of the crystal, pyrophosphate (PPi), is required for CPP crystals to be generated and that PPi in CPPD is analogous to the urate anion in gout.[14] Less is known about the influence of calcium levels and the extracellular matrix changes that are necessary for the generation of CPP crystals.[15] Probenecid may block PPi production by chondrocytes through its actions on the progressive ankylosis gene product commonly known as ANK. ANK is a putative PPi transporter.[16] Magnesium is a cofactor for PPi degrading enzymes and correction of low levels may increase PPi hydrolysis and reduce levels of PPi available for crystal formation. Drugs that increase alkaline phosphatase may also reduce PPi levels.[17] Ongoing work to understand PPi transport and the role of ANK in CPPD will ultimately result in novel therapies that block PPi production; however, at present, no therapies are available that clearly interfere with this stage of the disease. The presence of mineralized matrix likely alters cartilage biomechanics and may initiate or accelerate articular damage during this early phase.

In the next phase of this disease, CPPD crystals are mined or released from the cartilage surface and may elicit an inflammatory response though innate immune pathways[18] as well as by interacting with other inflammatory cells.[19] Colchicine and anti-inflammatory medications, particularly those targeted at interleukin (IL)-1β, may be useful in this phase of the disease. During the third phase of disease, crystals accelerate cartilage degeneration through mechanical strain and wear, and through other actions on articular chondrocytes and synoviocytes. Although no therapies are currently available to affect crystal interactions with cells, work in vitro with phospho-citrate[20] suggests the crystal–articular cell interaction may represent a rich source of potential therapeutic targets.

This section discusses the current recommendations for management of CPPD. An excellent review of CPPD management strategies based on a consensus from experts across Europe was recently published[21] that summarizes the commonly used medications for CPPD and clearly identifies multiple areas needing further study.

Acute CPPD

Acute CPPD is treated in a similar manner to acute gouty arthritis. The mainstays of pharmacologic therapy are intraarticular corticosteroids, nonsteroidal antiinflammatory drugs (NSAIDs), and colchicine. The relative effectiveness of these therapies has not been studied and, typically, therapeutic decisions are based on the safety of these interventions in the context of individual patient comorbidities and preferences of the provider. There is some evidence supporting the effectiveness of intraarticular corticosteroid injections in acute CPPD.[22] Oral colchicine is also commonly used, but has not been well studied. Because the dose recommendations for acute gout have dramatically changed the way colchicine is used, studies of similar low-dose short-term regimens in acute CPPD are warranted. The use of NSAIDs in acute CPPD is extrapolated from the gout literature but advanced patient age and common comorbidities in CPPD patients often increase the risk of these drugs. Oral corticosteroids have seen a resurgence in use for crystal arthropathies in general.[23] The IL-1β inhibitor, anakinra, has been useful in some patients with acute CPPD. A recent case series of 16 subjects who were otherwise refractory and intolerant of other treatments describes anakinra treatment of CPPD.[22] The mean number of injections was 15 (±42.9) and relapse occurred in one-third. Most subjects had a good response, but certainly the cost and side effects of this and similar medications may limit their widespread use. Similarly, canakinumab, an IL-1β inhibitor with a different mechanism of action than anakinra that has been tested in clinical trials for acute gout,[24] may also have some efficacy in CPPD.

Nonpharmacologic therapies are often used adjunctively in CPPD but, again, have not been rigorously compared with other therapies. Arthrocentesis, with or without lavage, may reduce the burden of both crystals and inflammatory mediators and would logically improve symptoms. Heat, ice, and rest may be useful and pain medications including narcotics may be indicated for short-term relief. Complementary or alternative treatments such as green tea polyphenols may eventually be useful based on their antiinflammatory effects in vitro.[25]

Chronic Inflammatory CPPD

The chronic inflammatory form of CPPD with either a polyarticular inflammatory presentation or an OA-like presentation with episodic inflammation can be particularly challenging to treat. These patients often suffer from frequent attacks and may have significant pain between attacks of inflammation. NSAIDs may help in those patients able to tolerate them. Systemic corticosteroids are also used and may be effective, despite serious long-term side effects. There is some weak evidence to support the use of long-term low-dose oral colchicine,[26] although its current cost makes this option more difficult for many patients. Long-term corticosteroids, despite the high risk of side effects, are necessary in some patients. There is some evidence supporting the use of methotrexate in patients with recurrent inflammatory attacks[27,28] and scattered case reports using IL-1β blockade.[29] Less evidence supports the use of hydroxychloroquine,[30] magnesium,[31] probenecid,[32] or other long-term antiinflammatory strategies.

If a single or a few large joints are involved in chronic CPPD, joint replacement may be helpful. A recent report suggests similar outcomes in unicompartmental knee arthroplasty in those with and without radiographic chondrocalcinosis.[33] Heat, ice, and physical therapy to maintain strength and flexibility in the muscles and soft tissues around the joints may also be useful adjuncts.

Chronic Noninflammatory CPPD

Chronic noninflammatory CPPD is typically managed with similar strategies used for the treatment of OA. The mainstays of pharmacologic therapy for OA include intraarticular corticosteroids, acetaminophen, NSAIDs, and pain medications.[34] Acetaminophen or NSAIDs, as tolerated, are first-line therapies for patients whose joint involvement precludes use of intraarticular corticosteroids. Hyaluronan injections are relatively contraindicated in CPPD because acute crystal arthritis has been associated with their use.[35] Colchicine may be useful in some patients with OA, but has not been well studied in chronic noninflammatory CPPD. Some patients may require more aggressive pain regimens, including narcotics. Whether recently approved therapies for OA such as duloxetine would be helpful in this form of CPPD is not-known. Emerging strategies include drugs that block nerve growth factor,[36] which may soon be available for patients suffering from OA and may have some efficacy in CPPD.

Heat, ice, and physical therapy are useful adjunctive strategies for some patients. Joint replacement surgery can be effective long-term treatment of large joint involvement.

Summary of CPPD

In summary, therapies are borrowed from acute gout, rheumatoid arthritis, and OA to manage various forms of CPPD. This underscores the need for more specific and effective pharmacologic therapies for CPPD. It is hoped that an improved understanding of the cause of CPPD will lead to the development of novel treatments or preventive strategies that interfere with the early stages of this disease before extensive joint damage occurs. Careful attention to diagnosis and large population-based studies of risk factors and current treatment patterns will provide an improved evidence base on which to make treatment decisions.

TREATMENT OF BCP-DEPOSITION DISEASES

BCP crystals deposit in a variety of diseased tissues, including musculoskeletal tissues: cartilage, synovial fluid, and periarticular structures. Three principal forms of BCP in joint fluids have been identified by Fourier transform infrared spectroscopy as hydroxyl-substituted apatite, octacalcium phosphate, and tricalcium phosphate.[37] The role of BCP crystals in causing disease in these tissues, although unproven, is suggested by clinical observations and in vitro studies. This section summarizes the available treatment strategies for combating the pathologic processes associated with BCP crystal deposits in tendons and joints.

Acute Calcific Tendinitis

Acute calcific tendinitis typically occurs around the shoulder joint, where it may present with acute severe pain, associated with large radiographically apparent calcific deposits (**Fig. 4**). It has been described in the hands and feet, as well as the shoulder. The cause of calcific tendinitis remains unclear.

Standard conservative treatment of acute calcific tendinitis involves treatment with NSAIDs, exercises, and injections. IL-1β inhibition has also seemed effective in a small open label series of five subjects treated with anakinra for 3 consecutive days.[38] For those cases refractory to standard treatment, several physical modality options exist. Ultrasound therapy is considered part of standard traditional conservative management providing short-term improvement in symptoms (but not long-term improvement at 9 months) and associated with no changes in the size of calcifications[39] compared with sham treatment.

Newer approaches to treatment are available. Extracorporeal shock wave therapy (ESWT) involves application of 0.06 to 0.55 mJ/mm^2 at 1000 to 6000 impulses per session to the calcified area. Conscious sedation or intravenous analgesia may be necessary for this procedure, which is often painful. The largest study of ESWT compared high-energy level with low-energy level and with sham shock waves. The design incorporated concomitant physiotherapy.[40] Both high-energy and low-energy ESWT

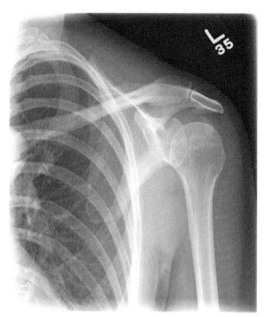

Fig. 4. Calcific tendinitis. A round radiodense deposit of calcium is seen in the supraspinatus tendon of this shoulder radiograph.

directed at the areas of calcification improved pain and shoulder function while reducing size of calcific deposits compared with placebo. Subjects receiving high-energy treatment fared better than those receiving low-energy therapy. A recent systematic review indicates a level of evidence B for this intervention.[41] Side effects included erythema at the site of treatment and hematomas. Conscious sedation is especially desirable in those with ongoing acute symptomatology before the shock-wave treatment. One form of ESWT, termed radial shock wave therapy, delivers pneumatic instead of ultrasound impulses. This mode of delivery seems to be less painful and equally effective.[42]

Needling of tendon calcifications, also known as barbotage, has long been used for treatment of acute calcific tendinitis,[43] often in combination with lavage. The rationale is that needling may decrease intratendon pressure and lavage removes some of the particulate matter that is inciting inflammation. For instance, an open study of fluoroscopic needling with saline lavage resulted in improvement in symptoms and a 50% decrease of radiographic calcium deposit size 6 months after procedure.[44] Interpretation of these results and those of most needling studies is complicated by the subjects having received intralesional or bursal glucocorticoid injections at the conclusion of the lavage procedure. Similarly, a longer term 1-year follow-up of ultrasound-guided needling, lavage, and steroid injection indicated an 89% complete or near complete resolution of calcifications and 91% of subjects had substantial improvement of symptoms and clinical findings.[45] Other case series have described similar outcomes for ultrasound-guided needling, lavage, and injection.[46] To assess the impact of the needling and lavage versus that of the steroid injection, a study compared glucocorticoid injection into the subacromial bursa alone with the combination of needling-lavage-subacromial injection.[47] Significantly more improvement was noted in the combination therapy than in the subacromial bursa injection alone. Needling and lavage added significant benefit to injection alone. Refinements to the needling and lavage approach have been identified. Two-needle lavage (one for inflow another for outflow) has been advocated and specifics of methodology have been recently reviewed.[48] Using warm saline solution lavage improves calcium deposit reduction, shortens the procedure time, and diminishes the frequency of bursitis after lavage compared with the use of lavage with room temperature saline.[49] Another "needling" technique is mesotherapy, defined as the intermittent injection of drugs into painful tissues. In a randomized controlled study, EDTA treatment was tested. Forty patients received mesotherapy weekly with an EDTA-containing solution along with interval pulsed-mode sonotherapy with an EDTA-containing sonographic gel 5 days weekly for 3 weeks. The comparator group of 40 subjects received injections not containing EDTA and sham ultrasound without EDTA and with the ultrasonic generator turned off. The EDTA treatment group had significant improvement in pain and shoulder function and a remarkable decrease in calcification at 4 weeks compared with the control group.[50]

Nonoperative treatments are usually successful. When surgery is necessary for refractory calcific tendinitis of the rotator cuff, debridement and concomitant subacromial decompression by acromioplasty is often advocated. However, a study comparing debridement alone with debridement plus subacromial decompression suggests that debridement alone is preferable.[51]

Acute Calcific Periarthritis of the Hand

Acute calcific periarthritis of the hand presents in much the same way as local infection, gout, acute CPPD, or palindromic rheumatism attacks. BCP crystals are noted in aspirates. It is typically a disease of premenopausal women and involves the hand,[52] although identical attacks may occur in the feet. Periarticular calcifications are often radiographically subtle. Its course is self-limited but recurrences are common. Treatment with either corticosteroid injection or NSAIDs has been described and either is thought to be effective. No controlled studies or large series of treatment are available due to its rarity and self-limited nature.

BCP-Associated Arthropathies

Milwaukee shoulder syndrome

The best characterized, but not the most common, form of joint disease associated with BCP deposition is the Milwaukee shoulder syndrome (MSS), comparable in many respects with the previous descriptions of cuff-tear arthropathy (**Fig. 5**).[53–55] This syndrome is a noninflammatory enzyme-driven destruction of articular structures, including articular cartilage and rotator cuff tendons, accompanied by large effusions. The unifying feature of MSS is the presence of BCP crystals in the joint fluid. One-half of affected patients have coexistent CPP crystals and one-half have involvement of joints other than the glenohumeral joints, notably the knees. Standard treatment has involved use of NSAIDs, analgesics, physical therapy, and intraarticular injections of glucocorticoids. Randomized controlled studies that validate this approach are lacking. The paucity of therapeutic studies of MSS results in part from lack of convenient assays for detecting and quantifying BCP crystals in joint fluids. Use of magnesium supplementation is anecdotal but may be helpful for BCP disease or the frequently attendant CPPD.[31,56] In the authors' clinic, repeated arthrocentesis with glucocorticoid injection seems to relieve pain and decrease effusions in some individuals but has not increased function. Other investigators have suggested treatment with tidal irrigation.[57,58] In the latter study, subjects with advanced radiographic changes fared less well than those with minor radiographic changes. Potentially, this treatment's efficacy depends on the removal of BCP crystals from joints that do not yet have

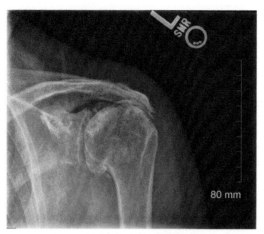

Fig. 5. MSS. Note the severe cartilage loss evidenced by the loss of glenohumeral joint space, subchondral sclerosis, and global joint degeneration in this radiograph from a patient with MSS.

extensive damage. When conservative strategies fail, surgical outcomes may be extrapolated from the literature surrounding the closely related entity of cuff tear arthropathy. Reverse total shoulder arthroplasty seems to have better outcomes than hemiarthroplasty.[59,60]

Musculoskeletal involvement with BCP crystals: targeting the crystals. The next approach?

Ultimately, successful treatment of the above conditions may necessitate either preventing crystal deposition or blocking the harmful biologic effects. A rationale for targeting BCP crystals in future approaches to treatment is provided below.

BCP Crystals Are Linked to Degenerative Joint Processes

BCP crystals have been uniformly detected in osteoarthritic hyaline cartilages removed from hip or knee joints at the time of arthroplasty.[2,61] In these studies, hyaline cartilage BCP deposits were not visible on standard preoperative radiographs but could be seen using digital-contact radiography on the surgical specimens. The degree of cartilage calcification correlated with the severity of OA both on preoperative radiographs and by histology of operative specimens. Markers of chondrocyte hypertrophy were prominent in the pathologic specimens. Control cartilage specimens from subjects undergoing amputation for malignancies did not contain BCP deposits, albeit the few control subjects were generally younger than the OA subjects. Thus, cartilage BCP deposits are intimately linked to advanced OA of sufficient severity to require joint replacement. These findings confirm and extend those of a previous study of cartilage calcification in consecutive postmortem knees, which also noted a correlation between presence of calcium phosphate mineral and histologic severity of OA.[62] Joint fluid studies also indicate frequent detection of BCP crystals in specimens taken from osteoarthritic joints.[1]

In Vitro Effects of BCP Crystals Suggest a Role in Inflammation and Degenerative Processes

In general, calcium-containing crystals elicit numerous biologic responses that may lead to tissue injury and inflammation. Among the responses are synthesis and release of several proteases. Proteases, including matrix metalloproteinases 1, 3, 8, 9, and 13, are released after exposing cells to BCP crystals.[63–65] At the same time these crystals down-regulate tissue inhibitor of metalloproteinase.[66] BCP crystals also elicit release of prostaglandin E2 and IL-1β from fibroblasts.[67] Nitric oxide production was enhanced in cells exposed to other calcium-containing crystals and will likely increase with BCP exposure.[18] BCP crystals are also mitogens, which results in proliferation of tissues such as synovium,[68] increasing the cell population that may secrete proteases and cytokines. The usefulness of targeting crystal formation and blockade of calcium crystal downstream effects has been tested in an animal model. The Hartley guinea pig model of OA features intraarticular BCP formation. Treatment of these animals with phosphocitrate, which blocks growth of BCP crystals and their biologic effects, attenuated the degenerative process in this animal model of OA.[69]

Summary of BCP-related Diseases

Current treatment approaches to BCP-related diseases differ little from the treatment of coexistent OA or tendon disease. However, specific procedures (vide supra) improve outcomes in patients with calcific tendinitis refractory to standard treatments. Promising avenues for ameliorating the pathologic effects of BCP crystals include use of magnesium, possible use of colchicine, and phosphocitrate compounds. Each of these can block crystal formation and/or biologic effects of calcium-containing crystals. Further studies would be facilitated by more convenient and standardized methods of identifying BCP crystals in biologic specimens, which would enable a more precise identification of the target population.

SUMMARY

In conclusion, calcium-containing crystals are commonly associated with painful musculoskeletal syndromes. A better understanding of why and how these crystal deposits occur, the use of more accurate diagnostic modalities, and randomized controlled trials of available therapies will lead to the development of more specific and effective management strategies for patients with these conditions.

REFERENCES

1. Derfus B, Kurian J, Butler J, et al. The high prevalence of pathologic calcium crystals in pre-operative knees. J Rheumatol 2002;29:570–4.
2. Fuerst M, Bertrand J, Lammers L, et al. Calcification of articular cartilage in human osteoarthritis. Arthritis Rheum 2009;60:2694–703.
3. Rosenthal A, Ryan L. Calcium pyrophosphate crystal deposition diseases, pseudogout, and articular chondrocalcinosis. In: WJ K, Moreland L, editors. Arthritis and allied conditions. Philadelphia: Lippincott Williams & Wilkins; 2004. p. 2373–96.
4. McCarty DJ. Diagnostic mimicry in arthritis: patterns of joint involvement associated with calcium pyrophosphate dihydrate crystal deposits. Ann Rheum Dis 1975;25:804–9.
5. Ishida T, Dorfman H, Bullough P. Tophaceous pseudogout (tumoral calcium pyrophosphate dihydrate crystal deposition disease). Hum Pathol 1995;26(6):587–93.
6. Williams C. Familial calcium pyrophosphate dihydrate deposition disease and the ANKH gene. Curr Opin Rheumatol 2003;15:326–31.

7. Jones AC, Chuck AJ, Arie EA, et al. Diseases associated with calcium pyrophosphate deposition disease. Semin Arthritis Rheum 1992;22(3):188–202.
8. Doherty M, Watt I, Dieppe P. Localised chondrocalcinosis in post-meniscetomy knees. Lancet 1982;1:1207–10.
9. Ryan L, McCarty D. Calcium pyrophosphate crystal deposition disease; pseudogout; articular chondrocalcinosis. In: McCarty D, editor. Arthritis and allied conditions. Philadelphia: Lea & Febiger; 1985. p. 1515–46.
10. Ivorra J, Rosas J, Pascual E. Most calcium pyrophosphate crystals appear as non-birefringent. Ann Rheum Dis 1999;58:582–4.
11. Rosenthal A, Mandel N. Identification of crystals in synovial fluids and joint tissues. Curr Rheumatol Rep 2001;3:11–6.
12. Frediani B, Filippou G, Falsetti P, et al. Diagnosis of calcium pyrophosphate dihydrate crystal deposition disease: ultrasonographic criteria proposed. Ann Rheum Dis 2005;64:638–40.
13. Beltran J, Marty-Delfaut E, Bencardino J, et al. Chondrocalcinosis of the hyaline cartilage of the knee: MRI manifestations. Skeletal Radiol 1998;27:369–74.
14. Ryan L, Rosenthal A. Metabolism of extracellular pyrophosphate. Curr Opin Rheumatol 2003;15:311–4.
15. Rosenthal A. Pathogenesis of calcium pyrophosphate crystal deposition disease. Curr Rheumatol Rep 2001;3:17–23.
16. Ho A, Johnson M, Kingsley D. Role of the mouse ank gene in tissue calcification and arthritis. Science 2000;289:265–70.
17. Tsui F, Las Heras F, Inman R, et al. Functional Roles of ANKH/Ank: insights from CPPDD-associated ANKH Mutations and the ank/ank Mouse. J Clin Rheumatol Musculoskelet Med 2010;1(1):50–5.
18. Liu-Brian R, Pritzker K, Firestein G, et al. TLR2 signaling in chondrocytes drives calcium pyrophosphate dihydrate and monosodium urate crystal-induced nitric oxide generation. J Immunol 2005;174:5016–23.
19. Pang L, Haves C, Buac K, et al. Pseudogout-associated inflammatory calcium pyrophosphate dihydrate microcrystals induce formation of neutrophil extracellular traps. J Immunol 2013;190(12):6488–500.
20. Nair D, Misra R, Sallis J, et al. Phosphocitrate inhibits a basic calcium phosphate and calcium pyrophosphate dihydrate crystal-induced mitogen-activated protein kinase cascade signal transduction pathway. J Biol Chem 1997;272:18920–5.
21. Zhang W, Doherty M, Pascual E, et al. EULAR recommendations for calcium pyrophosphate deposition. Part II: management. Ann Rheum Dis 2011;70:571–5.
22. Masuda I, Ishikawa K. Clinical features of pseudogout attack: a survey of 50 cases. Clin Orthop Relat Res 1987;229:173–81.
23. Werlen D, Gabay C, Vischer T. Corticosteroid therapy for the treatment of acute attacks of crystal-induced arthritis: an effective alternative to nonsteroidal antiinflammatory drugs. Rev Rhum Engl Ed 1996;63:248–54.
24. Schlesinger N, Mysler E, Lin H, et al. Canakinumab reduces the risk of acute gouty arthritis flares during initiation of allopurinol treatment: results of a double blind randomised study. Ann Rheum Dis 2011;70:1264–71.
25. Oliviero F, Sfriso P, Scanu A, et al. Epigallocatechin-3-gallate reduces inflammation induced by calcium pyrophosphate crystals in vitro. Front Pharmacol 2013;4(51):1–7.
26. Alvarellos A, Spilberg I. Colchicine prophylaxis in pseudogout. J Rheumatol 1986;13:804–5.
27. Andres M, Sivera F, Pascual E. Methotrexate is an option for patients with refractory calcium pyrophosphate crystal arthritis. J Clin Rheumatol 2012;18:234–6.

28. Chollet-Janin A, Finckh A, Dudler J, et al. Methotrexate as an alternative therapy for chronic calcium pyrophosphate deposition disease: an exploratory analysis. Arthritis Rheum 2007;56:688–92.
29. Diamantopoulos A, Brodin C, Hetland H, et al. Interleukin 1β blockade improves signs and symptoms of chronic calcium pyrophosphate resistant to treatment. J Clin Rheumatol 2012;18(6):310–1.
30. Rothschild B, Yakubov L. Prospective 6-month, double-blind trial of hydroxychloroquine treatment of CPDD. Compr Ther 1997;23:327–31.
31. Doherty M, Dieppe P. Double blind, placebo controlled trial of magnesium carbonate in chronic pyrophosphate arthropathy. Ann Rheum Dis 1983;42(Suppl): 106–7.
32. Trostle D, Schumacher H. Probenecid therapy of refractory CPPD deposition disease. Arthritis Rheum 1999;42(Suppl):S160.
33. Hernigou P, Pascale W, Pascale V, et al. Does primary or secondary chondrocalcinosis influence long-term survivorship of unicompartmental arthroplasty? Clin Orthop Relat Res 2012;470:1973–9.
34. Hochberg M, Altman R, April K, et al. American College of Rheumatology 2012 recommendations for the use of nonpharmacologic and pharmacologic therapies in osteoarthritis of the hand, hip and knee. Arthritis Care Res 2012;64(4): 465–74.
35. Ali Y, Weinstein M, Jokl P. Acute pseudogout following intra-articular injection of high molecular weight hyaluronic acid. Am J Med 1999;106(6):641–2.
36. Brown M, Murphy F, Radin D, et al. Tanezumab reduces osteoarthritis hip pain: results of a randomized double-blind controlled phase III trial. Arthritis Rheum 2013;65(7):1795–803.
37. McCarty D, Lehr J, Halverson P. Crystal populations in human synovial fluid. Arthritis Rheum 1983;26:1220.
38. Zufferey P, So A. A pilot study of IL-1 inhibition in acute calcific periarthritis of the shoulder. Ann Rheum Dis 2013;72:465–7.
39. Ebenbichler G, Erdogmus C, Resch K, et al. Ultrasound therapy for calcific tendinitis of the shoulder. N Engl J Med 1999;340:1533–8.
40. Gerdesmeyer L, Wagenpfeil S, Haake M, et al. Extracorporeal shock wave therapy for the treatment of chronic calcifying tendonitis of the rotator cuff. JAMA 2003;290:2573–80.
41. Lee SY, Cheng B, Grimmer-Somers K. The midterm effectiveness of extracorporeal shockwave therapy in the management of chronic calcific shoulder tendinitis. J Shoulder Elbow Surg 2011;20:845–54.
42. Cacchio A, Paoloni M, Barile A, et al. Effectiveness of radial shock-wave therapy for calcific tendinitis of the shoulder: single-blind randomized clinical study. Phys Ther 2006;86:672–82.
43. Patterson R, Darrach W. Treatment of acute bursitis by needle irrigation. J Bone Joint Surg Am 1937;19:993–1002.
44. Pfister J, Gerber H. Chronic calcifying tendinitis of the shoulder – Therapy by percutaneous needle aspiration and lavage: a prospective open study of 62 shoulders. Clin Rheumatol 1997;16:269–74.
45. del Cura J, Torre I, Zabala R, et al. Sonographically guided percutaneous needle lavage in calcific tendinitis of the shoulder: short- and long-term results. AJR Am J Roentgenol 2007;189:128–34.
46. Yoo J, Koh K, Park W, et al. The outcome of ultrasound-guided needle decompression and steroid injection in calcific tendinitis. J Shoulder Elbow Surg 2010; 19:596–600.

47. De Witte P, Selten J, Navas A, et al. Calcific tendinitis of the rotator cuff: a randomized controlled trial of ultrasound-guided needling and lavage versus subacromial corticosteroids. Am J Sports Med 2013;14:1665–73.
48. Sconfienza L, Vigano S, Martini C, et al. Double-needle ultrasound-guided percutaneous treatment of rotator cuff calcific tendinitis: tips and tricks. Skeletal Radiol 2013;42:19–24.
49. Sconfienza L, Bandirali M, Serafini G, et al. Rotator cuff calcific tendinitis: does warm saline solution improve the short-term outcome of double-needle US-guided treatment? Radiology 2012;262:560–6.
50. Cacchio A, De Blasis E, Desiati P, et al. Effectiveness of treatment of calcific tendinitis of the shoulder by disodium EDTA. Arthritis Care Res 2009;61:84–91.
51. Marder R, Heiden E, Kim S. Calcific tendonitis of the shoulder: is subacromial decompression in combination with removal of the calcific deposit beneficial? J Shoulder Elbow Surg 2011;20:955–60.
52. Wiper J, Garrido A. Acute calcific tendinitis. N Engl J Med 2008;359:2477.
53. McCarty D, Halverson P, Carrera G, et al. Milwaukee shoulder syndrome: association of microspheroids containing hydroxyapatite crystals, active collagenase, and neutral protease with rotator cuff defects, I. Clinical aspects. Arthritis Rheum 1981;24:464–73.
54. Halverson P, Cheung H, McCarty D, et al. Milwaukee shoulder: association of microspheroids containing hydroxyapatite crystals, active collagenase and neutral protease with rotator cuff defects: II. Synovial fluid studies. Arthritis Rheum 1981;24:474–83.
55. Neer C, Cragin E, Fukuda H. Cuff tear arthropathy. J Bone Joint Surg Am 1983; 65:1232–44.
56. Patel K, Weidnsaul D, Palma C, et al. Milwaukee shoulder with massive bilateral cysts: effective therapy for hydrops of the shoulder. J Rheumatol 1997;24: 2453–79.
57. Weiss J, Good A, Schumacher H. Four cases of "Milwaukee shoulder syndrome" with a description of clinical presentation and long term treatment. J Am Geriatr Soc 1985;33:202–5.
58. Epis O, Caporali R, Scire C, et al. Efficacy of tidal irrigation in Milwaukee shoulder syndrome. J Rheumatol 2007;34:1545–50.
59. Coe P, Greiwe R, Josh IR, et al. The cost-effectiveness of reverse total shoulder arthroplasty compared with hemiarthroplasty for rotator cuff arthropathy. J Shoulder Elbow Surg 2012;21:1278–88.
60. Young S, Zhu M, Walker C, et al. Comparison of functional outcomes of reverse shoulder arthroplasty with those of hemiarthroplasty in the treatment of cuff-tear arthropathy: a matched pair analysis. J Bone Joint Surg Am 2013;95:910–5.
61. Fuerst M, Niggemeyer O, Lammers L, et al. Articular cartilage mineralization in osteoarthritis of the hip. BMC Musculoskelet Disord 2009;10:166.
62. Gordon G, Villanueva T, Schumacher H, et al. Autopsy study correlating degree of osteoarthritis, synovitis and evidence of articular calcification. J Rheumatol 1984;11:681–6.
63. McCarthy G, Mitchell P, Struve J, et al. Basic calcium phosphate crystals cause coordinate induction and secretion of collagenase and stromelysin. J Cell Physiol 1992;153:140–6.
64. McCarthy G, Macius A, Christopherson P, et al. Basic calcium phosphate crystals induce synthesis and secretion of 92 kDa gelatinase (gelatinaseB/matrix metalloproteinase 9) in human fibroblasts. Ann Rheum Dis 1998;57: 56–64.

65. Reuben P, Wenger L, Cruz M, et al. Induction of metalloproteinase-8 in human fibroblasts by basic calcium phosphate crystals: effect of phosphocitrate. Connect Tissue Res 2001;42:1–12.

66. Bai G, Howell D, Howard G, et al. Basic calcium phosphate crystals up-regulate metalloproteinases but down-regulate tissue inhibitor of metalloproteinase-1 and -2 in human fibroblasts. Osteoarthr Cartil 2001;9:416–22.

67. Morgan M, Whelan L, Sallis J, et al. Basic calcium phosphate crystal-induced prostaglandin E2 production in human fibroblasts. Arthritis Rheum 2004;50: 1642–9.

68. Cheung H, Story M, McCarty D. Mitogenic effects of hydroxyapatite and calcium pyrophosphate dihydrate crystals on cultured mammalian cells. Arthritis Rheum 1984;27:668–74.

69. Cheung H, Sallis J, Demadis K, et al. Phosphocitrate blocks calcification-induced articular joint degeneration in a guinea pig model. Arthritis Rheum 2006;54:2452–61.

Long-Term Management of Gout
Nonpharmacologic and Pharmacologic Therapies

Yashaar Chaichian, MD, Saima Chohan, MD,
Michael A. Becker, MD*

KEYWORDS

- Gout • Hyperuricemia • Risk reduction • Urate-lowering therapy • Allopurinol
- Febuxostat • Uricosuric agents • Pegloticase

KEY POINTS

- Management of hyperuricemic individuals, whether asymptomatic or with gout, aims primarily at maintaining serum urate concentrations in a subsaturating range (usually <6 mg/dL), thus preventing or reversing the clinical consequences of urate crystal formation and deposition.
- Although nonpharmacologic (lifestyle) adjustments may lessen the risk for incident gout in hyperuricemic individuals and ameliorate the course of patients with established gout, pharmacologic urate-lowering therapy to achieve goal-range serum urate is, in most instances, required.
- Inhibition of xanthine oxidase (XO) activity with allopurinol at doses titrated to achieve goal-range serum urate levels remains the first-line urate-lowering pharmacotherapy in the US; febuxostat, an alternative XO inhibitor, or benzbromarone (where available) are suitable alternative first-line options, especially for patients at high-risk for allopurinol toxicity.
- Nonadherence to long-term medication use and inadequate monitoring/titration of urate-lowering therapies are important factors contributing to the suboptimal outcomes for patients with gout documented in many countries.
- For patients who have progressed to severe gout with impaired physical function or quality of life (because of either refractoriness to or intolerance of oral urate-lowering agents or inadequate previous therapy), the modified recombinant uricase, pegloticase, is a biological therapeutic option warranting consideration.

Disclosures: Y. Chaichian, MD and S. Chohan, MD: none; M.A. Becker, MD: consultant/advisory boards: Takeda Pharmaceuticals; Savient Pharmaceuticals; Ardea Biosciences/AstraZeneca Pharmaceuticals; BioCryst Pharmaceuticals; Metabolex Pharmaceuticals; Regeneron Pharmaceuticals; URL/Mutual Pharmaceuticals; royalties (for authorship and editing): UpToDate.
Section of Rheumatology, The University of Chicago, 5841 South Maryland Avenue, MC 0930, Chicago, IL 60637, USA
* Corresponding author.
E-mail address: mbecker@medicine.bsd.uchicago.edu

INTRODUCTION

The clinical signs and symptoms of gout reflect inflammatory responses to monosodium urate crystals deposited in tissues from extracellular fluids saturated for urate.[1] Hyperuricemia (defined as serum or plasma urate concentrations exceeding 6.8 mg/dL, the limit of urate solubility) is a necessary but not sufficient pathogenetic factor in gout, as shown by recent estimates of 8.3 million and 40 million persons for the respective prevalences of gout and asymptomatic hyperuricemia (hyperuricemia without clinical gout) in the American population.[2] Persons with gout or with asymptomatic hyperuricemia alone have considerably increased prevalences of significant chronic comorbidities (discussed later), which can affect the safety and efficacy of treatment of hyperuricemia and can, in turn, be affected by it.[3,4]

Treatment of acute gouty arthritis typically involves brief courses of antiinflammatory medication aimed at reducing the pain, duration, and disability of flares with acceptable benefit/risk ratios (see later discussion). However, antiinflammatory agents do not lower urate concentrations and are thus not appropriate for long-term management of established gout or prevention of incident gout. Instead, accomplishment of the latter aims center on nonpharmacologic and pharmacologic means to achieve and maintain serum urate levels in a subsaturating range, because persistent goal-range decrease of urate levels is accompanied over time by resolution and even reversal of the signs and symptoms of established gout.[5-9]

NONPHARMACOLOGIC APPROACHES TO CHRONIC GOUT: RISK REDUCTION

Among risk factors for the development of gout (**Table 1**), some such as age, gender, race, and ethnicity are not modifiable, whereas others are. Advanced age is strongly associated with increases in both the incidence and prevalence of gout.[10-13] The risk of gout is also higher in men than women at all ages, although this gap narrows after the female menopause.[11,13] Racial and ethnic disparities in gout risk have also been observed.[14-16]

Nonpharmacologic management of gout relies on lifestyle adjustments aimed at reducing the roles of modifiable risk factors in the expression or severity of gout. In addition to institution of appropriate pharmacologic or nonpharmacologic treatment of comorbid disorders, lifestyle adjustments should be considered and appropriately recommended to patients with gout (or asymptomatic hyperuricemia). It is thought that these initiatives promote overall health and may lead to sustained goal-range decrease in urate levels and/or lessen the burden of pharmacologic urate-lowering therapy (ULT). Lifestyle measures directly decrease urate levels by reducing the availability of uric acid

Table 1	
Nonmodifiable and modifiable risk factors for gout	
Nonmodifiable Risk Factors	**Modifiable Risk Factors**
Age	Hyperuricemia
Gender	Obesity
Race	Hypertension
Ethnicity	Hyperlipidemia
	Ischemic cardiovascular disease
	Diabetes mellitus
	Chronic kidney disease
	Dietary factors
	Medications that alter urate balance

precursors or by promoting urate excretion. Some may also play an indirect role by diminishing contributions of comorbid diseases to incident or established gout. Lifestyle adjustments include long-term weight reduction to ideal body mass; alcohol restriction; changes in dietary intake and composition; use of favorable and avoidance of unfavorable dietary supplements; and substitution, where possible, of hyperuricemia-inducing medications.

Obesity, hypertension, ischemic cardiovascular disease, type 2 diabetes, hyperlipidemia, and chronic kidney disease (CKD) are all associated with increased risk of gout.[3,14,17–21] For example, obesity is strongly associated with gout, and the degree of risk increases as the body mass index (BMI, calculated as weight in kilograms divided by the square of height in meters) increases.[3,17–20] In the Health Professionals Follow-up Study of 47,150 men without a previous history of gout, the relative risk of incident gout was 1.95 in men with BMI 25 to 29.9 kg/m^2 (compared with 1.00 when BMI was 21–22.9) and increased to 2.97 with BMI of at least 35.[20] In this study, weight loss was protective against the development of gout. Thus, beyond other health benefits, maintaining a BMI in the normal range is recommended to reduce the risk of gout.[22–24]

Alcohol consumption has also been associated with increased risk of gout in several observational studies.[16,25–27] Based on data from the largest prospective study, consumption of at least 2 beers daily confers the highest risk of gout (2.5-fold compared with no beer intake).[27] Gout risk also increases (to a lesser extent) with consumption of spirits, although drinking 2 glasses (118 mL, 4 oz) of wine daily does not seem to increase risk.

Various dietary constituents and additives are risk factors for gout, whereas others are neutral in terms of risk or may even be protective. Increased meat or seafood intake is associated with greater risk of gout.[28–30] Dairy intake, particularly low fat dairy, is associated with a significantly lower risk of gout, whereas moderate intake of purine-rich vegetables does not confer increased risk.[29] Higher levels of coffee consumption (including decaffeinated coffee, but not tea) significantly decrease the risk of gout.[31,32] There are conflicting data regarding fruits and gout risk, although frequent cherry consumption seems to reduce risk for recurrent gout attacks.[30,33,34] Whether this effect reflects a decrease in urate levels or an inflammation-suppressing effect of cherry constituents is uncertain. Among dietary additives, sucrose-sweetened juices and soft drinks containing high fructose corn syrup increase the risk of incident gout, whereas artificially sweetened (diet) soft drinks do not.[34,35] There is evidence that high levels of simple sugar ingestion operate at least in part independently of promoting obesity, perhaps by selectively impairing renal uric acid excretion mediated by glut9, a urate/glucose/fructose transporter encoded by genetically diverse alleles of the SLC2A9 gene.[36]

Several medications are also implicated as potential risk factors for the development of gout. Thiazide and loop diuretics increase the risk of incident gout.[17,20,21,26] In one study, diuretic use imparted a risk ratio of 2.39 in women and 3.41 in men for incident gout.[17] Diuretic medications are also implicated in increased risk for flare recurrence in patients with established gout.[37] Thus, substituting an affordable and comparably efficacious antihypertensive for a diuretic can be useful to reduce the risk of incident gout or the dose of urate-lowering medication needed to control hyperuricemia in patients with established gout. Cyclosporine, an important medication in the organ transplant population, is also associated with increased risk and severity of gout related to induction of renal urate retention.[38] Aspirin has a dose-dependent relationship to urate metabolism: high-dose aspirin (>2–3 g/d) is uricosuric and reduces serum urate, but lower-dose aspirin (<2 g/d) promotes renal uric acid retention.[39] Although aspirin is not recommended either for treatment of acute gout or for chronic ULT, it is usually continued when prescribed at very low doses (81–325 mg/d) for clot prophylaxis.[40]

PHARMACOLOGIC ULT

Nonpharmacologic approaches to gout management are important and should be emphasized with patients at each visit. Nevertheless, these measures are often either less than optimally adhered to or insufficient to achieve and maintain goal-range serum urate levels. As a result, most patients with gout require addition of pharmacologic ULT to achieve successful disease control.

CONSIDERATIONS IN THE USE OF PHARMACOLOGIC ULT
Indications for Pharmacologic ULT

The decision to initiate urate-lowering medication should be individualized, but most published treatment recommendations[22–24,41] recognize specific clinical indications for urate-lowering pharmacotherapy in patients with gout (**Box 1**). In contrast, there is less agreement regarding pharmacologic ULT for asymptomatic hyperuricemia, which is, for example, usually not recommended in the United States but is in Japan for patients with serum urate levels persistently greater than 9 mg/dL (or even lower in the presence of a comorbidity such as hypertension).[41] Whether pharmacologic ULT has favorable benefit to risk ratios with respect to gout or comorbid disease outcomes in asymptomatic hyperuricemia is an unanswered question.

Pharmacologic ULT: Initiation and Treatment Duration

Pharmacologic ULT has traditionally been initiated in the interval between attacks because of concern that immediate urate reduction might worsen or prolong an ongoing attack. Although a recent small trial found no significant difference in daily pain, recurrent flares, or levels of inflammatory markers between patients started on allopurinol during an attack and those beginning treatment 2 weeks later,[42] we

---

Box 1
Indications for pharmacologic ULT in patients with gout

Frequent and disabling gout attacks

- No exact definition is agreed on, although 2 or 3 attacks per year is often used as a treatment threshold; a lower threshold may be appropriate in patients with history of less frequent but more prolonged and severe gout attacks

Tophaceous gout

- Determined clinically or on radiographs

Chronic gouty arthropathy

- Joint or bone damage caused by gout; determined clinically or on radiographs

CKD

- Estimated glomerular filtration rate (eGFR) less than 60 mL/min/BSA (stage 3 or more severe CKD) or eGFR 60 to 90 mL/min/BSA plus evidence of renal structural damage (stage 2 CKD)

Recurrent nephrolithiasis

- With uric acid stones: failure of hydration and urinary alkalinization therapy
- With calcium oxalate stones: daily urinary uric acid excretion greater than 800 mg in men or greater than 750 mg in women

Patients undergoing chemotherapy or radiotherapy

- For treatment of lymphoproliferative, myeloproliferative, or large solid organ cancers

recommend the traditional approach, with only rare exception. The brief delay in starting what is usually lifelong treatment presents no discernible risk in long-term outcomes, and provides more opportunity to evaluate and counsel each patient with regard to the need for and optimal choice of ULT.[24]

Successful maintenance of goal-range serum urate levels usually results in reduction over time in gout symptoms, prompting many patients to question the need for continued therapy.[43] In several studies, no benefit and a clear risk of gout recurrence were found if ULT is discontinued.[44–46] In one study,[46] patients maintaining serum urate levels averaging 5 mg/dL during 5 years of treatment showed a longer time to gout recurrence than those maintaining levels nearer 7 mg/dL during treatment. Perez-Ruiz and colleagues[43] have suggested that once gout symptoms and signs have resolved for several years, the goal of ULT may be reset at a higher level in the subsaturating range, allowing lower-dose maintenance ULT.

Serum Urate Goals and Monitoring

The most widely recommended serum urate goal-range during ULT is less than 6 mg/dL, modestly less than the 6.8 mg/dL limit of urate solubility.[22–24,41] A goal serum urate of less than 5 mg/dL is recommended for patients with tophi because these lesions signify more advanced gout, and lower serum urate levels are associated with more rapid tophus resolution.[6,8] Slow reduction in serum urate (no more than 1 to 2 mg/dL per month) is also recommended to minimize gout flares in the early months of ULT.[22–24,47] This approach accords well with the important concept of urate-monitored titration of urate-lowering agents.

Monitoring of serum urate levels is also essential to ensure that goal-range urate concentrations are maintained and to guide urate-lowering drug dose adjustment when needed. We concur with recommendations for measurement of serum urate concentration 2 to 4 weeks after each dose adjustment and twice within the first 6 months after goal range is first achieved.[22–24] Once sustained goal-range decrease is confirmed, measurement of urate levels every 6 months for the next year and annually thereafter is sufficient, unless changes in comedication or lifestyle factors potentially altering urate levels have occurred.

Nonadherence

Nonadherence is an important limitation to chronic urate-lowering management. In a study tracking adherence to allopurinol therapy over 2 years in a managed care setting,[48] less than 20% of patients initiating treatment met adherence criteria. Adherence may be improved if patients are given an understandable rationale for long-term daily therapy, even though symptoms have resolved. An additional reason for nonadherence to treatment in patients with gout may be the paradoxic occurrence of flares early in ULT, a problem shared by all effective agents and largely mitigated by 6 months (or longer in patients with tophaceous gout) daily cotherapy with an antiinflammatory prophylaxis agent, such as colchicine (see article elsewhere in this issue by Schlesinger).[49]

Strategies Underlying Pharmacologic ULT

Uric acid is the obligate end product of purine metabolism in humans caused by a species-wide lack of the enzyme uricase.[50] As a result, extracellular fluid urate concentrations in humans are substantially higher than in nonprimate mammals and predispose to gout because of the limited solubility of uric acid and monosodium urate (the predominant ionized form of urate at physiologic pH). Under physiologic conditions, the total body urate content is soluble, nearly constant in amount, and determined by the balance between uric acid production (from catabolism of endogenous and dietary purines) and disposal by renal and gastrointestinal excretion. When this balance is disturbed by impaired renal uric acid clearance or excess uric acid production, soluble urate concentrations increase. This situation leads to urate saturation of extracellular fluids, increased risk for monosodium urate crystal formation and deposition, and the acute inflammatory and chronic destructive features of gout. In this light, currently used pharmacologic strategies for achieving and maintaining long-term decrease of urate levels in gout patients are rational and correspond mechanistically to the aims indicated in **Box 2**.

REDUCTION OF URIC ACID PRODUCTION: XANTHINE OXIDASE INHIBITORS

Xanthine oxidoreductase (XOR) is a complex dimeric enzyme existing in interconvertible oxidized (xanthine oxidase [XO]) and reduced (xanthine dehydrogenase) forms. XO is the form most closely associated with uric acid synthesis, catalyzing the terminal 2 steps in purine catabolism in humans: conversion of hypoxanthine to xanthine and xanthine to urate.[51] The 2 available XO inhibitors (XOIs) are allopurinol and febuxostat, with allopurinol the most widely used urate-lowering agent worldwide for nearly 50 years. In contrast to uricosuric agents, which are primarily indicated only in patients with impaired renal excretion of uric acid, XOIs are safe and efficacious in virtually all circumstances warranting ULT for gout. However, in some patients, safety considerations limit their use.

ALLOPURINOL
Mechanism of Action

Allopurinol and its major active metabolite, oxypurinol, are pyrazolopyrimidine analogues of the purine bases hypoxanthine and xanthine, respectively. Both competitively inhibit XO activity and decrease the rate of urate production, leading to increases in extracellular fluid hypoxanthine and xanthine concentrations.[51–53] Allopurinol is less specific for XO inhibition than febuxostat, because allopurinol, oxypurinol, and their metabolites have effects on several other steps in purine and pyrimidine metabolism.

Box 2
Pharmacologic urate-lowering strategies in the treatment of gout

Reduce urate production via inhibition of xanthine oxidase activity (xanthine oxidase inhibitors [XOIs])

- Allopurinol
- Febuxostat

Increase uric acid disposal by increasing renal uric acid clearance (uricosuric agents)

- Probenecid
- Benzbromarone
- Sulfinpyrazone

Convert uric acid to the soluble purine metabolite allantoin (modified recombinant uricase)

- Pegloticase

Combination XOI and uricosuric therapy

Dose and Indications

Allopurinol is approved at daily doses in the United States up to 800 mg[53] and in Europe up to 900 mg[54] for treatment of gout. Nevertheless, more than 90% of patients in these venues are prescribed daily doses of 300 mg or less.[55] Although the dose of allopurinol necessary to achieve goal-range serum urate levels varies among patients, recent studies show that a daily dose of 300 mg allopurinol is effective in achieving serum urate less than 6.0 mg/dL in only 40% to 50% of patients.[56–59] Thus, most patients treated with allopurinol in recent years may have been underdosed and likely undertreated, prompting recommendations for dose titration to goal-range serum urate levels.[22–24,54,60,61]

We initiate allopurinol treatment at 100 mg daily in patients with eGFR greater than 60 mL/min/BSA. The dose is uptitrated in 100-mg increments every 2 to 4 weeks until the minimum dose necessary to achieve and maintain goal serum urate levels is reached. The urate-lowering efficacy of an allopurinol dose can be determined within 2 to 3 weeks.[57] Although patients with extensive tophaceous deposits and higher baseline serum urate levels (>10 mg/dL) are likely to require a higher dose of allopurinol to achieve goal-range serum urate levels, refractoriness to allopurinol monotherapy is uncommon and is most often caused by nonadherence.

For patients with impaired renal function, we concur with recommendations[23,62] for reductions in allopurinol starting dose and dose adjustments, respectively, to less than 1.5 mg per mL/min eGFR and 50 mg daily every 4 weeks. These recommendations stem from recent evidence for the safety of slow allopurinol dose titration in patients with impaired GFR,[61] and from a retrospective analysis of 54 patients with allopurinol hypersensitivity syndrome[62] (AHS; see later discussion), which found that hypersensitivity reactions[63] were more likely to occur in patients with renal impairment in whom the initial dose of allopurinol exceeded 1.5 mg per mL/min eGFR. These studies suggest that cautious allopurinol dose increases, monitored to goal-range serum urate levels, are likely to be safe in patients with impaired renal function[23] despite prolongation of the half-life of oxypurinol and metabolites in CKD.[64] It is important for this major change in the recommendation for allopurinol dosing in chronic renal disease to be confirmed by careful observational studies, because future randomized controlled trials are unlikely to be undertaken. Until recently, permanent allopurinol dose reduction in moderate or more severe renal disease was widely used, as a result of which most such patients never reached goal-range decrease in serum urate levels or long-term resolution of gout symptoms.[60,65–67]

Side Effects

Most allopurinol-related skin rashes are mild, but skin rash can herald development of an allopurinol hypersensitivity reaction, including toxic epidermal necrolysis, Stevens-Johnson syndrome, and AHS (consisting of an erythematous rash, fever, hepatitis, eosinophilia, and acute renal failure).[63,68] These events occur in approximately 0.1% to 0.3% of treated patients in Western countries but carry with them substantial morbidity and mortality and, in our opinion, have adversely influenced allopurinol dosing worldwide toward therapeutically inadequate doses of this agent.

Risk factors for allopurinol hypersensitivity reactions include female gender, age, CKD, diuretic therapy, and recent initiation of allopurinol.[62–64] In addition, the HLA-B*5801 haplotype, which is most common in patients of Han Chinese, Korean, and Thai ancestry, confers a genetic risk for development of allopurinol hypersensitivity.[69–71] Screening of Korean patients with stage 3 and higher CKD and patients of Han Chinese or Thai ancestry (regardless of renal function) for HLA-B*5801 is recommended before initiating allopurinol.[23] Patients with the risk haplotype should be treated with an alternative urate-lowering agent. Although successful desensitization to allopurinol has been reported in patients with milder cutaneous allopurinol reactions,[72] desensitization protocols are cumbersome and recurrence of hypersensitivity reactions has been reported. We do not recommend desensitization in patients with previous features of serious allopurinol hypersensitivity.

Additional allopurinol side effects and drug-drug interactions are shown in **Table 1**.

FEBUXOSTAT
Mechanism of Action

Febuxostat is an orally administered thiazolecarboxylic acid derivative (rather than a purine base analogue), which selectively inhibits both oxidized and reduced forms of XOR by noncompetitive and uncompetitive mechanisms, thereby reducing serum urate levels and urinary uric acid excretion.[57–59,73] Febuxostat metabolism is mainly hepatic, and urinary excretion of febuxostat and its active metabolites is less than 10% of an administered dose. As with allopurinol, urate-lowering efficacy of febuxostat has been established in patients with gout with either uric acid overproduction or impaired renal uric acid clearance.[74]

Dose, Efficacy, and Indications

Randomized clinical trials have confirmed urate-lowering efficacy and safety for febuxostat (at once-daily doses ranging from 40 mg to 120 mg) compared with allopurinol (at doses most commonly prescribed in practice)[57–59] and placebo.[58] In initial trials,[57,58] urate-lowering efficacies of febuxostat 80 mg and 120 mg (assessed by proportion of patients achieving sustained decrease in serum urate levels from baseline ≥ 8 mg/dL to <6 mg/dL) were both superior to those of allopurinol (300 mg) and placebo in patients with normal or mildly impaired renal function. In another trial,[59] efficacy of febuxostat 40 mg daily was equivalent (noninferior) to that of allopurinol 300 mg daily. In this trial, the urate-lowering efficacies of febuxostat (both 40 mg and 80 mg) were superior to that of allopurinol in patients with reduced renal function (eGFR 31–89 mL/min/BSA), and no additional safety signals were detected, confirming that renal dose reduction was unnecessary for febuxostat in patients with mild or moderate renal impairment. None of these comparative 6-month or 12-month trials of oral XOI therapies established differences in clinical efficacy markers, such as flare rate or tophus reduction, despite trends to improvement with both agents in the year-long trial.[57] From data from these trials and extended safety and efficacy studies of up to 3 and 5 years duration,[7,75] febuxostat has been approved for treatment of the hyperuricemia of gout in many countries but at varying daily doses, a situation of some importance, because the urate-lowering efficacy of febuxostat increases significantly with dose increments from 40 mg to 80 mg and from 80 mg to 120 mg.[57–59]

Febuxostat is an attractive therapeutic option in patients failing to achieve target serum urate with allopurinol. Although 2012 American College of Rheumatology guidelines recommend either allopurinol or febuxostat as first-line urate-lowering therapies,[23] primarily because cost was not considered, the longer clinical experience with allopurinol and its significantly lower cost in the United States prompt us to recommend allopurinol as the usual first-line urate-lowering agent for patients without contraindications. However, there are circumstances in which febuxostat may be a preferable first-line agent. First, unlike allopurinol, febuxostat clearly does not require dose adjustment in the setting of mild or moderate renal impairment. Although upward titration of allopurinol dose has recently been recommended in patients with stage 2 and higher renal impairment,[23,61] this recommendation has not, in our opinion, been sufficiently validated with regard to safety.[23,76] Second, compared with allopurinol, febuxostat has fewer drug-drug interactions that may limit urate-lowering efficacy or safety. Third, in patients who have had (or are at high risk for) an allopurinol hypersensitivity reaction and are thus not candidates for allopurinol treatment, febuxostat may be an effective and well-tolerated ULT.[77]

Side Effects and Drug Interactions

In the qualifying clinical trials,[7,75,77] numerically (but not significantly) more cardiovascular events were documented during febuxostat than allopurinol treatment (0.74 [0.95% confidence interval (CI) 0.36–1.37] vs 0.60 [0.95% CI 0.16–1.53] events per 100 patient years, respectively). However, an increased cardiovascular risk was not confirmed in a larger trial[59] comparing daily febuxostat (40 mg or 80 mg) with allopurinol treatment, and no mechanistic hypotheses or temporal relationships relating the drug to cardiovascular events were identified. A febuxostat/allopurinol comparative cardiovascular outcomes trial is in progress.[78] Additional side effects and drug interactions of febuxostat are presented in **Table 2**.

INCREASE RENAL EXCRETION OF URIC ACID: URICOSURIC AGENTS PROBENECID, BENZBROMARONE, SULFINPYRAZONE
Indications and Efficacy

In 85% to 90% of patients with gout, impaired renal uric acid clearance is the major mechanism resulting in hyperuricemia.[81] Uricosuric drugs are weak organic acids that promote uric acid clearance by inhibiting proximal tubule urate anion transporters that mediate urate reabsorption.[82–84] Thus, these agents should provide a rational approach to decreasing urate levels in most patients with gout. However, since allopurinol was introduced into clinical practice in 1966, uricosuric drug treatment has been used sparingly in the United States, where probenecid is the only potent drug of this

Table 2
Important side effects and drug interactions for allopurinol and febuxostat

	Allopurinol	Febuxostat
Side effects	Acute gout flare Liver function test abnormalities Drug fever, diarrhea, leukopenia, thrombocytopenia, or rash Hypersensitivity reaction (toxic epidermal necrolysis, Stevens-Johnson syndrome, AHS)	Acute gout flare Liver function test abnormalities Cardiovascular events Numerically higher incidence compared with allopurinol in clinical trials[78]
Drug interactions	Azathioprine and 6-mercaptopurine Increased risk of bone marrow suppression[79] If concomitant use unavoidable, either drug can be dose-reduced by ≥50% with close surveillance Cyclophosphamide Increased risk of bone marrow suppression[80] Ampicillin Increased risk of rash	Azathioprine and 6-mercaptopurine Increased risk of bone marrow suppression Safety of dose reduction in setting of febuxostat unclear

class currently available. Among reasons for this discrepancy are: a smaller range of patients with gout (compared with XOIs) for whom uricosuric agents are appropriate (they are not first-line agents for patients with uric acid overproduction or a history of or high risk for urolithiasis[22–24]); the urate-lowering efficacy of probenecid is markedly reduced in patients with moderate or more severe renal impairment; the need for multiple daily dosing of probenecid; and concerns about probenecid drug-drug interactions. Uricosuric therapy is more commonly used in countries where benzbromarone, a highly effective, single-daily-dose agent[85,86] is available, including those with populations having a substantial frequency of the HLA-B*5801 risk haplotype for severe allopurinol adverse reactions.

Dosing

The starting, typically effective, and maximum daily doses of each of the potent uricosuric agents are summarized in **Table 3**, along with side effects and drug interactions.

Adjunctive Agents with Uricosuric Properties

Losartan[88] and fenofibrate[88,89] have modest uricosuric properties and can be useful adjuncts in the ULT of patients with gout with hypertension or hyperlipidemia, disorders for which they are respectively indicated. The uricosuric effect of losartan is unique among angiotensin II receptor blockers and is maximal at 50 mg to 100 mg/d.[88] Vitamin C may also have a mild but persistent urate-lowering effect at doses as low as 500 mg daily.[90]

Table 3
Summary of potent uricosuric agents

	Probenecid	Benzbromarone	Sulfinpyrazone
Starting dose	250 mg twice daily	25 to 50 mg daily	50 mg twice daily
Typical effective dose (maximum dose)	500 mg 2 times daily (2000 mg daily)	100 mg daily (200 mg daily)	100–200 mg 3–4 times daily (800 mg daily)
Side effects	Acute gout flare Gastrointestinal intolerance Rash Urolithiasis	Acute gout flare Gastrointestinal intolerance Rash Urolithiasis Rare severe hepatotoxicity reported[86]	Acute gout flare Gastrointestinal intolerance Rash Urolithiasis
Drug interactions	Penicillin, penicillamine,[87] ampicillin, aspirin	—	—
Limitations	Ineffective when eGFR <60 mL/min	Not available in United States	Not available in United States Ineffective when eGFR <60 mL/min
Contraindications	Patients at risk for urolithiasis or uric acid nephropathy (relative contraindication) Cystinuria	Patients at risk for urolithiasis or uric acid nephropathy (relative contraindication)	Patients at risk for urolithiasis or uric acid nephropathy (relative contraindication)

CONVERSION OF URIC ACID TO ALLANTOIN: RECOMBINANT URICASE THERAPY

Most patients with gout can achieve target serum urate levels (and control of symptoms) using 1 or a combination of oral urate-lowering agents. However, there are patients who, because of intolerance of oral agents or previous ULT failure or under-treatment, do not achieve this goal and are at risk for developing the defining features of refractory chronic gout. Biological ULT with a recombinant uricase is a promising approach to preventing or even reversing disease progression in many of these patients.[8]

PEGLOTICASE
Mechanism of Action

Pegloticase is a modified porcine recombinant uricase covalently linked to multiple strands of monomethoxypoly(ethylene glycol) to prolong uricolytic activity and reduce immunogenicity.[91] Within hours of an initial 8-mg intravenous (IV) pegloticase infusion, plasma or serum urate levels decrease to very low or undetectable levels and remain subsaturating for several weeks. The concentration gradient between intravascular and extravascular soluble urate is hypothesized to draw extracellular soluble urate into the circulation for rapid degradation to allantoin, a soluble and readily excreted product of uricase action. Repeated pegloticase infusions thus promote resorption of urate crystal deposits in tissues and reduce the body urate pool, with subsidence of the crystal-induced inflammatory and destructive processes mediating the clinical events of gout.

Dose and Efficacy Data

Pegloticase is approved in the United States[92] for the treatment of chronic gout refractory to conventional (oral) therapy. Treatment involves biweekly IV infusions of pegloticase (8 mg), usually for a minimum of 6 months but with no maximum duration of treatment yet defined. Urate-lowering and clinical efficacy data for pegloticase come from the results of 2 replicate 6-month randomized placebo-controlled trials[8] involving a total of 212 patients with refractory chronic gout, defined by: baseline serum urate 8.0 mg/dL or greater; clinically active gouty arthritis or arthropathy or tophaceous gout; and failure to achieve serum urate levels of less than 6 mg/dL either because of allopurinol treatment failure or intolerance. Patients were randomly assigned to 3 groups, which received either pegloticase every 2 weeks or every 4 weeks or placebo. Pegloticase responders were patients maintaining plasma urate levels of less than 6.0 mg/dL for 80% of the time during trial months 3 and 6.

Pooled results from the replicate trials showed responder rates in the biweekly and monthly pegloticase groups (42% and 35%, respectively) significantly higher than placebo-treated patients (0%). In addition, pegloticase-treated patients achieved prespecified clinical end points significantly more often than those receiving placebo. These end points included complete resolution of at least 1 tophus, reduction in proportion of patients with gout flare, pain reduction, and improved physical function and quality of life.[8] From overall trends to less frequent urate-lowering efficacy and more frequent adverse events with monthly than with biweekly treatment, only biweekly pegloticase infusion is currently recommended.[8,92]

Although all patients showed goal-range decrease in urate levels with the initial pegloticase infusion, many lost the urate-lowering response in the first few months of treatment.[8] A major factor in loss of responsiveness appeared to be the development of high-titer (empirically defined) pegloticase antibody, which occurred in nearly 40% of treated patients and was highly correlated with loss of the urate-lowering response. The immunogenicity of pegloticase had additional clinical significance, because patients with high-titer pegloticase antibody were also more likely to have adverse reactions to pegloticase infusion (infusion reactions [IRs]) than patients with low or no antibody titers. Of major importance was the finding that loss of urate-lowering responsiveness to pegloticase preceded the first IR in more than 90% of biweekly pegloticase-treated patients suffering an IR. That is, preinfusion serum urate levels exceeding 6.0 mg/dL seem to be an early and easily determined surrogate marker for immune-mediated loss of pegloticase responsiveness and for IR risk. This observation was the basis for 2 recommendations aimed at mitigation of IRs: to monitor the course of pegloticase treatment by measuring serum urate levels immediately preceding all infusions after the first; and to discontinue pegloticase treatment if preinfusion serum urate levels exceed 6 mg/dL on 2 successive occasions.[92]

Side Effects

There was a high frequency of adverse events in the 6-month pegloticase trials, but gout flares and IRs (some fulfilling criteria for anaphylaxis), were the most common occurrences.[8] However, in an open-label extension study[93] in which treatment was continued for up to 30 months, no new safety signals emerged. Although the extended treatment study was not a randomized controlled trial, sustained urate-lowering efficacy and continued clinical improvement were observed in most patients who sustained the urate-lowering response during the initial 6-month trial.

Indications and Limitations

Pegloticase treatment should be considered for patients with gout refractory to or intolerant of oral ULTs, including XOIs and uricosuric agents, either alone or in combination. The rapidity of clinical improvement (in months rather than years, as with oral agents) in patients with persistent urate-lowering responses to pegloticase[8] is particularly attractive in patients with tophaceous deformities or complications (eg, infection, compression neuropathy) or severe gout-related compromise of lifestyle. As a result, expansion of consideration for use of this agent in such patients previously untreated or undertreated with oral ULT is reasonable. Treatment with pegloticase is contraindicated with glucose-6-phosphate dehydrogenase deficiency and has not been studied in patients receiving dialysis for end-stage renal disease. Pegloticase should not be used in conjunction with another urate-lowering agent because cotreatment could compromise monitoring serum urate levels for the loss of pegloticase urate-lowering efficacy and the increased risk of IR.[92] The cost of pegloticase therapy is substantial and is likely to be a limiting factor in availability.

CHOOSING A URATE-LOWERING AGENT

Oral monotherapy with an approved XOI or uricosuric agent at a dose titrated to achieve and maintain serum urate at a prespecified subsaturating goal level established for the individual patient often results within months to several years in a decrease and cessation of acute gout flares and prevention or resolution of tophi. Factors determining the choice of agent chosen for first-line therapy in an individual patient may include the range of agents approved and thus available to the clinician in the practice venue; the dose range recommended for each approved agent in that

---

Box 3
Recommendations for chronic pharmacologic ULT in patients with gout

- The XOI, allopurinol, is the first-line ULT of choice for most patients

- For patients preferring febuxostat to allopurinol or at high risk for allopurinol toxicity, ULT with febuxostat is an appropriate first-line choice

- Until the safety of doses of allopurinol greater than 300 mg/d is formally established (particularly in patients with moderate or more severe CKD), febuxostat should be considered an appropriate (although more costly) first-line XOI agent

- In patients intolerant of or failing to reach goal-range serum urate levels with allopurinol, a trial of febuxostat ULT is an appropriate second-line choice

- Uricosuric agents provide a mechanistic alternative to XOIs for ULT in most patients with gout whose hyperuricemia results from impaired renal uric acid clearance

- In some countries, benzbromarone is the first-line ULT of choice; however, probenecid, the only potent uricosuric drug available in the United States, requires multiple daily dosing and has reduced efficacy in patients with moderate or more severe renal impairment

- Despite exclusion of uric acid overproducers and urinary tract stone formers from first-line uricosuric therapy, a more potent drug of this class with fewer limitations and safety concerns would be an attractive choice for first-line status

- In patients with gout and hypertension or hyperlipidemia, combining an XOI with either of the mildly uricosuric agents losartan or fenofibrate, respectively, may expedite achievement of goal-range serum urate levels at a reduced XOI dose

- Combination therapy using an XOI and a potent uricosuric agent is infrequently required when first-line monotherapy is pursued to the highest approved dose but may be an effective second-line therapeutic choice

- Combination treatment is a provisional recommendation (particularly with regard to probenecid, in the absence of larger randomized controlled trials than performed to date[94]), although the results of studies with benzbromarone are encouraging

- We limit use of combination ULT to patients in whom first-line oral urate-lowering monotherapies fail to achieve the serum urate goal range, or patients with disease severity requiring rapid clinical benefit unlikely to occur unless very low urate levels are achieved

- In patients with advanced gout refractory to or intolerant of conventional (oral) treatment, biological ULT with pegloticase should be a consideration, especially when progressive gout is accompanied by manifestations mandating more rapid clinical benefit than has been shown with available oral agents

For all oral urate-lowering agents, dose titration monitored to serum urate goal range and appropriate for the individual patient is assumed.

---

venue; limitations on choice or dose of an agent set by the comorbidities frequent in gout patients; and the history of previous ULT outcomes. With these considerations in mind, our usual approach to the choice of urate-lowering agent follows the description in **Box 3**.

REFERENCES

1. Wortmann RL. Gout and hyperuricemia. Curr Opin Rheumatol 2002;14:281–6.
2. Zhu Y, Pandya BJ, Choi HK. Prevalence of gout and hyperuricemia in the US general population: the National Health and Nutrition Examination Survey 2007-2008. Arthritis Rheum 2011;63:3136–41.

3. Choi HK, Mount DB, Reginato AM. Pathogenesis of gout. Ann Intern Med 2005; 143:499–516.

4. Feig DI, Kang DH, Johnson RJ. Uric acid and cardiovascular risk. N Engl J Med 2008;359:1811–21.

5. Shoji A, Yamanaka H, Kamatani N. A retrospective study of the relationship between serum urate level and recurrent attacks of gouty arthritis: evidence for reduction of recurrent gouty arthritis with antihyperuricemic therapy. Arthritis Rheum 2004;51:321–5.

6. Perez-Ruiz F, Calabozo M, Pijoan JI, et al. Effect of urate-lowering therapy on the velocity of size reduction in tophi in chronic gout. Arthritis Rheum 2002;47:356–60.

7. Becker MA, Schumacher HR, MacDonald PA, et al. Clinical efficacy and safety of successful long term urate lowering with febuxostat or allopurinol in subjects with gout. J Rheumatol 2009;36:1273–82.

8. Sundy JS, Baraf HS, Yood RA, et al. Efficacy and tolerability of pegloticase for the treatment of chronic gout in patients refractory to conventional treatment: two randomized controlled trials. JAMA 2011;306:711–20.

9. Pascual E, Sivera F. The required for disappearance of urate crystals from synovial fluid after successful hyperuricemic treatment relates to the duration of gout. Ann Rheum Dis 2007;66:1056–8.

10. Mikuls TR, Farrar JT, Bilker WB, et al. Gout epidemiology: results from the UK General Practice Research Database, 1990-1999. Ann Rheum Dis 2005;64:267–72.

11. Arromdee E, Michet CJ, Crowson CS, et al. Epidemiology of gout: is the incidence rising? J Rheumatol 2002;29:2403–6.

12. Roubenoff R, Klag MJ, Mead LA, et al. Incidence and risk factors for gout in white men. JAMA 1991;266:3004–7.

13. Wallace K, Riedel A, Joseph-Ridge N, et al. Increasing prevalence of gout and hyperuricemia over 10 years among older adults in a managed care population. J Rheumatol 2004;31:1582–7.

14. Hochberg MC, Thomas J, Thomas DJ, et al. Racial differences in the incidence of gout. The role of hypertension. Arthritis Rheum 1995;38:628–32.

15. Rose BS. Gout in Maoris. Semin Arthritis Rheum 1975;5:121–45.

16. Chang SJ, Ko YC, Wang TN, et al. High prevalence of gout and related risk factors in Taiwan's Aborigines. J Rheumatol 1997;24:1364–9.

17. Bhole V, de Vera M, Rahman MM, et al. Epidemiology of gout in women: fifty-two-year followup of a prospective cohort. Arthritis Rheum 2010;62:1069–76.

18. Chen SY, Chen CL, Shen ML, et al. Trends in the manifestations of gout in Taiwan. Rheumatology (Oxford) 2003;42:1529–33.

19. Chen SY, Chen CL, Shen ML. Manifestations of metabolic syndrome associated with male gout in different age strata. Clin Rheumatol 2007;26:1453–7.

20. Choi HK, Atkinson K, Karlson EW, et al. Obesity, weight change, hypertension, diuretic use, and risk of gout in men: the Health Professionals' Follow-Up Study. Arch Intern Med 2005;165:742–8.

21. Suppiah R, Dissanayake A, Dalbeth N. High prevalence of gout in patients with type 2 diabetes: male sex, renal impairment, and diuretic use are major risk factors. N Z Med J 2008;121:43–50.

22. Zhang W, Doherty M, Bardin T, et al. EULAR evidence based recommendations for gout. Part II: management. Report of a task force of the EULAR Standing Committee for International Clinical Studies Including Therapeutics (ESCISIT). Ann Rheum Dis 2006;65:1312–24.

23. Khanna D, Fitzgerald JD, Khanna PP, et al. 2012 American College of Rheumatology guidelines for the management of gout. Part 1: systemic nonpharmacologic and pharmacologic therapeutic approaches to hyperuricemia. Arthritis Rheum 2012;64:1431–46.

24. Becker MA. Prevention of recurrent gout. In: Basow DS, editor. UpToDate. Waltham (MA): UpToDate; 2014.

25. Choi HK, Atkinson K, Karlson EW, et al. Alcohol intake and risk of incident gout in men: a prospective study. Lancet 2004;363:1277–81.

26. Lin KC, Lin HY, Chou P. The interaction between uric acid level and other risk factors on the development of gout among asymptomatic hyperuricemic men in a prospective study. J Rheumatol 2000;27:1501–5.

27. Lyu LC, Hsu CY, Yeh CY, et al. A case-control study of the association of diet and obesity with gout in Taiwan. Am J Clin Nutr 2003;78:690–701.

28. Shulten P, Thomas J, Miller M, et al. The role of diet in the management of gout: a comparison of knowledge and attitudes to current evidence. J Hum Nutr Diet 2009;22:3–11.

29. Choi HK, Atkinson K, Karlson EW, et al. Purine-rich foods, dairy and protein intake, and the risk of gout in men. N Engl J Med 2004;350:1093–103.

30. Williams PT. Effects of diet, physical activity and performance, and body weight on incident gout in ostensibly healthy, vigorously active men. Am J Clin Nutr 2008;87:1480–7.

31. Choi HK, Curhan G. Coffee, tea, and caffeine consumption and serum uric acid level: the third national health and nutrition examination survey. Arthritis Rheum 2007;57:816–21.

32. Choi HK, Willett W, Curhan G. Coffee consumption and risk of incident gout in men: a prospective study. Arthritis Rheum 2007;56:2049–55.

33. Zhang Y, Neogi T, Chen C, et al. Cherry consumption and decreased risk of recurrent gout attacks. Arthritis Rheum 2012;64:4004–11.

34. Choi HK, Curhan G. Soft drinks, fructose consumption, and the risk of gout in men: a prospective study. BMJ 2008;336:309–12.

35. Choi JW, Ford ES, Gao X, et al. Sugar-sweetened soft drinks, diet soft drinks, and serum uric acid level: the Third National Health and Nutrition Examination Survey. Arthritis Rheum 2008;59:109–16.

36. Dalbeth N, House ME, Gamble GD, et al. Population-specific influence of SLC2A9 genotype on the acute hyperuricaemic response to a fructose load. Ann Rheum Dis 2013;72(11):1868–73.

37. Hunter DJ, York M, Chaisson CE, et al. Recent diuretic use and the risk of recurrent gout attacks: the online case-crossover study. J Rheumatol 2006;33:1341–5.

38. Abbot KC, Kimmel PL, Dharnidharka V, et al. New-onset gout after kidney transplantation: incidence, risk factors and implications. Transplantation 2005;80: 1383–91.

39. Yu TF, Gutman AB. Study of the paradoxical effects of salicylate in low, intermediate and high dosage on the renal mechanisms for excretion of urate in man. J Clin Invest 1959;38:1298–315.

40. Caspi D, Lubart E, Graff E, et al. The effect of mini-dose aspirin on renal function and uric acid handling in elderly patients. Arthritis Rheum 2000;43:103–8.

41. Yamanaka H. Japanese guideline for the management of hyperuricemia and gout: second edition. Nucleosides Nucleotides Nucleic Acids 2011;30:1018–29.

42. Taylor TH, Mecchella JN, Larson RJ, et al. Initiation of allopurinol at first medical contact for acute attacks of gout: a randomized clinical trial. Am J Med 2012; 125:1126–34.

43. Perez-Ruiz F, Herrero-Beites AM, Carmona L. A two-stage approach to the treatment of hyperuricemia in gout: the "dirty dish" hypothesis. Arthritis Rheum 2011; 63:4002–6.
44. Van Lieshout-Zuidema MF, Breedveld FC. Withdrawal of longterm antihyperuricemic therapy in tophaceous gout. J Rheumatol 1993;20:1383–5.
45. Gast LF. Withdrawal of longterm antihyperuricemic therapy in tophaceous gout. Clin Rheumatol 1987;6:70–3.
46. Perez-Ruiz F, Atxotegi J, Hernando I, et al. Using serum urate levels to determine the period free of gouty symptoms after withdrawal of long-term urate-lowering therapy: a prospective study. Arthritis Rheum 2006;55:786–92.
47. Yamanaka H, Togashi R, Hakoda M, et al. Optimal range of serum urate concentrations to minimize risk of gouty attacks during anti-hyperuricemic treatment. Adv Exp Med Biol 1998;431:13–8.
48. Sarawate CA, Patel PA, Schumacher HR, et al. Serum urate levels and gout flares: analysis from managed care data. J Clin Rheumatol 2006;12:61–5.
49. Borstad GC, Bryant LR, Abel MP, et al. Colchicine for prophylaxis of acute flares when initiating allopurinol for chronic gouty arthritis. J Rheumatol 2004;31:2429–32.
50. Wu XW, Muzny DM, Lee CC, et al. Two independent mutational events in the loss of urate oxidase during hominoid evolution. J Mol Evol 1992;34:78–84.
51. Harrison R. Structure and function of xanthine oxidoreductase: where are we now? Free Radic Biol Med 2002;33:774–97.
52. Day RO, Graham GG, Hicks M, et al. Clinical pharmacokinetics and pharmacodynamics of allopurinol and oxypurinol. Clin Pharmacokinet 2007;46:623–44.
53. US National Library of Medicine DailyMed: FDA information: allopurinol tablet. Available at: http://dailymed.nlm.nih.gov/dailymed/search.cfm?startswith=allopurinol. Accessed August 24, 2013.
54. Jordan KM, Cameron JS, Snaith M, et al. British Society for Rheumatology and British Health Professionals in Rheumatology guideline for the management of gout. Rheumatology (Oxford) 2007;46:1372–4.
55. Sarawate CA, Brewer KK, Yang W, et al. Gout medication treatment patterns and adherence to standards of care from a managed care perspective. Mayo Clin Proc 2006;81:925–34.
56. Perez-Ruiz F, Alonso-Ruiz A, Calabozo M, et al. Efficacy of allopurinol and benzbromarone for the control of hyperuricemia: a pathogenetic approach to the treatment of primary chronic gout. Ann Rheum Dis 1998;57:545–9.
57. Becker MA, Schumacher HR Jr, Wortmann RL, et al. Febuxostat compared with allopurinol in patients with hyperuricemia and gout. N Engl J Med 2005;353:2450–61.
58. Schumacher HR Jr, Becker MA, Wortmann RL, et al. Effects of febuxostat versus allopurinol and placebo in reducing serum urate in subjects with hyperuricemia and gout: a 28-week, phase III, randomized, double-blind, parallel-group trial. Arthritis Rheum 2008;59:1540–8.
59. Becker MA, Schumacher HR, Espinoza LR, et al. The urate-lowering efficacy and safety of febuxostat in the treatment of the hyperuricemia of gout: the CONFIRMS trial. Arthritis Res Ther 2010;12:R63.
60. Dalbeth N, Kumar S, Stamp L, et al. Dose adjustment of allopurinol according to creatinine clearance does not provide adequate control of hyperuricemia in patients with gout. J Rheumatol 2006;33:1646–50.
61. Stamp LK, O'Donnell JL, Zhang M, et al. Using allopurinol above the dose based on creatinine clearance is effective and safe in patients with chronic gout, including those with renal impairment. Arthritis Rheum 2011;63:412–21.

62. Stamp LK, Taylor WJ, Jones PB, et al. Starting dose is a risk factor for allopurinol hypersensitivity syndrome: a proposed safe starting dose of allopurinol. Arthritis Rheum 2012;64:2529–36.
63. Arellano F, Sacristan JA. Allopurinol hypersensitivity syndrome: a review. Ann Pharmacother 1993;27:337–43.
64. Hande KR, Noone RM, Stone WJ. Severe allopurinol toxicity. Description and guidelines for prevention in patients with renal insufficiency. Am J Med 1984;76:47–56.
65. Dalbeth N, Stamp L. Allopurinol dosing in renal impairment: walking the tightrope between adequate urate lowering and adverse events. Semin Dial 2007;20:391–5.
66. Keenan RT. Safety of urate-lowering therapies: managing the risks to gain the benefits. Rheum Dis Clin North Am 2012;38:663–80.
67. Chao J, Terkeltaub R. A critical reappraisal of allopurinol dosing, safety, and efficacy for hyperuricemia in gout. Curr Rheumatol Rep 2009;11:135–40.
68. Lupton G, Odom R. Severe allopurinol hypersensitivity syndrome. J Am Acad Dermatol 1979;72:1361–8.
69. Jung JW, Song WJ, Kim YS, et al. HLA-B58 can help the clinical decision on starting allopurinol in patients with chronic renal insufficiency. Nephrol Dial Transplant 2011;26:3567–72.
70. Tassaneeyakul W, Jantararoungtong T, Chen P, et al. Strong association between HLA-B*5801 and allopurinol-induced Stevens-Johnson syndrome and toxic epidermal necrolysis in a Thai population. Pharmacogenet Genomics 2009;19:704–9.
71. Hung SI, Chung WH, Liou LB, et al. HLA-B*5801 allele as a genetic marker for severe cutaneous adverse reactions caused by allopurinol. Proc Natl Acad Sci U S A 2005;102:4134–9.
72. Fam AG, Lewtas J, Stein J, et al. Desensitization to allopurinol in patients with gout and cutaneous reactions. Am J Med 1992;93:299–304.
73. US National Library of Medicine DailyMed: FDA information: febuxostat tablet. Available at: http://dailymed.nlm.nih.gov/dailymed/search.cfm?startswith=febuxostat. Accessed August 24, 2013.
74. Goldfarb DS, MacDonald PA, Hunt B, et al. Febuxostat in gout: serum urate response in uric acid overproducers and underexcretors. J Rheumatol 2011;38:1385–9.
75. Schumacher HR Jr, Becker MA, Lloyd E, et al. Febuxostat in the treatment of gout: five-year findings of the FOCUS Efficacy and Safety Study. Rheumatology 2009;48:188–94.
76. Reinders MK, Haagsma C, Jansen TL, et al. A randomized controlled trial on the efficacy and tolerability with dose escalation of allopurinol 330-600 mg/day versus benzbromarone 100-200 mg/day in patients with gout. Ann Rheum Dis 2009;68:892–7.
77. Chohan S. Safety and efficacy of febuxostat treatment in subjects with gout and severe allopurinol adverse reactions. J Rheumatol 2011;38:1957–9.
78. ClinicalTrials.gov. Cardiovascular safety of febuxostat and allopurinol in patients with gout and cardiovascular comorbidities (CARES). Available at: http://www.clinicaltrials.gov/ct2/show/NCT01101035?term=allopurinol+febuxostat&rank=4. Accessed September 21, 2013.
79. Gearry RB, Day AS, Barclay ML, et al. Azathioprine and allopurinol: a two-edged interaction. J Gastroenterol Hepatol 2010;25:653–5.
80. Witten J, Frederiksen PL, Mouridsen HT. The pharmacokinetics of cyclophosphamide in man after treatment with allopurinol. Acta Pharmacol Toxicol (Copenh) 1980;46:392–4.

81. Puig JG, Torres RJ, de Miguel E, et al. Uric acid excretion in normal subjects: a nomogram to assess the mechanisms underlying purine metabolic disorders. Metabolism 2012;61:512–8.

82. Enomoto A, Kimura H, Chairoungdua A, et al. Molecular identification of a renal urate anion exchanger that regulates blood urate levels. Nature 2002;417: 447–52.

83. Anzai N, Ichida K, Jutabha P, et al. Plasma urate level is directly regulated by a voltage-driven urate efflux transporter URATv1 (SLC2A9) in humans. J Biol Chem 2008;283:26834–8.

84. Dalbeth N, Merriman T. Crystal ball gazing: new therapeutic targets for hyperuricemia and gout. Rheumatology (Oxford) 2009;48:222–6.

85. Reinders MK, van Roon EN, Jansen TL, et al. Efficacy and tolerability of urate-lowering drugs in gout: a randomised controlled trial of benzbromarone versus probenecid after failure of allopurinol. Ann Rheum Dis 2009;68:51–6.

86. Lee MH, Graham GG, Williams KM, et al. A benefit-risk assessment of benzbromarone in the treatment of gout. Was its withdrawal from the market in the best interest of patients? Drug Saf 2008;31:643–65.

87. Yu TF, Roboz J, Johnson S, et al. Studies on the metabolism of D-penicillamine and its interaction with probenecid in cystinuria and rheumatoid arthritis. J Rheumatol 1984;11:467–70.

88. Takahashi S, Moriwaki Y, Yamamoto T, et al. Effects of combination treatment using anti-hyperuricemic agents with fenofibrate and/or losartan on uric acid metabolism. Ann Rheum Dis 2003;62:572–5.

89. Feher MD, Hepburn AL, Hogarth MB, et al. Fenofibrate enhances urate reduction in men treated with allopurinol for hyperuricemia and gout. Rheumatology (Oxford) 2003;42:321–5.

90. Choi HK, Gao X, Curhan G. Vitamin C intake and the risk of gout in men: a prospective study. Arch Intern Med 2009;169:502–7.

91. Sherman MR, Saifer MG, Perez-Ruiz F. PEG-uricase in the management of treatment-resistant gout and hyperuricemia. Adv Drug Deliv Rev 2008;60:59–68.

92. Krystexxa TM. Prescribing information 2013. Available at: http://krystexxa.com/pdfs/krystexxa prescribing information.pdf. Accessed September 21, 2013.

93. Becker MA, Baraf HS, Yood RA, et al. Long-term safety of pegloticase in chronic gout refractory to conventional treatment. Ann Rheum Dis 2013;72:1469–74.

94. Stocker SL, Graham GG, McLachlan AJ, et al. Pharmacokinetic and pharmacodynamic interaction between allopurinol and probenecid in patients with gout. J Rheumatol 2011;38:904–10.

Emerging Therapies for Gout

N. Lawrence Edwards, MD[a],*, Alexander So, PhD, FRCP[b]

KEYWORDS

- Gout • Urate-lowering therapy • Febuxostat • Pegloticase • Lesinurad • Ulodesine
- Interleukin-1 inhibitor • Melanocortin

KEY POINTS

- The most commonly used dose of allopurinol achieves urate reduction to the minimal target of less than 6.0 mg/dL in only 35% to 40% of gouty patients.
- The new generation of uricosuric agents, when used in combination with current xanthine oxidase inhibitors, results in synergistic urate lowering not achievable by oral monotherapy.
- Activation of the NLRP3-inflammasome and its promotion of interleukin-1β production are central to the pain and inflammation of gout. Interrupting this pathway is an effective way of treating gout-driven pain.
- Corticotropin and other melanocortin peptides are effective in treating gout inflammation by interacting with the melanocortin receptors on macrophages.

The prevalence of gout worldwide has been steadily increasing over the past several decades. It has been estimated that in the United States 8.3 million people, or almost 3% of the population, suffer from gout, and 12% to 15% have hyperuricemia.[1] Similar statistics are found in most developed countries. This expanding market would be enough to draw the interest of the pharmaceutical industry, but other factors have come into play. Over the past 10 years clinicians have been inundated with studies showing how inadequate the traditional approaches to this destructive arthritis have been. The time-honored therapies for treating the pain and inflammation of gout include nonsteroidal anti-inflammatories (NSAIDs), colchicine, and oral corticosteroids. Yet in the few controlled trials conducted with these agents, one finds that patients can expect to still have 50% of their acute pain after 36 to 48 hours of treatment regardless of which agent is used.[2,3] Given the severity of acute gout symptoms, 50% reduction still leaves patients in considerable pain. Patients, physicians, and the pharmaceutical industry recognize a large unmet need for better and more specific anti-inflammatory approaches to gout.

[a] Department of Medicine, University of Florida College of Medicine, 1600 South West Archer Road, Gainesville, FL 32610-0277, USA; [b] Service de Rhumatologie, CHUV, Avenue Pierre Decker, Lausanne 1011, Switzerland
* Corresponding author.
E-mail address: edwarnl@medicine.ufl.edu

Rheum Dis Clin N Am 40 (2014) 375–387
http://dx.doi.org/10.1016/j.rdc.2014.01.013
0889-857X/14/$ – see front matter © 2014 Elsevier Inc. All rights reserved.

Similarly, deficiencies in the use and efficacy of urate-lowering therapies (ULTs) have also been brought to light by recent studies. Allopurinol and probenicid had been the mainstays of gout therapy since the 1960s. Intolerance to these drugs usually meant that the gout patient would go untreated, and over years would slowly advance to a chronic crippling form of arthritis. The concept of treating the serum urate level (sUA) to a target was not widely held by the medical profession until this approach was strongly endorsed by the European League Against Rheumatism, and more recently in the American College of Rheumatology (ACR) guidelines on managing gout.[4,5] Data from the early febuxostat trials by Takeda Pharmaceuticals demonstrated the inadequacy of the most commonly used dose of allopurinol (300 mg/d) in bringing patients' sUA levels down to the target of less than 6.0 mg/dL, with only 35% to 40%, achieving even this minimal target.[6] Again, the need for more aggressive treatment, as well as safer and more effective alternatives to allopurinol, was made apparent by study after study.[7]

This article strives to outline the current therapies under development for the management of gout. In general, these agents build on a wealth of new information about the mechanism of gouty inflammation and urate elimination that was unknown a decade ago.

URATE-LOWERING THERAPIES

Reducing sUA levels to below the solubility limit of urate in body fluids (ie, <6.8 mg/dL) has long been recognized as the definitive treatment for gout. The generally agreed therapeutic target of less than 6.0 mg/dL is safely below the solubility threshold, and will certainly prevent new crystallization of urate and further expansion of the body's urate burden. Many studies support the concept that decreasing the sUA level to less than 6.0 mg/dL will, over time, reduce gout symptoms, shrink tophaceous deposits, and improve the quality of life.[8] It has also been demonstrated that these good outcomes can be achieved more rapidly if the sUA level is pushed even lower than the minimal target of less than 6.0 mg/dL.[9]

Allopurinol was approved by the Food and Drug Administration (FDA) in 1966, and clinicians have a lot of experience with its efficacy and toxicity profiles, although this is only true for daily doses of 300 mg or less. Although it is approved in doses of up to 800 mg/d, little is known about the safety of allopurinol in the higher dose ranges. Two new ULTs were introduced in the past 5 years. The new xanthine oxidase inhibitor, febuxostat, was approved in 2009 as an alternative for patients intolerant to allopurinol or for those who could not be adequately dosed with allopurinol because of chronic kidney disease. Febuxostat has a simpler dose escalation schedule than allopurinol, and was recommended in the recent ACR gout management guidelines as a first-line agent to accompany allopurinol.[5]

Savient's pegylated uricase, pegloticase, was approved by the FDA in 2010 for use in patients with severe, recalcitrant gout. It is the first parenteral therapy for gout, and has shown dramatic ability to lower serum urate and promote tophus resorption in subjects with advanced disease.

ULTs currently in development include lesinurad, arhalofenate, ulodesine, and levotofisopam.

Lesinurad (RDEA594)

Lesinurad is a uricosuric agent in development for the chronic management of gout and hyperuricemia. It was discovered by Ardea Biosciences as a major metabolite of a candidate nonnucleoside reverse transcriptase inhibitor, RDEA809, and was found to be the compound responsible for the urate-lowering effect observed in their study subjects. Lesinurad has been demonstrated to inhibit both the URAT-1 and OAT4 transporters in the renal tubule (**Fig. 1**).

Two phase 2b trials were conducted on gout patients including subjects with mild and moderate renal impairment.[10] Study 202 enrolled patients with sUA of at least 8.0 mg/dL while not on other urate-lowering therapy. Study 203 enrolled patients with sUA of at least 6.0 mg/dL despite 10 weeks on a stable dose of allopurinol before starting lesinurad. Increased renal excretion of uric acid was demonstrated for lesinurad doses of 200, 400 and 600 mg daily, with no attributable serious adverse events. Gout patients with mild to moderate renal impairment in these two Phase 2b trials derived sUA lowering to an extent similar to that for patients with normal renal function.

Another multicenter open-label trial (RDEA599-111) investigated the efficacy and safety of lesinurad in combination with febuxostat.[11] All subjects received either 40 or 80 mg febuxostat daily for 7 days followed by combination treatment with lesinurad, 400 mg daily for 7 days (**Fig. 2**), then combination treatment with lesinurad 600 mg daily for 7 days (data not shown). The combination of lesinurad and febuxostat produced substantial additive urate lowering, with nearly 100% of subjects achieving sUA targets of less than 6.0 mg/dL, less than 5.0 mg/dL, and less than 4.0 mg/dL. This study demonstrated that combining drugs with complementary mechanisms of

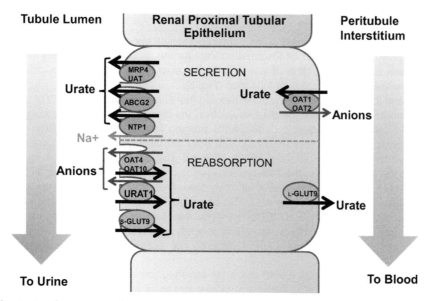

Fig. 1. Renal transport of urate in proximal tubule of kidney. Serum urate reaches the tubule lumen by glomerular filtration and by secretion through the proximal tubular epithelium. Secretion of urate is facilitated in the luminal direction by MRP4, UAT, ABCG2, and NTP1, and at the basolateral membrane by OAT1 and OAT3. Reabsorption of urate from the tubular lumen is facilitated by URAT1, OAT4, OAT10, and the short isoform of GLUT9, and at the basolateral membrane by the long isoform of GLUT9. ABCG2, adenosine triphosphate–binding cassette transporter; GLUT, glucose transporter; MRP, multidrug resistance–related protein; NTP, sodium phosphate transport protein; OAT, organic acid transporters; URAT, uric acid. (*Adapted from* Basseville A, Bates SE. Gout, genetics and ABC transporters. F1000 Biol Rep 2011;3:23.)

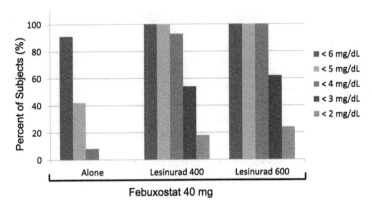

Fig. 2. Lesinurad in combination with febuxostat shows additive urate-lowering effects in gouty subjects. RDEA594-11 multicenter, open-label study (n = 12) of febuxostat, 40 mg/d alone or in combination with 400 mg/d or 600 mg/d lesinurad. Target serum urate levels of less than 6 mg/dL to less than 2 mg/dL are shown. Measurements are made 12 hours after dose.

action produced significantly greater reductions in sUA than increasing the dose of a single agent.

Ulodesine (BCX4208)

Ulodesine is an oral once-daily novel purine nucleoside phosphorylase (PNP) inhibitor being developed by BioCryst Pharmaceuticals for the chronic management of gout. Ulodesine blocks production of uric acid at the step higher in the purine catabolic pathway than xanthine oxidase inhibition (**Fig. 3**).

A phase 2 placebo-controlled, dose-ranging trial of the efficacy and safety of ulodesine monotherapy involved 24 gout subjects in the placebo group and 85 gouty subjects divided into 5 ulodesine dosing arms ranging from 40 to 240 mg daily.[12] The serum urate targets of less than 6.0, less than 5.0, and less than 4.0 mg/dL were achieved by 30%, 21%, and 0% of the 80 mg/d ulodesine group, respectively, and by 77%, 54%, and 23% of the 240 mg/d ulodesine group. Adverse events for all doses of ulodesine were not significantly different from those for placebo, but the higher doses did result in more diarrhea (20%) and rash (13%). Despite dose-related decreases in $CD4^+$, $CD8^+$, and $CD20^+$ lymphocytes, there was no observed increase in infection. This finding was a theoretical concern because the inborn error in purine metabolism resulting from PNP deficiency is associated with a combined immunodeficiency.

A separate phase 2 trial tested the urate-lowering effects of combining low-dose ulodesine (20, 40, and 80 mg/d) with various doses of allopurinol (**Fig. 4**, data for 80 mg ulodesine not shown).[13] Synergistic reduction in serum urate was observed with the ulodesine and allopurinol combination, with 100% of subjects taking 40 mg/d ulodesine and 300 mg/d allopurinol achieving the target sUA of less than 6.0 mg/dL.

Levotofisopam

The investigational drug, levotofisopam, is the s-enantiomer of racemic tofisopam, a 2,3-benzodiazepine derivative approved in more than 20 countries outside the United States for anxiety and autonomic instability. Two phase 1 studies were performed by

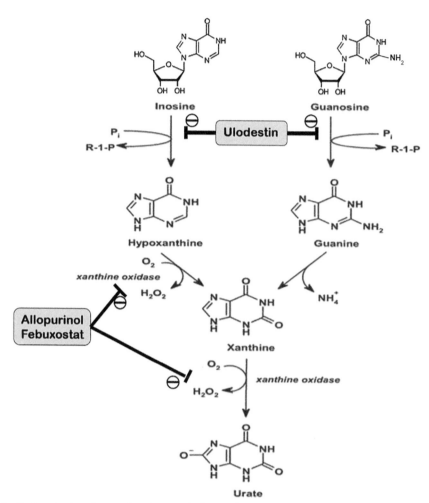

Fig. 3. Terminal pathway of purine catabolism in humans. The breakdown of purine nucle-osides and bases is regulated by 2 enzymes. Purine nucleoside phosphorylase allows the catabolism of the nucleosides, inosine and guanosine, to their respective purine bases, hypoxanthine and guanine. Hypoxanthine is converted to xanthine by xanthine oxidase while guanine is decimated to xanthine by guanase. Xanthine is further reduced to uric acid by xanthine oxidase.

Velos Pharmaceuticals in 2006 before its merger with Pharmos Corporation. Healthy volunteers in the United Kingdom and the Netherlands showed urate-lowering capability with acceptable safety and tolerability.

An open-label phase 2a trial of levotofisopam, 50 mg 3 times a day for 7 days, was carried out in 13 gouty subjects.[14] At day 7, the mean serum urate reduction was 48.8% (range 31%–65%) with an absolute reduction of 3.9 mg/dL (range 2.3–5.3 mg/dL). All 13 subjects achieved the target urate level of less than 6.0 mg/dL while 77% and 54% achieved the targets of less than 5.0 mg/dL and less than 4.0 mg/dL, respectively.

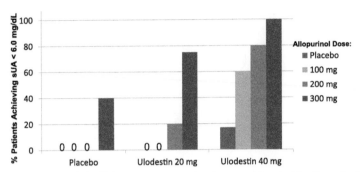

Fig. 4. Ulodesine synergistically lowers serum urate when combined with allopurinol in gouty subjects. Percentage of patients achieving the target sUA level of less than 6.0 mg/dL is shown for ulodesine and allopurinol dosing groups.

DUAL-ACTING ANTI-INFLAMMATORY AND URATE-LOWERING THERAPY
Arhalofenate (MBX-102)

While developing this PPAR-γ modulator for glycemic control, Cymabay Therapeutics (formerly Metabolex) noted several metabolic properties that made it attractive for the management of acute and chronic gout. In test subjects arhalofenate was noted to have uricosuric properties and was subsequently shown to inhibit the uric acid transporters URAT-1, OAT4, and OAT10.[15] In studies on isolated mouse macrophages, arhalofenate was able to block monosodium urate (MSU) crystal–induced production of pro–interleukin (IL)-1β mRNA and other nuclear factor (NF)-κB–dependent inflammatory mediators by PPAR-γ transrepression.[16] The potential of a potent, oral IL-1β inhibitor combined with uricosuric effects is exciting for gout management, and awaits human trials.

Four phase 2 trials of 3 to 6 months' duration have been carried out in healthy volunteers and diabetic subjects using 600 mg arhalofenate daily. Even though most subjects in these studies were normouricemic, substantial uricosuria was still demonstrated, with decreases in serum urate generally ranging from 20% to 40%. Of note, unlike probenicid, which loses its uricosuric effects as renal function deteriorates, there was no observed decrement in the uricosuria of arhalofenate as kidney function declines.

ANTI-INFLAMMATORY THERAPIES

To understand the inflammation of acute gout and its treatment, it is useful to have an overview of the mechanisms that come into play when crystals are shed and enter into contract with cells. **Fig. 5** summarizes the interpretation of the sequence of events that is triggered, and the actions of therapies on the different stages. Based on both experimental and clinical observations, IL-1β is the cytokine that is located at the start of the inflammatory cascade in gout. The NLRP3-inflammasome is essential for the production of IL-1β when macrophages are incubated with MSU or calcium pyrophosphate dihydrate crystals.[17,18] Although the inflammasome is not the only pathway that generates IL-1β during MSU-induced inflammation, there is general agreement that many of the observed inflammatory phenomena are accounted for by this mechanism.[19] These findings quickly led to the testing of IL-1 inhibitors in an animal model of gout and in a small open clinical study, which showed that the IL-1 receptor antagonist (IL-1RA) anakinra was very effective in relieving the acute symptoms of gouty arthritis.[18] The current experience with IL-1 inhibitors in gout is summarized in **Table 1**. Anakinra

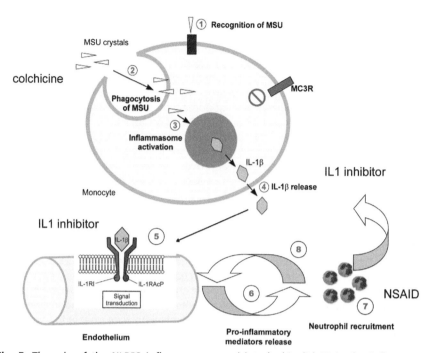

Fig. 5. The role of the NLRP3 inflammasome and interleukin (IL)-1β in the inflammatory cascade of acute gout. The different steps of crystal recognition and stimulation of proinflammatory cytokine release by synovial macrophages and the sites of known inhibitors. (1) Monosodium urate (MSU) contact with surface toll-like receptors. (2) Phagocytosis and uptake of MSU crystals. (3) inflammasome activation. (4) IL-1β release extracellularly. (5) IL-1 binding to endothelial IL-1R1 to modulate cell adhesion. (6) Release of inflammatory mediators from leukocytes (neutrophils and mast cells). (7) Neutrophil recruitment to the inflammatory site. (8) Further release of inflammatory mediators from leukocytes.

Table 1
Summary of key studies with known anti–interleukin-1 agents

Agent	Study	References
Anakinra	1. Open-label study of acute gout, 10 patients	18
	2. Open-label study, 26 patients	21
	3. Open study, 10 patients	25
Rilonacept	1. RCT, 10 patients with chronic gouty arthritis	3
	2. RCT, prevention of gout flares on initiating allopurinol, 241 patients	38
	3. RCT, acute gout, 225 patients	30
Canakinumab	1. RCT phase II dose-finding study vs triamcinolone acetate, 200 patients	39
	2. RCT, canakinumab vs triamcinolone acetate in acute gout, 456 patients	28
	3. RCT, canakinumab vs colchicine in prevention of acute flares on initiating allopurinol, 200 patients	32

Abbreviation: RCT, randomized controlled trial.

has a half-life of 4 to 6 hours, and was originally developed for the treatment of rheumatoid arthritis. Its specificity as an IL-1 inhibitor has led investigators and clinicians to test its efficacy in diseases that are, or are suspected to be, IL-1 mediated (see Ref.[20] for a review). Two other compounds have been developed for the IL-1 inhibiting potential. Canakinumab, a fully humanized immunoglobulin G1 (IgG1) monoclonal antibody, is specific for IL-1β with a half-life of around 28 days. Rilonacept (or IL-1 Trap) is a fusion protein formed by the ligand-binding domain of the extracellular part of IL-1R1 and IL-1 receptor accessory protein (IL-1RAcP) linked to the Fc portion of human IgG1 (half-life of 9 days). Both molecules have been approved for the treatment of CAPS (cryopyrin-associated periodic syndrome), an IL-1 mediated autoinflammatory syndrome, and canakinumab has been approved for use in the treatment of acute gout in Europe. Other IL-1 inhibitors are in development, but have not yet gained regulatory approval for use in gout.

Anakinra

The published clinical studies have evaluated the efficacy of IL-1 inhibitors in various clinical situations. Anakinra was evaluated in open clinical studies and in case reports.[18,21–27] Different dose regimens have been used, but most patients were treated with 100-mg daily injections for 2 to 3 days. The characteristics of the patient population treated were also varied, ranging from patients who had severe renal impairment, including one case with a renal transplant, to patients who were unable to tolerate or had contraindications to standard treatments such as colchicine and NSAIDs. In the larger case series, more than 60% of patients reported a very satisfactory and rapid resolution of symptoms of acute gout.[21] However, not all patients responded, and it is unclear as to what is the cause of unresponsiveness. The overall impression is that anakinra is effective in this setting, and is able to control the acute attacks that are refractory to corticosteroids.

Canakinumab and Rilonacept

Controlled studies were performed in 2 settings: first in patients who had an acute attack of gout, and second in patients who were at risk of an acute attack as they were beginning ULT. Canakinumab was evaluated as treatment for acute attack in 2 published studies (phase 2 and 3) in patients who had contraindications or were unresponsive to either colchicine or NSAIDs. Most of these patients have known comorbidities that are commonly found in the gouty population (hypertension and renal impairment being the major ones). A single dose of canakinumab (150 mg) was effective in relieving pain and symptoms of acute gout, and was superior to the comparator drug triamcinolone (a corticosteroid) in terms of its rapid onset of action and reduction of subsequent gout flares.[28] Rilonacept was initially assessed in the setting of chronic gouty arthritis in a pilot study and was reported to be effective[29]; in a subsequent study of acute gout, when rilonacept was compared with indomethacin or the combination of rilonacept and indomethacin, it was not shown to be superior to the comparator.[30] In the prevention of acute flares in patients who had been started on ULT, both canakinumab and rilonacept were shown to be superior to the comparator (colchicine in the case of canakinumab and placebo in the case of rilonacept) in the reduction of flares.[31,32]

The use of canakinumab in acute gout is approved in Europe by the European Medicines Agency for patients who have contraindications or are refractory to colchicine and NSAIDs, and in whom corticosteroids are contraindicated also. There has been concern about potential infections when patients are subjected to IL-1 inhibition, but there has been no documentation of significant toxicity in the trials performed to date.

Corticotropin and Melanocortins

The melanocortin-3 receptor (MC3R) is a member of the melanocortin receptor family of 7-transmembrane G-protein–coupled receptors that are widely expressed. On macrophages, MC3R transmits an anti-inflammatory signal that leads to reduced activities of NF-κB and heme oxygenase 1 (**Fig. 6**). In experimental studies, the inflammatory effects of MSU crystals were significantly reduced when the MC3R agonist γ-MSH was administered in the peritonitis model of inflammation.[33] Corticotropin and MSH are natural ligands for this receptor, and the action of corticotropin as an anti-inflammatory agent may in part be mediated by this mechanism, besides its ability to stimulate the secretion of adrenal corticosteroid. In a clinical case series reporting the experience from one center, more than 180 patients received at least one injection of 1 mg of corticotropin as treatment of acute gout. In this study, the investigators reported a very rapid clinical response (1 day) in more than 70% of patients, and the treatment was well tolerated.[34] This promising approach needs to be investigated in future controlled clinical studies, as it may be a valuable addition to therapeutic options in gout.

Caspase Inhibitors

Caspases (caspase-1 and -5) are necessary for the intracellular processing of pro–IL-1β secretion, and its inhibition will block IL-1β secretion. Synthetic caspase inhibitors have been developed to inhibit apoptosis and IL-1 secretion, with initial hopes that

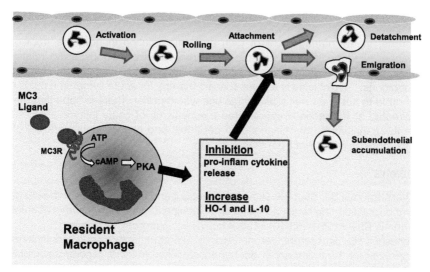

Fig. 6. Reversal of IL-1β–induced neutrophil migration in gout through MC3R activation. A proposed mechanism for the shut-off mechanism in gouty inflammation involves the interaction of corticotropin or other melanocortin peptides with the melanocortin-3 receptor (MC3R) on the surface of resident synovial macrophages. This process results in the accumulation of cyclic adenosine monophosphate (cAMP) and activation of protein kinase A (PKA), which leads to inhibition of IL-1β and other proinflammatory cytokines, thus shutting down neutrophil migration into the joint. PKA also leads to an increase in the anti-inflammatory cytokines heme oxygenase 1 and IL-10.

it may be effective in rheumatoid arthritis. However there are only scant reports documenting their clinical efficacy in humans, even though these inhibitors were effective in animal models of inflammation.[35] One potential problem with these inhibitors might be cross-reactivity with other caspases, which would lead to adverse effects in other organ systems outside the target one. If a truly selective inhibitor that inhibited only IL-1β processing is discovered, it may have an impact on acute gout.

SUMMARY

The available armamentarium for managing gout has doubled over the past 5 years, yet there are still unmet needs in treating this common form of arthritis. The additions of febuxostat and pegloticase offer a much-needed expansion to gouty patients with recalcitrance or intolerance to the traditional approaches of allopurinol and probenicid. Even with these new additions, however, gout remains poorly treated. In truth, the greatest obstacle to better gout management does not reside with ineffective medications but rather rests in the perennial problems of: (1) lack of understanding of the disease process by both patients and physicians; (2) lack of universal acceptance of established treatment guidelines; and (3) lack of recognition that gout is a serious condition with real physical and social consequences.[36] Even if these 3 obstacles could be overcome, not all gout patients would achieve optimal outcomes without more potent approaches to urate-lowering and anti-inflammatory therapy.

This article reviews the exciting new therapies on the horizon. More potent approaches to lowering uric acid and thereby hastening the elimination of the excess urate burden associated with gout may soon be possible with combination of currently available xanthine oxidase inhibitors and the new forms of uricosuric or PNP inhibitors. In the studies presented it seems clear that using 2 drugs with different mechanisms of urate lowering is more effective, and may be safer than the use of higher doses of a single agent.

Likewise, in the management of pain and inflammation in gout the traditional approaches need modification. NSAIDs and corticosteroids are nonspecific, relatively impotent, and contraindicated in many patients with gout because of comorbid medical conditions.[37] Colchicine is a more specific therapy for acute symptoms but is still not as rapid to act or as well tolerated as one would prefer. There is hope that therapies directed at the recently appreciated mechanisms of gouty inflammation, such as the IL-1β inhibitors, the melanocortin peptides, and caspase inhibitors will offer patients more prompt relief from their suffering.

REFERENCES

1. Zhu Y, Pandya BJ, Choi HK. Prevalence of gout and hyperuricemia in the US general population: the National Health and Nutrition Examination Survey 2007-2008. Arthritis Rheum 2011;63(10):3136–41.
2. Janssens HJ, Janssen M, van de Lisdonk EH, et al. Use of oral prednisolone or naproxen for the treatment of gout arthritis: a double-blind, randomized equivalence trial. Lancet 2008;371(9627):1854–60.
3. Terkeltaub RA, Furst DE, Bennett K, et al. High vs low dosing of oral colchicine for early acute gout flare: twenty-four hour outcome results of the first randomized, placebo-controlled, dose comparison colchicine trial. Arthritis Rheum 2010; 62(4):1060–8.
4. Zhang W, Doherty M, Pascual E, et al. EULAR Committee for International Clinical Studies including Therapeutics. EULAR evidence based recommendations for gout. Part II. Management report of a Task Force of the EULAR Standing

Committee for International Clinical Studies including Therapeutics (ESCISIT). Ann Rheum Dis 2006;65:1312–24.

5. Khanna D, Fitzgerald JD, Khanna PP, et al. American College of Rheumatology. 2012 American College of Rheumatology guidelines for management of gout. Part 1: systematic nonpharmacologic and pharmacologic therapeutic approaches to hyperuricemia. Arthritis Care Res 2012;64(10):1431–46.

6. Becker MA, Schumacher HR Jr, Wortmann RL, et al. Febuxostat compared with allopurinol in patients with hyperuricemia and gout. N Engl J Med 2005;353: 2450–61.

7. Edwards NL. Quality of care in patients with gout: why is management suboptimal and what can be done about it? Curr Rheumatol Rep 2011;13(2):154–9.

8. Perez-Ruiz F, Liote F. Lowering serum uric acid levels: what is the optimal target for improving clinical outcomes in gout? Arthritis Rheum 2007;57:1324–8.

9. Perez-Ruiz F, Calabozo M, Pijoan JI, et al. Effect of urate-lowering therapy on the velocity of size reduction of tophi in chronic gout. Arthritis Care Res 2002;47: 356–60.

10. Perez-Ruiz F, Sundy J, Krishnan E, et al. Efficacy and safety of Lesinurad (RDEA594), a novel uricosuric agent, given in combination with allopurinol in allopurinol-refractory gout patients: randomized, double-blind, placebo-controlled, Phase 2B study. Ann Rheum Dis 2011;70(Suppl 3):104.

11. Fleishmann R, Shen Z, Yeh LT, et al. Lesinurad (DEA594), a novel uricosuric agent, in combination with febuxostat shows significant additive urate-lowering effects in gout patients with 100% response achieved for all combination dose regimens. Ann Rheum Dis 2011;70(Suppl 3):188.

12. Fitzpatrick D, Drummond W, Pappas J, et al. Effects of a purine nucleoside phosphorylase inhibitor, BCX4208, on serum uric acid concentrations in patients with gout. ACR/ARHP Annual Meeting. 2010. Abst 150.

13. Hollister AS, Becker M, Terkeltaub R, et al. BCX4208 shows synergistic reductions in serum uric acid in gout patients when combined with allopurinol. Ann Rheum Dis 2011;70(Suppl 3):183.

14. O'Day R, Williams KM, Graham GG. Urate-lowering therapy: uricosurics. Future Medicine 2013;174–88. http://dx.doi.org/10.2217/ebo.13.104.

15. Gregoire F, Zhang F, Clarke HJ, et al. MBX-102/JNJ39659100, a novel peroxisome proliferator-activated receptor-ligand with weak transactivation activity retains antidiabetic properties in the absence of weight gain and edema. Mol Endocrinol 2009;23:975–88.

16. Giamarellos-Bourboulis EJ, Mouktarond M, Bodar E, et al. Crystals of monosodium urate monohydrate enhance lipopolysaccharide-induced release of interleukin 1β by mononuclear cells through a caspase 1-mediated process. Ann Rheum Dis 2009;68:273–8.

17. Martinon F, Petrilli V, Mayor A, et al. Gout-associated uric acid crystals activate the NALP3 inflammasome. Nature 2006;440:237–41.

18. So A, DeSmedt T, Revaz S, et al. A pilot study of IL-1 inhibition by anakinra in acute gout. Arthritis Res Ther 2007;9:R28.

19. Joosten LA, Ea HK, Netea MG, et al. Interleukin-1β activation during acute joint inflammation: a limited role for the NLRP3 inflammasome in vivo. Joint Bone Spine 2010;78(2):107–10.

20. Lachmann HJ, Quartier P, So A, et al. The emerging role of interleukin-1β in auto-inflammatory disease. Arthritis Rheum 2011;63:314–24.

21. Ghosh P, Cho M, Rawat G, et al. Treatment of acute gouty arthritis in complex hospitalized patients with anakinra. Arthritis Care Res (Hoboken) 2013;65:1381–4.

22. Direz G, Noel N, Guyot C, et al. Efficacy but side effects of anakinra therapy for chronic refractory gout in a renal transplant recipient with preterminal chronic renal failure. Joint Bone Spine 2012;79:631.

23. Tran AP, Edelman J. Interleukin-1 inhibition by anakinra in refractory chronic tophaceous gout. Int J Rheum Dis 2011;14:e33–7.

24. Funck-Brentano T, Salliot C, Leboime A, et al. First observation of the efficacy of IL-1ra to treat tophaceous gout of the lumbar spine. Rheumatology (Oxford) 2011;50:622–4.

25. Chen K, Fields T, Mancuso CA, et al. Anakinra's efficacy is variable in refractory gout: report of ten cases. Semin Arthritis Rheum 2010;40:210–4.

26. Singh D, Huston KK. IL-1 inhibition with anakinra in a patient with refractory gout. J Clin Rheumatol 2009;15:366.

27. Gratton SB, Scalapino KJ, Fye KH. Case of anakinra as a steroid-sparing agent for gout inflammation. Arthritis Rheum 2009;61:1268–70.

28. Schlesinger N, Alten RE, Bardin T, et al. Canakinumab for acute gouty arthritis in patients with limited treatment options: results from two randomized, multicenter, active-controlled, double-blind trials and their initial extensions. Ann Rheum Dis 2012;71(11):1839–48.

29. Terkeltaub R, Sundy J, Schumacher HR, et al. The IL-1 inhibitor rilonacept in treatment of chronic gouty arthritis: results of a placebo-controlled, cross-over pilot study. Ann Rheum Dis 2009;68:1613–7.

30. Terkeltaub RA, Schumacher HR, Carter JD, et al. Rilonacept in the treatment of acute gouty arthritis: a randomized, controlled clinical trial using indomethacin as the active comparator. Arthritis Res Ther 2013;15:R25.

31. Mitha E, Schumacher HR, Fouche L, et al. Rilonacept for gout flare prevention during initiation of uric acid-lowering therapy: results from the PRESURGE-2 international, phase 3, randomized, placebo-controlled trial. Rheumatology (Oxford) 2013;52:1285–92.

32. Schlesinger N, Mysler E, Lin HY, et al. Canakinumab reduces the risk of acute gouty arthritis flares during initiation of allopurinol treatment: results of a double-blind, randomized study. Ann Rheum Dis 2011;70:1264–71.

33. Getting SJ, Kaneva M, Bhadresa Y, et al. Melanocortin peptide therapy for the treatment of arthritic pathologies. ScientificWorldJournal 2009;9:1394–414. http://dx.doi.org/10.1100/sw2009.163.

34. Daoussis D, Antonopoulos I, Yiannopoulos G, et al. ACTH as first line treatment for acute gout in 181 hospitalized patients. Joint Bone Spine 2013;80: 291–4.

35. Wannamaker W, Davies R, Namchuk M, et al. (S)-1-((S)-2-{[1-(4-amino-3-chloro-phenyl)-methanoyl]-amino}-3,3-dimethyl-butanoyl)-pyrrolidine-2-carboxylic acid ((2R,3S)-2-ethoxy-5-oxo-tetrahydro-furan-3-yl)-amide (VX-765), an orally available selective interleukin (IL)-converting enzyme/caspase-1 inhibitor, exhibits potent anti-inflammatory activities by inhibiting the release if IL-1β and IL-18. J Pharmacol Exp Ther 2007;321:509–16.

36. Edwards NL, Sundy JS, Forsythe A, et al. Work productivity loss due to flares in patients with chronic gout refractory to conventional therapy. J Med Econ 2011; 14(1):10–5.

37. So A. Developments in the scientific and clinical understanding of gout. Arthritis Res Ther 2008;10:221–6.

38. Schumacher HR Jr, Evans RR, Saag KG, et al. Rilonacept (interleukin-1 trap) for prevention of gout flares during initiation of uric acid-lowering therapy: Results

from a phase III randomized, double-blind, placebo-controlled, confirmatory efficacy study. Arthritis care & Research 2012;64:1462–70.

39. So A, De Meulemeester M, Pikhlak A, et al. Canakinumab for the treatment of acute flares in difficult-to-treat gouty arthritis: Results of a multicenter, phase II, dose-ranging study. Arthritis and Rheumatism 2010;62:3064–76.

Index

Rheum Dis Clin N Am 40 (2014) 389–399
http://dx.doi.org/10.1016/S0889-857X(14)00024-6
0889-857X/14/$ – see front matter © 2014 Elsevier Inc. All rights reserved.

rheumatic.theclinics.com

Moving?

Make sure your subscription moves with you!

To notify us of your new address, find your **Clinics Account Number** (located on your mailing label above your name), and contact customer service at:

Email: journalscustomerservice-usa@elsevier.com

800-654-2452 (subscribers in the U.S. & Canada)
314-447-8871 (subscribers outside of the U.S. & Canada)

Fax number: 314-447-8029

Elsevier Health Sciences Division
Subscription Customer Service
3251 Riverport Lane
Maryland Heights, MO 63043

*To ensure uninterrupted delivery of your subscription, please notify us at least 4 weeks in advance of move.

ELSEVIER

Printed and bound by CPI Group (UK) Ltd, Croydon, CR0 4YY

03/10/2024

01040409-0006